AF413081

Scarless
Wound Healing

BASIC AND CLINICAL DERMATOLOGY

Series Editors

ALAN R. SHALITA, M.D.

*Distinguished Teaching Professor and Chairman
Department of Dermatology
State University of New York
Health Science Center at Brooklyn
Brooklyn, New York*

DAVID A. NORRIS, M.D.

*Director of Research
Professor of Dermatology
The University of Colorado
Health Sciences Center
Denver, Colorado*

1. Cutaneous Investigation in Health and Disease: Noninvasive Methods and Instrumentation, *edited by Jean-Luc Lévêque*
2. Irritant Contact Dermatitis, *edited by Edward M. Jackson and Ronald Goldner*
3. Fundamentals of Dermatology: A Study Guide, *Franklin S. Glickman and Alan R. Shalita*
4. Aging Skin: Properties and Functional Changes, *edited by Jean-Luc Lévêque and Pierre G. Agache*
5. Retinoids: Progress in Research and Clinical Applications, *edited by Maria A. Livrea and Lester Packer*
6. Clinical Photomedicine, *edited by Henry W. Lim and Nicholas A. Soter*
7. Cutaneous Antifungal Agents: Selected Compounds in Clinical Practice and Development, *edited by John W. Rippon and Robert A. Fromtling*
8. Oxidative Stress in Dermatology, *edited by Jürgen Fuchs and Lester Packer*
9. Connective Tissue Diseases of the Skin, *edited by Charles M. Lapière and Thomas Krieg*
10. Epidermal Growth Factors and Cytokines, *edited by Thomas A. Luger and Thomas Schwarz*
11. Skin Changes and Diseases in Pregnancy, *edited by Marwali Harahap and Robert C. Wallach*
12. Fungal Disease: Biology, Immunology, and Diagnosis, *edited by Paul H. Jacobs and Lexie Nall*
13. Immunomodulatory and Cytotoxic Agents in Dermatology, *edited by Charles J. McDonald*

ADDITIONAL VOLUMES IN PREPARATION

Scarless Wound Healing

edited by

Hari G. Garg
Harvard Medical School
at Massachusetts General Hospital
Charlestown, Massachusetts

Michael T. Longaker
New York University School of Medicine
New York, New York

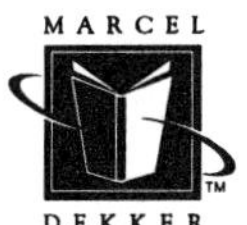

MARCEL DEKKER, INC. NEW YORK · BASEL

ISBN: 0-8247-0285-9

This book is printed on acid-free paper.

Headquarters
Marcel Dekker, Inc.
270 Madison Avenue, New York, NY 10016
tel: 212-696-9000; fax: 212-685-4540

Eastern Hemisphere Distribution
Marcel Dekker AG
Hutgasse 4, Postfach 812, CH-4001 Basel, Switzerland
tel: 41-61-261-8482; fax: 41-61-261-8896

World Wide Web
http://www.dekker.com

The publisher offers discounts on this book when ordered in bulk quantities. For more information, write to Special Sales/Professional Marketing at the headquarters address above.

Current printing (last digit):
10 9 8 7 6 5 4 3 2 1

PRINTED IN THE UNITED STATES OF AMERICA

To my wife and our daughter and son,
for their support, generous love, and unfailing patience.

Hari G. Garg

To my mother, my wife, and my son,
for their loyal support, generous love, and unfailing patience.

Michael T. Longaker

Series Introduction

During the past decade there has been a vast explosion in new information relating to the art and science of dermatology as well as fundamental cutaneous biology. Furthermore, this information is no longer of interest only to the small but growing specialty of dermatology. Scientists from a wide variety of disciplines have come to recognize both the importance of skin in fundamental biological processes and the broad implications of understanding the pathogenesis of skin disease. As a result, there is now a multidisciplinary and worldwide interest in the progress of dermatology.

With these factors in mind, we have undertaken to develop this series of books specifically oriented to dermatology. The scope of the series is purposely broad, with books ranging from pure basic science to practical, applied clinical dermatology. Thus, while there is something for everyone, all volumes in the series will ultimately prove to be valuable additions to the dermatologist's library.

The latest addition to the series, edited by Hari G. Garg and Michael T. Longaker, is both timely and pertinent. The editors have assembled authors who are well known as plastic, reconstructive, cosmetic, maxillofacial, and general surgeons; dermatologists; and glyco- and chemical biologists. We trust that this volume will be of broad interest to scientists and clinicians alike.

Alan R. Shalita
SUNY Health Science Center
Brooklyn, New York

Preface

The significance of the concept of scarless healing is one which takes some insight to fully appreciate. Scarring is the consequence of a complex series of physico-chemical processes whereby a discontinuity in connective tissue integrity—a wound—heals. Postnatal healing involves a rapid but random deposition of structural elements to rebuild the tissue defect. The organization of this repair tissue, however, never achieves the high level of complexity exhibited by the cellular and matrix elements in the surrounding normal tissue. Nowhere is this more apparent than in human skin and, in particular, when skin has been extensively damaged as in a major burn. The deformity, the disability, and the despair that result from these injuries even today are a salutary reminder of where we are in the state of our practical understanding and control of clinical wound healing.

The skin is a highly elaborate structure that serves many functions, from protection through perception, and through complex physiological roles. The skin is the great interface between the self and the outer world. It is far more than just a physical construct, it is a highly complex physio-socio-biological construct. We begin to think in terms of perfection when we consider the softness and beauty of human skin.

The skin is the largest and most visible organ in the body and is endowed with many subtle properties. Scarless healing in the skin is a subject of intense investigation in both academic and commercial research departments. Excellent progress has been made in wound healing but it is not currently possible to prevent repair defects. This book provides an inspiring overview from authors who look at specific aspects of cell and matrix interactions. They give a very personal insight into the state of development in research in this fundamental area of biomedical investigation.

The 15 chapters in this book present a sequence leading from the alterations in the composition and organization of the matrix in the scar tissues following postnatal injury, through the role of different macromolecules in wound repair, recent advances in embryonic wound healing, and characteristics of fetal wound repair, and, finally, to artificial covering materials for wounds.

The first chapter, by Garg, Warren, and Siebert, focuses on the chemistry of scarring. Changes in the amounts, distribution, and composition of proteoglycans in different types of scars that develop in adult wound healing are discussed. The rapid progress in this area has provided significant information about the formation of normal, hypertrophic or keloid scars. It has been found that the sulfonation of proteoglycans increases in different scars to different degrees and that chlorate ions eliminate sulfation to various degrees depending on the concentration of chlorate ions. In Chapter 2 Silbert describes modification of proteoglycan sulfonation as a potential remedy for scarring.

The repair of injury is orchestrated by insoluble and soluble effectors. In Chapter 3 Gallo, Kainulainen, and Bernfield discuss the evidence demonstrating that syndecans may control the wound repair process. The integrin family has emerged as a critical player, as it is involved in all phases of repair after an injury. Integrins act as structural molecules important in cell adhesion, function, and signal processing. In Chapter 4 Xu and Clark address the issue of integrin regulation in tissue repair.

Collagen is the major component of skin, and a considerable amount of research has been done to establish a relationship between disorganization of collagen in scars and changes in the composition of types of collagen. In Chapter 5 Ehrlich reviews the collagen considerations in scarring and regenerative repair.

Hyaluronan increases immediately after an injury and returns to normal levels after about three weeks. The molecular weight of hyaluronan present in the early stages of the repair process appears to determine the type of scarring formed after healing. In Chapter 6 Savani, Bagli, Harrison, and Turley review the role of hyaluronan/receptor interactions in wound repair. In Chapter 7 Balazs and Larsen focus on developments involving hyaluronan that are aimed toward perfect skin generation.

In order to understand defects in the repair process after an injury, it is important to know the molecular and cellular biology of fibroproliferative disorders. In Chapter 8 Kim, Levinson, Gittes, and Longaker present the molecular mechanisms involving keloid biology. In Chapter 9 Bauer, Tredget, Scott, and Ghahary summarize the molecular and cellular biology of dermal fibroproliferative disorders.

In comparison to postnatal wound healing, early-gestation fetal wounds heal without any defect, but what is the importance of this for people? Research in this area has provided insights for adult wound healing with minimal defects. Transforming growth factor beta 1,2 has been detected only in neonatal and adult wounds, not in fetal wounds. In Chapter 10 Shah, Rorison, and Ferguson describe the role of transforming growth factors β in cutaneous scarring. In Chapter 11 Shaw discusses recent advances in the study of embryonic wound healing. In

Chapter 12 Chin, Stelnicki, Gittes, and Longaker summarize the characteristics of fetal wound healing.

In order to avoid outside infection during the healing process, temporary covering of the wound is important. Several materials have been developed to cover the wound area. In Chapter 13 Yannas gives facts about and models of induced organ regeneration in skin and peripheral nerves. In Chapter 14 Orgill, Park, and Demling review clinical use of skin substitutes. Finally, in Chapter 15, Burns and Barry describe the usefulness of hyaluronan-based membrane for the prevention of postsurgical adhesions.

In summary, this book presents significant information in the field of wound healing with its ultimate goal of scarless healing and also discusses the limitations of the research done in this area.

The information in this book provides an overview for all surgeons, particularly plastic surgeons, and dermatologists concerning developments in the wound repair process aimed toward scarless healing, which is the ultimate goal. It also delivers to medical students and nonspecialist researchers in the area of wound healing up-to-date information on scarless repair.

Hari G. Garg
Michael T. Longaker

Contents

Contributors

Darius J. Bagli, M.D., C.M., F.R.C.S.C.   Department of Anatomy and Cell Biology, University of Toronto and The Hospital for Sick Children, Toronto, Ontario, Canada

Endre A. Balazs, M.D.   Biomatrix, Inc., Ridgefield, New Jersey

Kevin J. Barry, M.S.   Department of Clinical Affairs, Genzyme Corporation, Cambridge, Massachusetts

Barbara S. Bauer, M.Sc.   Division of Plastic and Reconstructive Surgery and Critical Care, Department of Surgery, University of Alberta, Edmonton, Alberta, Canada

Merton Bernfield, M.D.   Division of Development and Newborn Medicine, The Children's Hospital, and Department of Dermatology, Harvard Medical School, Boston, Massachusetts

James W. Burns, Ph.D.   Department of Biosurgical Product Development, Genzyme Corporation, Cambridge, Massachusetts

Gyu S. Chin, M.D.   Department of Surgery, New York University School of Medicine, New York, New York

Richard A. F. Clark, M.D.   Department of Dermatology, School of Medicine, State University of New York at Stony Brook, Stony Brook, New York

Robert Demling, M.D.   Department of Surgery, Harvard Medical School, and Burn Center, Brigham and Women's Hospital, Boston, Massachusetts

H. Paul Ehrlich, Ph.D.   Department of Plastic and Reconstructive Surgery, Milton S. Hershey Medical Center, Hershey, Pennsylvania

Mark W. J. Ferguson, C.B.E., B.D.S., F.F.D., Ph.D.   Division of Cells, Immunology, and Development, School of Biological Sciences, University of Manchester, Manchester, England

Richard L. Gallo, M.D., Ph.D.   Department of Medicine and Pediatrics, University of California, San Diego, and San Diego VA Medical Center, San Diego, California

Hari G. Garg, Ph.D., D.Sc.   Pulmonary Research Laboratory, Department of Medicine, Harvard Medical School at Massachusetts General Hospital, Charlestown, Massachusetts

Aziz Ghahary, Ph.D.   Divisions of Plastic and Reconstructive Surgery and Critical Care, Department of Surgery, University of Alberta, Edmonton, Alberta, Canada

George K. Gittes, M.D.   Department of Surgery, New York University School of Medicine, New York, New York

Rene E. Harrison, M.Sc.   University of Toronto and The Hospital for Sick Children, Toronto, Ontario, Canada

Varpu Kainulainen, Ph.D.   Turku Centre for Biotechnology, Turku, Finland

William J. H. Kim, Ph.D.   Department of Surgery, New York University Medical Center, New York, New York

Nancy E. Larsen, Ph.D.   Biomatrix, Inc., Ridgefield, New Jersey

Howard Levinson, M.D.   Department of Surgery, New York University Medical Center, New York, New York

Michael T. Longaker, M.D., F.A.C.S.   Department of Surgery, New York University School of Medicine, New York, New York

Dennis P. Orgill, M.D., Ph.D.   Department of Surgery, Harvard Medical School, and Burn Center, Brigham and Women's Hospital, Boston, Massachusetts

Christine Park, M.D.   Department of Surgery, Harvard Medical School, and Burn Center, Brigham and Women's Hospital, Boston, Massachusetts

Patricia Rorison, M.B.Ch.B., F.R.C.S.(Ed)   Division of Cells, Immunology, and Development, School of Biological Sciences, University of Manchester, Manchester, England

Rashmin C. Savani, M.D., M.B.Ch.B.   University of Pennsylvania School of Medicine and Children's Hospital of Philadelphia, Philadelphia, Pennsylvania

Paul G. Scott, Ph.D.   Divisions of Plastic and Reconstructive Surgery and Critical Care, Department of Surgery, University of Alberta, Edmonton, Alberta, Canada

Mamta Shah, Ph.D., F.R.C.S.(Plast)   Division of Cells, Immunology, and Development, School of Biological Sciences, University of Manchester, Manchester, England

Alison M. Shaw, M.Sc., F.R.C.S.   Department of Plastic and Reconstructive Surgery, St. Andrew's Centre for Plastic Surgery and Burns, Broomfield Hospital, Chelmsford, Essex, England

John W. Siebert, M.D., P.C.   Institute of Reconstructive Plastic Surgery, New York University Medical Center, New York, New York

Jeremiah E. Silbert, M.D.   Division of Rheumatology/Immunology/Allergy, Brigham and Women's Hospital and Harvard Medical School, Boston, and VA Medical Center, Bedford, Massachusetts

Eric J. Stelnicki, M.D.   Department of Surgery, New York University School of Medicine, New York, New York

Edward E. Tredget, M.D., M.Sc., F.R.C.S.(C)   Division of Plastic Surgery, Department of Surgery, University of Alberta, Edmonton, Alberta, Canada

Eva A. Turley, Ph.D.   Division of Cardiovascular Research, University of Toronto and The Hospital for Sick Children, Toronto, Ontario, Canada

Christopher D. Warren, Ph.D.   Department of Biochemistry, Eunice Kennedy Shriver Center for Mental Retardation, Boston, Massachusetts

Jiahua Xu, Ph.D.   Department of Dermatology, School of Medicine, State University of New York at Stony Brook, Stony Brook, New York

Ioannis V. Yannas, Ph.D.   Department of Mechanical Engineering and Material Science Engineering, Massachusetts Institute of Technology, Cambridge, Massachusetts

1
Chemistry of Scarring

Hari G. Garg
Harvard Medical School at Massachusetts General Hospital,
Charlestown, Massachusetts

Christopher D. Warren
Eunice Kennedy Shriver Center for Mental Retardation,
Boston, Massachusetts

John W. Siebert
Institute of Reconstructive Plastic Surgery, New York University
Medical Center, New York, New York

I. SCAR FORMATION

Following an injury, the skin has a tremendous capacity to heal. When the injury involves the skin, with disruption of the dermis, the repair process entails removal of the damaged tissue and laying down of a new extracellular matrix (ECM) over which epidermal continuity can be reestablished. This process of repair and the subsequent reorganization of the dermal matrix is known as scar formation and maturation. A scar can be identified morphologically by a lack of specific organization of cellular and matrix elements when compared with surrounding uninjured skin. If the process of reorganization of the dermal repair matrix is very efficient, little or no scarring will result; this is demonstrated in fetal wound healing (1–9). The histopathological examination of normal skin and normal, hypertrophic, and keloid scars (Fig. 1) shows that collagen is disorganized in all the scar tissues. Collagen nodules are present in hypertrophic scar tissue and thick hyalinized collagen bundles are present in keloid scar tissues (10–13).

Clinical properties of different types of scars, namely normal, hypertrophic, and keloid are summarized in Table 1.

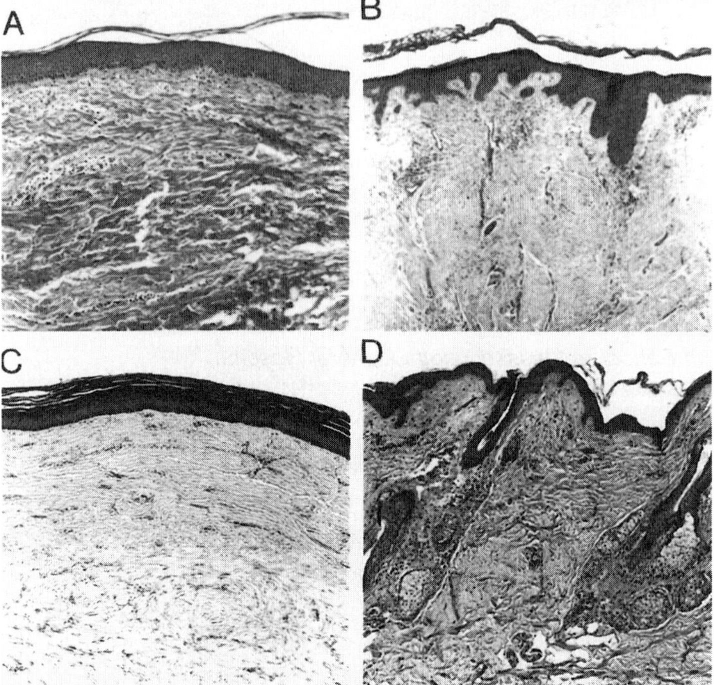

Figure 1 Microscopic findings of an excised normal scar tissue (A), an excised hyper-trophic scar tissue (B), an excised keloid scar tissue (C), and normal human skin (D), stained with hematoxylin and eosine or trichrome.

Table 1 Clinical Properties of Different Scar Tissues

Scar	Clinical properties
Normal	White or pink; indented below skin surface
Hypertrophic	White, pink or red; slightly raised, firm, and follow wound borders
Keloid	Deep red or purple; very raised, firm, and extended beyond wound borders

II. COMPOSITION OF DERMIS

The dermis in normal skin is composed primarily of collagen; this represents about 80% of the dry weight of the tissue (14). The remainder of the dermis is composed of lipid, elastin, and small amounts of small proteoglycans (PGs), hyaluronan (HA), and structural glycoproteins. Two major types of collagen (Types I and III) have been shown to be present in the dermis (15,16) as well as smaller quantities of basement membrane collagen (17). The so-called acid structural glycoproteins (18) are an ill-defined class of constituents which, due to their solubility characteristics, are thought to be closely associated with the collagen bundles in the ECM. Several types of PGs/glycosaminoglycans (GAGs), namely, chondroitin 4- and/or 6-sulfate, dermatan sulfate, heparan sulfate, and heparin, have been shown to be present in the dermis (19–22). In addition to there being a complex mixture of macromolecular constituents in the dermis there is also a heterogenous distribution of these components.

III. PROCESS INVOLVED IN INJURY REPAIR

Following an injury, a sequence of processes are set in motion to restore the epithelial covering and the mechanical and other functions of the skin (23,24). The would healing process is considered to occur in three stages (Fig. 2). After an initial acute phase that involves clot formation and the invasion of inflammatory cells into the wound area, there is a proliferative phase during which time a highly vascular connective tissue matrix is established. During this phase the synthesis of new matrix constituents occurs, contraction decreases the area of the wound, and epithelialization establishes a cover. There is then an extended remodeling phase involving both the resorption and synthesis of components and the reorganization of these constituents to form the healed skin. The fibroblasts present in the healed skin tissue are the tissue elements responsible for the biosynthesis of the matrix structural components. It is these events that occur in the remodeling phase that determine the extent of the defects of repair of the skin (type of scarring).

IV. PROTEOGLYCANS IN DERMIS

The dermis contains different types of glycoaminoglycans (25) that are associated with the collagen-rich extracellular matrix. The GAGs present in the greatest amounts are hyaluronan, which is distributed throughout the dermis extracellular matrix but with higher concentrations near the surface, and dermatan sulfate (DS)

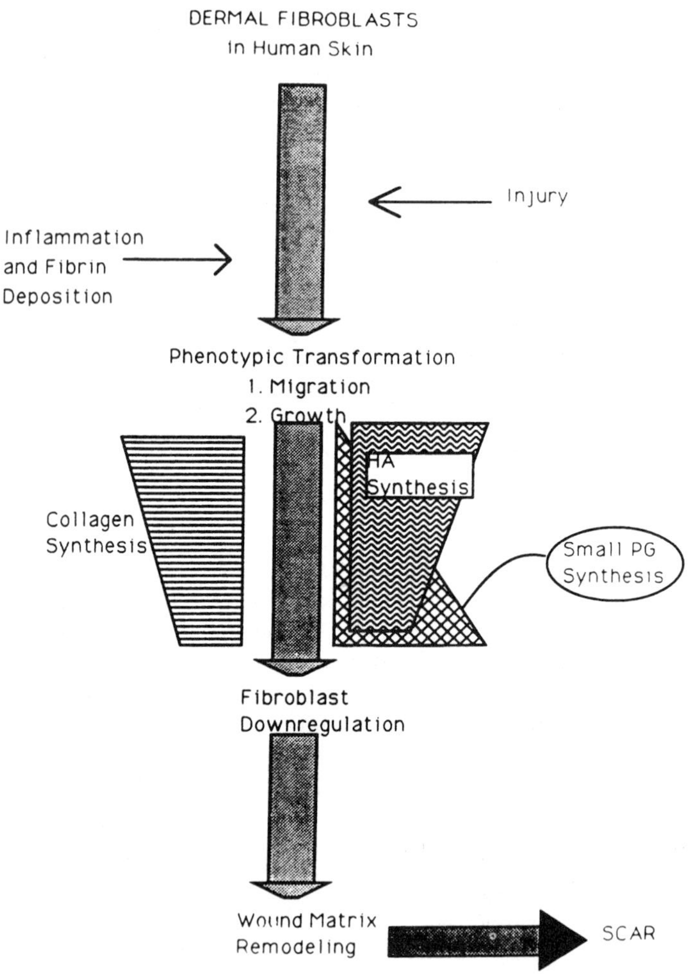

Figure 2　Schematic representation of adult wound healing process.

which is fairly evenly distributed throughout the dermis (26,27). In addition, smaller quantities of chondroitin sulfate (CS), heparan sulfate (HS), and heparin (HP) are present (28,29). All these GAGs are built of repeating disaccharide units of acidic (D-glucuronic/L-iduronic acid) and basic (D-galactosamine/D-glucosamine) sugar residues (30). The molecular formulas of these disaccharide units present in different GAGs are given in Figure 3.

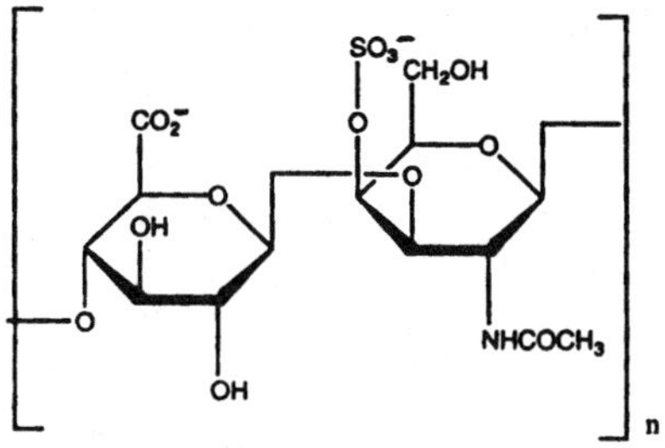

Chondroitin 4-sulfate (CS-4S)

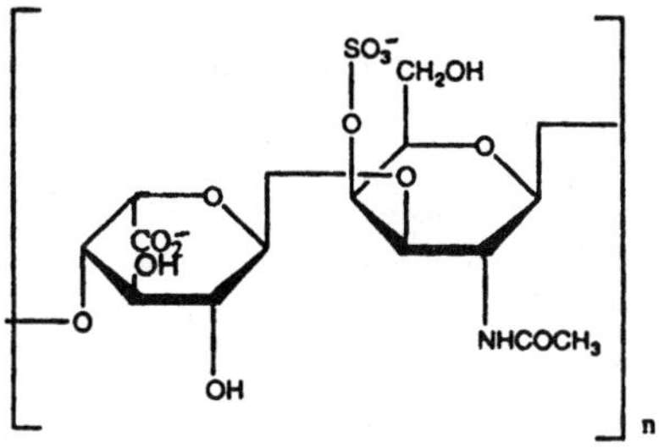

Dermatan sulfate (DS)

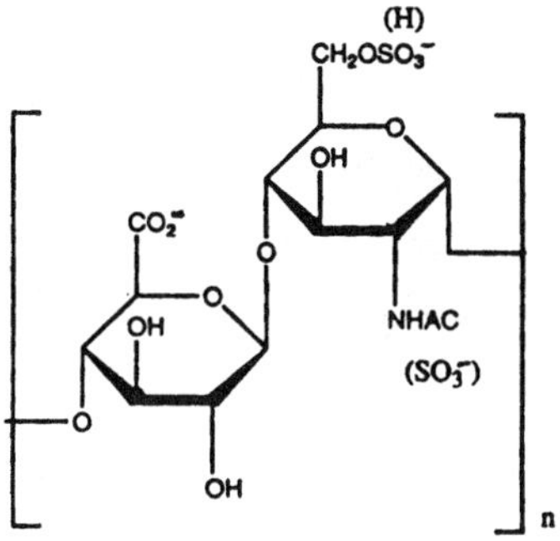

Heparan sulfate (HS)

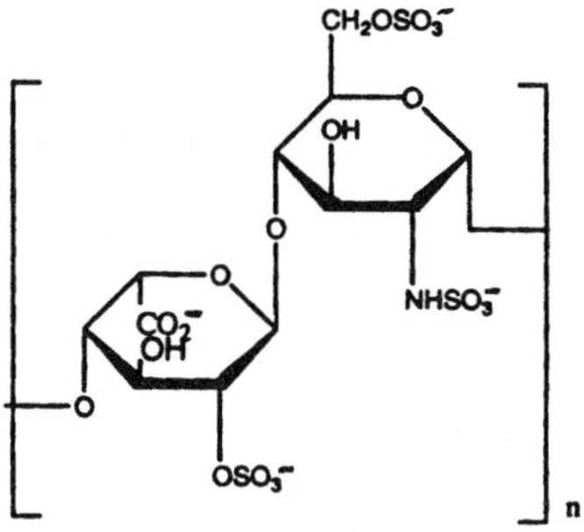

Heparin (HP)

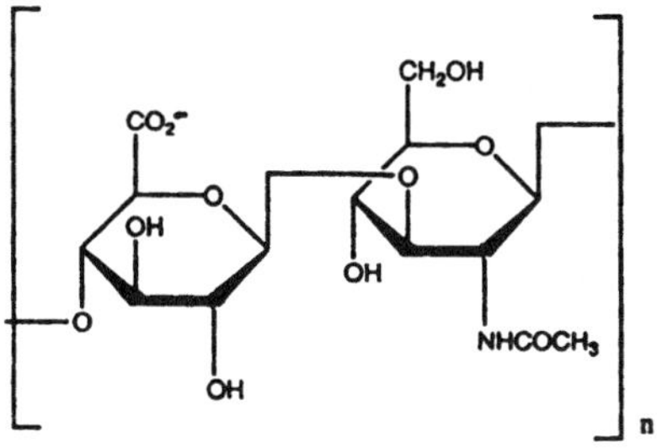

Hyaluronan (HA)

Figure 3 Disaccharide units of different glycosaminoglycans, namely, hyaluronan, chondroitin 4-sulfate, dermatan sulfate, heparan sulfate, and heparin.

A. Isolation and Fractionation of Proteoglycans from Skin and Scar Tissues

The general scheme employed to isolate the proteoglycans from skin/scar tissues is given in Figure 4. In addition to that extraction procedure, two additional methods are also used. The second method uses tissue that has been chopped by hand and the third method is that in which the tissue is repeatedly extracted with acetone and the air-dried tissue is ground in a Wiley mill (31–34). After extraction of the tissue followed by centrifugation, the supernatant is dialyzed successively against distilled water (until free from Cl ions), and finally with 6 M urea in 50 mM sodium acetate, pH 5.8 (buffer A). The dialyzed extract is applied directly to a DEAE (diethylaminoethyl)-cellulose column. The column is then

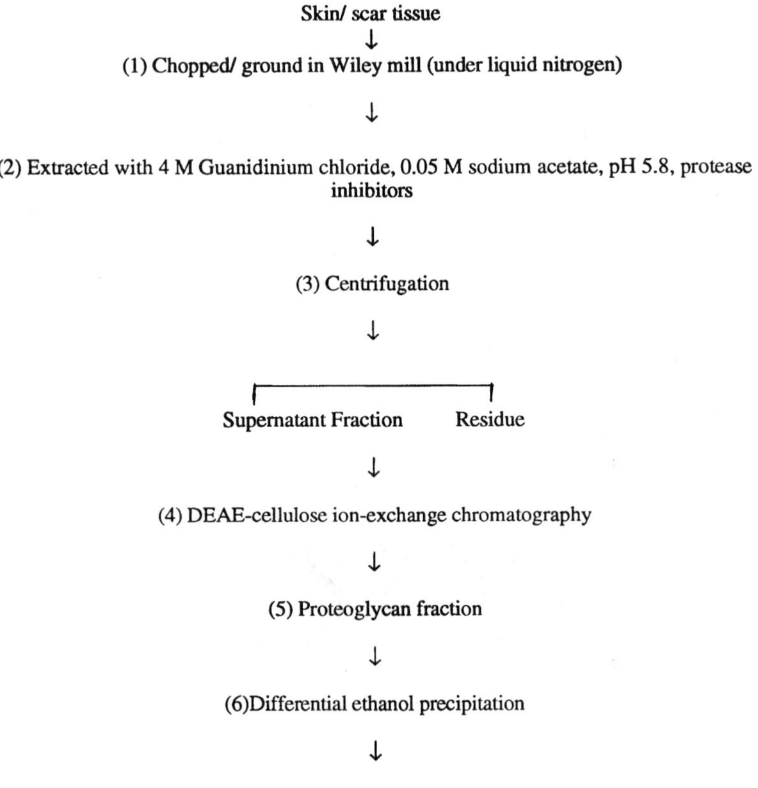

Figure 4 Flow diagram showing steps in the isolation of skin/scar proteoglycans.

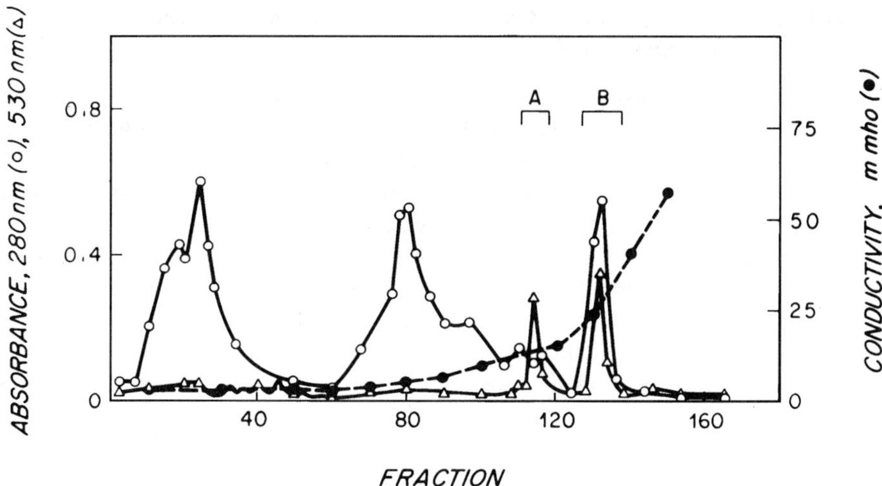

Figure 5 DEAE-cellulose chromatography of constituents extracted from scar tissue. The column fractions are analyzed for the protein content [absorbance 280 nm (O)], conductivity (●), and the uronic acid content (△).

eluted in sequence with: (1) buffer A, (2) a linear gradient of buffer A-0.2 M NaCl in Buffer A, and (3) a linear gradient of 0.2 M NaCl-2 M NaCl in buffer A (31). The column fractions are analyzed to determine protein content and uronic acid content according to Bitter and Muir (35). The elution profile is shown in Figure 5. The column fractions A and B contained hyaluronan and proteoglycans, respectively. The amounts of hyaluronan (fraction A) and proteoglycans (fraction B) from healed skins are given in Table 2.

Table 2 Yield of Hyaluronan (Fraction A) and Proteoglycans (Fraction B) from Two Different Types of Scars

Healed skin	Fractions[a]	
	A	B
Normal scar	206 + 59	445 + 144
Hypertrophic scar	249 + 49	679 + 256

[a]mg/g weight of dry tissue.
Source: Ref. 31.

B. Distribution of Proteoglycans by Cellulose Acetate Plate Electrophoresis

The analysis, by cellulose acetate plate electrophoresis (36) of the distribution of the proteoglycans in different types of scar tissues developed in healed skin, shows that changes do occur in the patterns of proteoglycans from different types of scar tissues (31,33,35). The electrophoretic patterns of normal scar, with and without treatment with chondroitinase AC, are shown in Figure 6.

The distribution of proteoglycans present in different types of scar tissues, namely, normal, hypertrophic, and keloid scars, and normal skin is given in Table 3. Hypertrophic scar contains the dermatan sulfate proteoglycans in larger amounts, whereas normal skin contains more hyaluronan compared to other tissues. Depletion of hyaluronan in scar tissues indicates that hyaluronan plays some

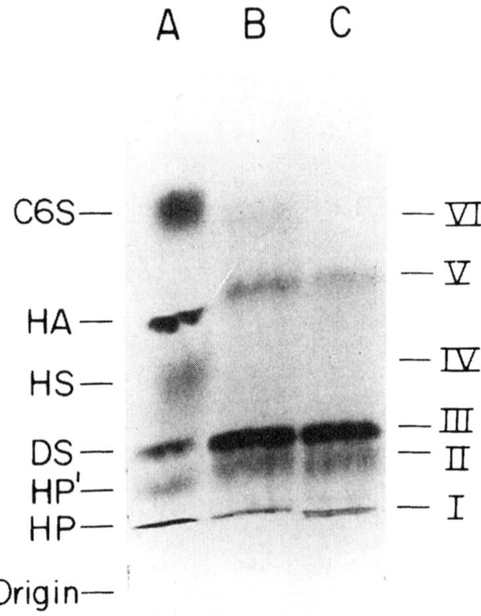

Figure 6 Cellulose acetate plate electrophoresis of proteoglycans. A mixture of reference glycosaminoglycans (C6S, chondroitin 6-sulfate, DS, dermatan sulfate, HA, hyaluronan, HS, heparan sulfate, and HP/HP', heparin) are applied in column A. The proteoglycans from normal scar are shown in column B, and after enzymatic treatment of the normal scar proteoglycans with chondroitinase AC in column C.

Table 3 Relative Quantities of Individual Proteoglycans Expressed As a Percentage of Total Proteoglycans

Tissue type	Percentage[a]					
	HP	HP'	DS	HS	HA	CS
Normal skin	8.02	10.9	33.2	13.7	22.10	12.1
Normal scar	8.46	9.48	38.61	13.97	14.29	15.16
Hypertrophic scar	7.33	4.07	44.89	16.09	10.71	16.92
Keloid scar	5.55	6.53	33.07	12.60	15.21	27.03

[a]CS, chondroitin sulfate; DS, dermatan sulfate; HA, hyaluronic acid; HP and HP', heparin (HP' has a greater electrophoretic mobility than HP); HS, heparan sulfate.

role in scarring. It is reported that a fetal wound heals without scarring at an early stage of gestation when no sulfated proteoglycans are present in the extracellular matrix. Appearance of the sulfated proteoglycans in the later stages of gestation corresponds to the appearance of scarring (Table 4) (37).

Dermatan sulfate and chondroitin sulfate proteoglycans are then separated by differential ethanol precipitation. The PGs fraction is dissolved in 4 M Gdm.Cl buffer and ethanol is added to achieve a concentration of 20% (v/v) ethanol. The mixture is kept overnight at 4°C and the precipitate is collected by centrifugation.

Table 4 Speciation of Proteoglycans from Fetal Sheep Skin

Gestational age in days	Percentage[a]				
	HP	DS	HS	HA	CS
80	6			94	
90	4			96	
105	4			96	
110	4	1		95	
115	4			96	
120	4	4	3	89	
125	7	3		90	
130	3	6	4	87	
135	3	8	2	87	
140	4	15	6	75	1
145	3	3	5	88	1

[a]See footnote of Table 3 for abbreviations.

Additional ethanol is added to a concentration of 30% (v/v) and again the precipitate is collected by centrifugation. This procedure is repeated at ethanol concentrations of 40, 50, and 75% (v/v) (32).

V. AMINO ACID AND CARBOHYDRATE COMPOSITION OF DERMATAN SULFATE PROTEOGYCANS

The amino acid composition of pure single-band dermatan sulfate proteoglycans obtained by differential ethanol precipitation of the above PGs varies (Table 5). Carbohydrate and other chemical composition (Table 6) also shows differences between scar tissues and normal skin and between different types of scars. Sulfation of normal scar DS PGs is lower than in hypertrophic scar (38).

Table 5 Amino Acid Composition of Dermatan Sulfate Proteoglycans in Human Skin and Scar Tissues

	Skin		Scar		
Amino acid[a]	Epidermis (33)	Dermis (33)	Normal (32)	Hypertrophic (32)	Keloid (34)
Aspartic acid	145	170	112	107	119
Threonine	50	36	46	40	53
Serine	87	91	72	76	81
Glutamic acid	109	138	104	114	140
Proline	73	124	97	88	84
Glycine	84	107	88	109	64
Alanine	49	56	68	65	51
Half-cystine	ND[b]	3	12	14	ND[b]
Valine	58	63	64	47	53
Methionine	11	1	20	9	14
Isoleucine	45	3	32	40	31
Leucine	121	45	99	90	140
Tyrosine	12	61	16	22	15
Phenylalanine	41	5	37	46	34
Lysine	67	21	65	66	53
Histidine	26	8	24	23	22
Arginine	36	39	44	44	46

[a]Residues per 1000 residues.
[b]ND, not detected.

Table 6 Carbohydrate and Sulfate Ester Composition (% w/w) of Dermatan Sulfate Proteoglycans in Human Skin and Scar Tissues

| | Skin | | Scar | |
| | Epidermis (33) | Dermis (33) | Normal (32) | Hypertrophic (32) |
Carbohydrate component				
Xylose	0.49	0.38	0.59	0.43
Mannose	1.19	0.19	0.38	0.23
Galactose	1.26	0.96	1.61	1.77
N-Acetylneuraminic acid	1.25	Trace	0.20	0.23
N-Acetylglucosamine	0.64	Trace	0.26	0.25
N-Acetylgalactosamine	11.10	20.33	23.1	23.8
Iduronic acid	6.36	13.34	13.13	13.24
Glucuronic acid	0.96	0.83	1.72	1.53
Sulfate % (w/w)	5.5	NA[a]	8.6	8.8
Δ-Di-4-sulfate	94.69	93.56	91.0	92.0
Δ-Di-6-sulfate	3.86	ND[b]	4.0	2.0
Δ-Di-0-sulfate	1.46	1.41	Trace	4.0
Δ-Di-di-sulfate			5.0	2.0

[a] NA, not available.
[b] ND, not detected.

VI. NH₂-TERMINAL AMINO ACID SEQUENCING OF DERMATAN SULFATE PROTEOGLYCANS

The NH_2-terminal amino acid sequences of dermatan sulfate proteoglycans from human skin and scar tissues are summarized in Table 7 (32,33). The A_1-A_{23} sequence is: NH_2Asp-Glu-Ala-B-Gly-Ile-Gly-Pro-Glu-Val-Pro-Asp-Asp-Arg-Asp-Phe-Glu-Pro-Ser-Leu-Gly-Pro-Val.

VII. COPOLYMERIC CHONDROITIN SULFATE-DERMATAN SULFATE PROTEOGLYCAN IN KELOID AND HYPERTROPHIC SCARS

In comparison with human hypertrophic or keloid scars, relatively small amounts of copolymeric CS-DS PGs are found in normal human skin and normal scar tissues. Therefore, copolymeric CS-DS PGs could not be isolated from normal skin or normal scar tissues. Single-band pure CS-DS PGs from human hypertro-

Table 7 Amino Acid Sequences of Dermatan Sulfate Proteoglycans in Human Skin and Scars

Residue number	Scar		Skin	
	Normal (32)	Hypertrophic (32)	Epidermis (33)	Dermis (33)
1	Asp	Asp	Asp	Asp
2	Glu	Glu	Glu	Glu
3	Ala	Ala	Ala	Ala
4	ND[a]	ND[a]	ND[a]	ND[a]
5	Gly	Gly	Gly	Gly
6	Ile		Ile	Ile
7	Gly		Gly	Gly
8	Pro		Pro	Pro
9	Glu		Glu	Glu
10	Val		Val	Val
11	Pro		Pro	Pro
12	Asp		Asp	Asp
13	Asp		Asp	Asp
14	Arg		Arg	Arg
15	Asp		Asp(?)[b]	Asp(?)[b]
16	Phe		Phe	Phe
17	Glu		Glu	Glu
18	Pro			Pro
19	Ser			Ser(?)[b]
20	Leu			Leu
21	Gly			
22	Pro			
23	Val			

[a] ND, not detected.
[b] (?), Uncertain result.

phic (39) and keloid (34) scars have been isolated and characterized. Their properties are given in Table 8.

There are differences in the properties of the two macromolecules from hypertrophic and keloid scar tissues. The protein core of coplymeric CS-DS PG is similar in size and has a similar NH_2-terminal amino acid sequence to dermatan sulfate proteoglycans. This suggests that the C-5 epimerase activity necessary to convert D-glucuronic acid to L-iduronic acid has low activity in hypertrophic and keloid tissues in comparison with normal skin and normal scar tissues. The glycosaminoglycan chains of the copolymeric CS-DS PGs have other properties in common with DS PGs from the same tissue, e.g., they are mainly 4-sulfated.

Table 8 Carbohydrate and Sulfate Ester Composition of Hypertrophic and Keloid Scar Copolymeric Chondroitin-Dermatan Sulfate Proteoglycans and 4′,5′-Unsaturated Disaccharide Released from Proteoglycans Following Treatment with Chondroitinase ABC

	Scar	
Carbohydrate components (% w/w)	Hypertrophic (39)	Keloid (34)
2-Amino-2-deoxy-glucose	1.7	2.1
2-Amino-2-deoxy-galactose	12.7	12.6
Hexuronic acid	11.0	11.0
Hexose	4.7	4.1
N-acetylneuraminic acid	4.1	3.5
Sulfate ester	10.6	13.7
Δ-Di-4-sulfate	53	96
Δ-Di-6-sulfate	38	ND[a]
Δ-Di-0-sulfate	8.5	ND[a]

[a]ND, not detected.

VIII. ASSESSMENT OF BIGLYCAN AND DECORIN IN DERMATAN SULFATE PROTEOGLYCAN PREPARATIONS

Two different species of dermatan sulfate proteoglycans, namely biglycan (PG-I) and decorin (PG-II) have been found in bovine skin and other connective tissues (40,41). The difference between the two proteoglycans is that biglycan has two glycosaminoglycan chains in most cases whereas decorin contains only one (Fig. 7).

The position of attachment of these chains to the protein core also differs. Decorin has been shown to bind to both collagen (42–44) and fibronectin (45–47), although studies have suggested that some species of biglycan may reside at the cell surface (48–50). Some studies have also suggested that by binding to other extracellular matrix macromolecules, small PGs can influence cell adhesion and migration (47,51), as well as collagen fibrillogenesis (52,53). It has also been found that the protein core of the PGs has the ability to inhibit fibrillogenesis (52). Furthermore, proteoglycans have been found to increase the tensile strength of extended collagen fibers (54).

Efforts to separate the two types of PGs in dermatan sulfate proteogycan from human skin and scar tissues remain unsuccessful. Therefore, in order to determine whether hypertrophic scarring is, in part, a result of changes in the

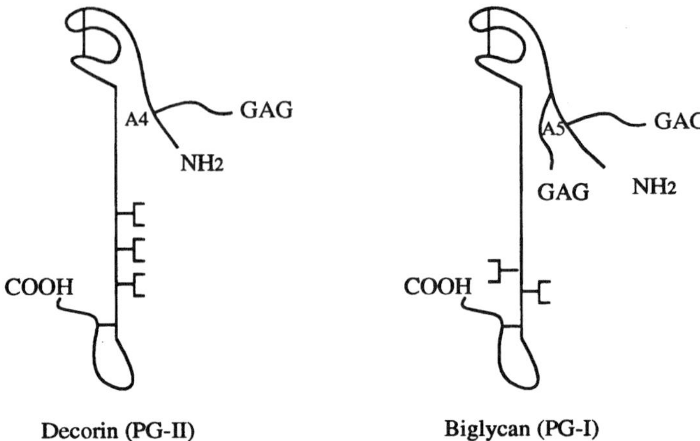

Figure 7   Structure of decorin (PG-II) and biglycan (PG-I); figure not drawn to scale.

population of PG-I and PG-II in dermatan sulfate proteoglycans, NH_2-terminal sequencing of different human skin and scar dermatan sulfate proteoglycans has been investigated (55). The difference in N-terminal amino acids is that the biglycan has Ala at position A_7, while decorin has Ile at position A_6. The data assessing PG-I and PG-II in different DS PGs are summarized in Table 9.

The above sequencing data for the dermatan sulfate proteoglycans from different human skin and scar tissues indicate that the quantities of two types of small PGs, biglycan and decorin, in hypertrophic scar tissue, differ significantly in dermatan sulfate proteoglycan in comparision with DS PGs from normal skin and normal scar tissues. This difference in amounts of biglycan and decorin in

Table 9   Assay of Biglycan and Decorin in Dermatan Sulfate Proteoglycan Preparations from Skin and Different Types of Scars (55)

Dermatan sulfate proteoglycan from tissue	Amount (estimated)[a]	
	Biglycan	Decorin
Epidermis	1	19
Dermis	1	13
Normal scar	1	27
Hypertrophic scar	1	2

[a]Based on the yields (pmol) of Ile (cycle 6) and Ala (cycle 7) obtained during amino acid sequence analysis followed by Edman degradation.

hypertrophic scar tissue may be a proximal cause of altered collagen fibrils, or may result in alterations in the sequestration of growth factors, which would then result in changes in collagen that affect the appearance of the scar. Furthermore, these data show a relationship between an increased amount of PG-I and scarring, the nature of which is unclear at present time. Additional research is needed to characterize this connection.

IX. ALTERATIONS OF DERMATAN SULFATE PROTEOGLYCANS DURING SCAR MATURATION

Alterations in properties of DS PGs at two different stages of maturation (i.e., 2–5 years after an injury: changing, stable, and immature; and 5+ years: unchanging, stable, and mature) (56) have been detected and are summarized in Table 10 (57). The major changes in maturation are: (1) The size of the glycosaminoglycan chains in DS PGs of both types of scar tissues decreases and (2) the degree of epimerization of the C-5 of D-glucuronic acid residues (conversion to L-iduronic acid) increases.

X. SYNTHESIS OF PROTEOGLYCANS BY EXPLANT CULTURE

The synthesis of proteoglycans by normal human skin and by normal and hypertrophic scars has been compared by explant culture. Newly synthesized proteoglycans were labeled with $[^{35}S]Na_2SO_4$ and the results are summarized in Table 11.

Significant differences are found in the proportions of $[^{35}S]$-radiolabel incorporated into tissues from skin and different types of scar and also in the accumulation of $[^{35}S]$-proteoglycans. The incorporation of $[^{35}S]$ radioactivity corresponds to the synthesis of proteoglycans, which occurs in two phases. The initial phase (0–3 hr) is when proteoglycan synthesis is fast, and there is a later phase (3–18 hr), when the incorporation of the $[^{35}S]$-sulfate is slow. Results for the synthesis of proteoglycans show that hypertrophic scar tissue and culture medium contain higher proportions of DS and CS PGs in comparison with normal skin and normal scar tissues. These results suggest that abnormal (hypertrophic) scarring is related to a change in the level of proteoglycan synthesis during the injury repair process (58).

Comparison of the effects of interleukin-1β on proteoglycan synthesis by human skin and scar explant cultures is given in Table 12. The data suggest that the synthesis of proteoglycans can be modified by treatment with interleukin-1β (59).

Table 10 Chemical Composition of Dermatan Sulfate Proteoglycan Preparations from Mature and Immature Human Hypertrophic and Normal Scars

Component % (w/w)	Hypertrophic scar		Normal scar	
	Mature (5+ yr after injury)	Immature (2–5 yr after injury)	Mature (5+ yr after injury)	Immature (2–5 yr after injury)
IdoA-Gal NAc (SO$_4$)	90	80	88	79
GlcA-Gal NAc (SO$_4$)	<5	<12	<10	<12
Hexuronic acid	15.2	17.2	15.2	16.3
Hexose	2.5	2.2	2.1	2.3
N-acetylneuraminic acid	0.2	0.5	0.3	0.2
Sulfate ester	9.3	9.1	8.2	8.0
Protein	20.2	22.8	19.6	21.4
Δ-Di-4-sulfate	92	91	90	92
Δ-Di-6-sulfate	2	4	6	4
Δ-Di-0-sulfate	ND[a]	3	ND[a]	ND[a]

[a]ND, not detected.
Source: Ref. 57.

Table 11 Percentage Distribution of Labeled Macromolecules in Human and Scar Explant—[^{35}S] Incorporated in 1 g Wet Tissue

Tissue	Medium	Extractable[a]	Nonextractable[b]
Normal skin			
1 hr	6.1	89	4.9
3 hr	5.8	90.2	3.2
5 hr	3.7	89.7	6.6
18 hr	7.8	86.1	6.1
Normal scar			
1 hr	9.0	62.3	28.7
3 hr	6.5	73.5	20.0
5 hr	10.2	67.0	22.8
18 hr	11.8	66.8	21.4
Hypertrophic scar			
1 hr	52.4	28.4	19.2
3 hr	39.8	36.3	23.9
5 hr	57.8	22.0	20.2
18 hr	64.4	14.2	21.4

[a] Extractable: [^{35}S]-labeled proteoglycans extracted from the tissue with 0.15 M NaCl and 4 M Gdm.Cl buffers.
[b] Nonextractable: [^{35}S]-labeled proteoglycans could not be extracted and remained in the tissue.
Source: Ref. 58.

Table 12 Effect of Interleukin-1β (IL-1β) on the Synthesis and Release of [^{35}S]-Labeled Proteoglycans by Human Skin and Normal Scar Explant Cultures: Percentage Incorporated [^{35}S] Radioactivity per g Wet Weight Tissue

	Human tissue		
Distribution of [^{35}S] proteoglycans[a]	Normal skin	+ IL-1β	Normal scar + IL-1β
Medium	29.4	36.2	9.9	11.4
Extractable[b]	48.0	42.5	52.1	56.1
Nonextractable[b]	22.6	21.3	38.0	32.5

[a] Cultures were labeled with [^{35}S]Na$_2$SO$_4$.
[b] See footnote to Table 11.
Source: Ref. 59.

XI. SUMMARY AND CONCLUSIONS

In summary, the following structural changes in proteoglycans occur in different types of scar formation following an injury: (1) change in the size of the glycosaminoglycan side chains, (2) alterations in the degree and location of sulfation, (3) changes in the size of the protein core, (4) alterations in the degree of D-glucuronic acid to L-iduronic acid epimerization, and (5) differences in the proportions of PG-I and PG-II.

In conclusion, proteoglycans, particularly dermatan sulfate proteoglycans having apparent abnormality in their structure, play an important role in the formation of an aberrant skin architecture during injury repair. This results in morphological consequences resulting in scarring.

REFERENCES

1. Burrington JD. Wound healing in the fetal lamb. J Ped Surg 1971; 6:423–528.
2. Gross AN. Interuterine healing of fetal rat oral mucosal, skin and cartilage wounds. J Oral Pathol 1977; 6:35–43.
3. Robinson BW, Gross AN. Intrauterine healing of fetal rat cheek wounds. Cleft Palate J 1981; 18:251–255.
4. Rosewell AR. The intra-uterine healing of foetal muscle wound: experimental study in the rat. Br J Plast Surg 1984; 37:635–642.
5. Adzick NS, Harrison MR, Glick Pl, Beckstead JH, Villa RL, Scheuenstuhl H, Goodson III, WH. Comparison of fetal, newborn, and adult healing by histologic, enzyme-histochemical and hydroxyproline determination. J Pediatr Surg 1985; 20:315–319.
6. Hallock GG. In uterocleft lip repair in A/J mice. Plast Reconstr Surg 1985; 75:785–788.
7. Hallock GG, Rice DC, McClure HM. In utero lip repair in the rhesus monkey: an update. Plast Reconstr Surg 1987; 80:855–858.
8. Krummel TM, Nelson JM, Dieglemann RF, Lindblad WJ, Salzberg AM, Greenfield LJ, Cohen IK. Fetal response to injury in the rabbit, J Pediatr Surg 1987; 22:640–644.
9. Siebert JW, Burd DAR, McCarthy JG, Weinzweig J, Ehrlich P. Fetal wound healing: a biochemical study of scarless healing. Plast Reconstr Surg 1990; 85:495–502.
10. Rockwell WB, Cohen IK, Ehrlich HP. Keloids and hypertrophic scars. Plast Reconstr Surg 1989; 84:827–837.
11. Rudolph R. Widespread scars, hypertrophic and keloids. Clin Plast Surg 1987; 14:253–260.
12. Muir IFK. On the nature of keloids and hypertrophic scars. Br J Plast Surg 1990; 43:61–69.
13. Murray JC, Pollack SV, Pinnell SR. Keloids and hypertrophic scars. Clin Dermatol 1984; 2:121–133.

14. Pearce RH, Grimmer BJ. Age and the chemical constitution of normal human dermis. J Invest Dermatol 1972; 58:347–361.
15. Epstein EH Jr, Munderloh NH. Human skin collagen. Presence of type I and type III at all levels of the dermis. J Biol Chem 1978; 253:1336–1337.
16. Epstein EH Jr. $[\alpha1(III)]_3$ human skin collagen. Release by pepsin digestion and preponderence in fetal life. J Biol Chem 1974; 249:3225–3231.
17. Gay S, Kresina TF, Gay R, Miller EJ, Montes LF. Immunohistochemical demonstration of basement membrane collagen in normal human skin and in psoriasis. J Cutan Pathol 1979; 6:91–95.
18. Timpl R, Wolff I, Weiser M. A new class of structural proteins from connective tissue. Biochem Biophys Acta 1968; 168:168–170.
19. Davidson EA, Small W. Metabolism in vivo of connective-tissue mucopolysaccharides. II. Chondroitin sulfate B and hyaluronic acid of skin. Biochim Biophys Acta 1963; 69:453–458.
20. Szirmai JA, Tyssonnsk EVB, Gardell S. Microchemical analysis of glycosaminoglycans, collagen, total protein and water in histological layers of nasal septum cartilage. Biochim Biophys Acta 1964; 136:331–350.
21. Barker SA, Crickshank DND, Webb T. Mucopolysaccharide in rat skin. Part I. Isolation and identification. Carbohydr Res 1965; 1:52–61.
22. Schiller S. Isolation of heparitin sulfate from skin of normal rats. Biochem Biophys Acta 1966; 124:215–217.
23. Pollack SV. Wound healing, a review. I. The biology of wound healing. J Dermatol Surg Oncol 1979; 5:389–393.
24. Hunt TK. Disorders of wound healing. World J Surg 1980; 4:271–277.
25. Pearce RH, Grimmer BJ. The nature of the ground substance. In: Montagna W, Bentley JP, Dobson RL, eds. Advances in the Biology of Skin. Vol. X. The Dermis. New York: Appleton-Century-Crofts, 1970:89–101.
26. Hoffman P, Linker A, Meyer K. The acid mucopolysaccharides of connective tissues. II. Further experiments on chondroitin sulfates. Arch Biochem Biophys 1957; 69:435–440.
27. Tajima S, Nagai Y. Distribution of macromolecular components in calf dermal connective tissue. Connect Tissue Res 1980; 7:65–71.
28. Meyer K, Davidson EA, Linker A, Hoffman P. The acid mucopolysaccharides of connective tissue. Biochim Biophys Acta 1956; 21:506–518.
29. Schiller S, Glover GA, Dorfman A. A method for the separation of acid mucopolysaccharides: its application to the isolation of heparin from the skin of rats. J Biol Chem 1961; 236:983–987.
30. Garg HG, Lyon N. Structure of collagen fibril-associated, small proteoglycans of mammalian origin. Adv Carbohydr Chem Biochem 1991; 49:239–261.
31. Swann DA, Garg HG, Jung W, Hermann H. Studies on human scar tissue proteoglycans. J Invest Dermatol 1985; 84:527–531.
32. Swann DA, Garg HG, Hendry CJ, Hermann H, Siebert E, Sotman S, Stafford W. Isolation and partial characterization of dermatan sulfate proteoglycans from postburn scar tissues. Coll Relat Res 1988; 8:295–313.
33. Garg HG, Burd DAR, Swann DA. Small dermatan sulfate proteoglycans in human epidermis and dermis. Biomed Res 1989; 10:197–207.

34. Garg HG, Lippay EW, Burd DAR. Purification and characterization of iduronic acid-rich and glucuronic acid-rich proteoglycans implicated in human post-burn keloid scar. Carbohydr Res 1990; 207:295–305.

35. Bitter T, Muir HM. A modified uronic acid carbazole reaction. Anal Biochem 1962; 4:330–334.

36. Cappelletti R, DelRosso M, Chiarugi VP. A new electrophoretic method for the complete separation of all known glycosaminoglycans in a monodimensional run. Anal Biochem 1979; 99:311–315.

37. Freund RM, Siebert JW, Cabrera RC, Longaker MT, Eidelman Y, Adzick NS, Garg HG. Serial quantitation of hyaluronan and sulfated glycosaminoglycans in fetal sheep skin. Biochem Molec Biol Int 1993; 29:773–783.

38. Longas M, Garg HG. Sulfate composition of dermatan sulfate from scar tissue. Carbohydr Res 1992; 237:319–324.

39. Garg HG, Siebert EP, Swann DA. Isolation and some structure analyses of a copolymeric chondroitin sulfate-dermatan sulfate proteoglycan from post-burn, human hypertrophic scar. Carbohydr Res 1990; 197:159–169.

40. Rosenberg LC, Choi HU, Tang L-H, Johnson TL, Pal S, Webber C, Reiner A, Poole AR. Isolation of dermatan sulfate proteoglycans from mature bovine articular cartilages. J Biol Chem 1985; 260:6304–6313.

41. Choi HU, Johnson TL, Paul S, Tang L-H, Rosenberg L, Neame PJ. Characterization of the dermatan sulfate proteoglycans, DS-PGI and DS-PGII, from bovine articular cartilage and skin isolated by octyl-sepharose chromatography. J Biol Chem 1989; 264:2876–2884.

42. Scott JE, Orford CR. Dermatan sulfate rich proteoglycan associates with rat tail-tendon collagen at the d band in the gap region. Biochem J 1981; 197:213–216.

43. Oldberg Å, Ruoslahti E. Interactions between chondroitin sulfate proteoglycan, fibronectin and collagen. J Biol Chem 1982; 257:4859–4863.

44. Scott PG, Winterbottom N, Dodd CM, Edwards E, Pearson CH. A role for disulfide bridges in the protein core interaction of proteodermatan sulfate and collagen. Biochem Biophys Res Commun 1986; 138:1348–1354.

45. Yamagata M, Yamada KM, Yoneda M, Suzuki S, Kimata K. Chondroitin sulfate proteoglycan (PG-M-like proteoglycan) is involved in the binding of hyaluronic acid to cellular fibronectin. J Biol Chem 1986; 261:13526–13535.

46. Schmidt G, Robenek H, Harrach B, Glössl J, Nolte V, Hörmann H, Richter H, Kresse H. Interaction of small dermatan sulfate proteoglycan from fibroblasts with fibronectin. J Cell Biol 1987; 104:1683–1691.

47. Lawandowska K, Choi HU, Rosenberg LC, Zardi L, Culp LA. Fibronectin-mediated adhesion of fibroblasts: inhibition by dermatan sulfate proteoglycan and evidence for a cryotic glycosaminoglycan-binding domain. J Cell Biol 1987; 105:1443–1454.

48. Yanagishita M, Hascall VC. Proteoglycan synthesized by rat ovarian granulosa cells in culture. Isolation, fractionation, and characterization of proteoglycan associated with cell layer. J Biol Chem 1984; 259:10260–10269.

49. Hedman K, Christner J, Julkunen I, Vaheri A. Chondroitin sulfate at the plasma membranes of culture fibroblasts. J Cell Biol 1983; 97:1288–1293.

50. Oldberg Å, Hayman EG, Ruoslahti E. Isolation of a chondroitin sulfate proteoglycan from a rat yolk sac tumor and immunochemical demonstration of its cell surface localization. J Biol Chem 1981; 256:10847–10852.

51. Brennan MJ, Oldberg Å, Hayman EG, Ruoslahti E. Effect of a proteoglycan produced by rat tumor cells on their adhesion to fibronectin-collagen substrata. Cancer Res 1983; 43:4302–4307.
52. Vogel KG, Paulsson M, Heinegård D. Specific inhibition of type I and type II collagen fibrillogenesis by small proteoglycan of tendon. Biochem J 1984; 223:587–597.
53. Scott JE, Orford CR, Hughes EW. Proteoglycan-collagen arrangements in developing rat tail tendon. An electron-microscopical and biochemical investigation. Biochem J 1981; 195:573–581.
54. Garg AK, Berg RA, Siver FH, Garg HG. Effect of proteoglycans on type I collagen fibre formation. Biomaterials 1989; 10:413–419.
55. Garg HG, Siebert JW, Garg A, Neame PJ. Inseparable iduronic acid-rich-containing proteoglycan PG (IdoA) preparations of human skin and post-burn scar tissues: evidence for elevated levels of PG (IdoA) in hypertrophic scar by N-terminal sequencing. Carbohydr Res 1996; 284:223–228.
56. Engrav LH. Some thoughts on hypertrophic scars: reply. Plast Reconstr Surg 1988; 82:1107.
57. Garg HG, Siebert JW, Garg A, Neame PJ. Iduronic acid-rich proteoglycans (PG IdoA) and human post-burn scar maturation: isolation and characterization. Carbohydr Res 1995; 267:105–113.
58. Garg HG, Lippay LW, Carter EA, Donelan MB, Remensnyder JP. Proteoglycan synthesis in human skin and burn scar explant culture. Burns 1991; 17:452–457.
59. Garg HG, Lippay EW, Donelan MB, Remensnyder JP. Comparision of the effects of interleukin-1β on proteoglycan synthesis by human skin and post-burn normal scar explant cultures. Biochem Molec Biol Int 1993; 31:583–591.

2

Modification of Proteodermatan/ Chondroitin Sulfation and Its Potential for Affecting Scarring

Jeremiah E. Silbert
Brigham and Women's Hospital and Harvard Medical School, Boston, and VA Medical Center, Bedford, Massachusetts

I. INTRODUCTION

Proteoglycans appear to be key matrix components in scarring after an injury (see Chapter 1), although their roles have not been well defined. Their role in skin and other tissues in relation to structure (1) can be divided into two main types of function, consisting of relatively nonspecific charge and size effects of the glycosaminoglycan components, and specific interactions directly due to the microstructure of the glycosaminoglycans and/or the structure of the core proteins. Usually, but not always, the glycosaminoglycans serve as the functional "business ends" while the core proteins serve to direct transport and channeling for biosynthesis, placement, and maintenance in appropriate locations.

General glycosaminoglycan functional characteristics of the first type relate to length of chains, degree of charge on individual polysaccharide chains, and density of charge provided by number of chains. In this fashion, versican, the large matrix proteoglycan (10–20 chondroitin sulfate chains) of skin as well as other tissues, functions in salt and water balance, as a macromolecular filter, and as a cushion to physical pressures. The highly polyanionic structure controls a large "domain," so that a volume of water many times the volume of the proteoglycan itself can be contained within the external limits of the molecule. In this domain, small noncharged molecules move freely, but large molecules, such as proteins, are excluded by the nature of the highly charged glycosaminoglycan chains. Under pressure, some of the water can be expressed from the domain, and with release of pressure the water reoccupies the space. Together with hyaluronan, which has a high viscosity in dilute solution, versican helps provide support for other components of tissues. Perlecan, the large heparan sulfate proteoglycan of basement membrane, can also be considered as having functions of filtration related to overall size and charge, although specific glycosaminoglycan microstructure may play an important role in some of its functions.

Cell surface proteoglycans, such as the syndecans and glypican, which contain heparan sulfate and/or dermatan/chondroitin sulfate, generally function by the second type of interaction, with the glycosaminoglycan "business ends" recognizing and interacting with matrix or other cells or as receptors or facilitators for extracellular substances (2). For example, syndecan-1, a small proteoglycan which contains both heparan sulfate and dermatan/chondroitin sulfate, has been implicated in attachment of epithelial cells to matrix by interacting both with matrix substances such as fibronectin and with the actin cytoskeleton (3). These functions generally depend upon the microstructure of the glycosaminoglycan, best exemplified by the highly specific pentasaccharide structure in heparan sulfate of cell surface syndecan-4 (ryudocan) which interacts with antithrombin III to provide anticoagulation for hemostasis (4). Cell surface heparan sulfate serves multiple other functions related to cell–cell, cell–matrix, and cell–solute interactions with substances such as fibronectin, laminin, and thrombospondin. These may be the most interactive of the proteoglycans with involvement in angiogenesis (5), attachment (6–9), migration, growth, and differentiation (3,8–10). It is likely that the fine structure of heparan sulfate with a vast variety of sulfate localization, variable N-sulfation, and iduronate content, provides the specificity for these interactions.

The core proteins of decorin and biglycan, small matrix proteoglycans having one and two dermatan sulfate chains, respectively, interact with collagen and/or growth factors such as TGFβ. The dermatan sulfate of decorin attached to collagen interacts in an antiparallel fashion with dermatan sulfate of decorin attached to an adjacent collagen, providing a bridge for positioning and maintaining collagen fibril organization (11). Since chondroitin sulfate will not provide such bridging, the microstructure due to degree and localization of dermatan sulfate epimerization controls function, while the core protein makes the attachment to the collagen. Dermatan sulfate microstructure has also been shown to provide the specific interaction for function in binding and activating heparin cofactor II in hemostasis (12,13).

Susceptibility to degradation is an additional functional consideration for dermatan/chondroitin glycosaminoglycan microstructure, since variable stability and turnover of glycosaminoglycans may depend upon their susceptibility to enzymatic degradation.

Thus, the detailed positions and degrees of epimerization, sulfation, and stability of glycosaminoglyans provide multiple specificities for function, including potential effects upon wound healing. It is possible that modifications of dermatan/chondroitin sulfate, possibly affecting the quality of healing, could be achieved by the simple, easy procedure of changing the availability of sulfate. The key to this lies in the high concentrations of sulfate necessary for full epimerization and sulfation during biosynthesis in vivo, the order in which specific sulfate residues are affected, and the variability among individuals concerning dietary sulfate and the capacity for skin to produce sulfate from sulfhydryl-containing amino acids. Modification in the availability of sulfate would not likely be of practical use for affecting heparan sulfation since full sulfation can occur at much lower concentrations than the high sulfate concentrations required for dermatan/chondroitin sulfation.

II. STRUCTURE OF DERMATAN/CHONDROITIN SULFATE

As described in Chapter 1, these glycosaminoglycans consist of repeating sulfated disacccharides containing *N*-acetylgalactosamine* (GalNAc) alternating with glucuronate (GlcA) for chondroitin and a mixture of variable amounts of iduronate (IdceA) and GlcA for dermatan, which can be considered as a variant of chondroitin containing any amount of IdceA. In the case of pig skin dermatan sulfate, it was found that the GlcA-containing regions were in short clusters alternating with clusters of IdceA-containing regions (14). Chondroitin sulfate chains usually have a mixture of nonsulfated GalNAc, GalNAc 4-sulfate (4S) and GalNAc 6-sulfate (6S), with a small amount of GalNAc 4,6-disulfate (4,6S) which is found almost exclusively as a chain terminal structure (15). Degrees of sulfation, and ratios of 4S to 6S are highly variable between individuals and tissues. There may also be small amounts of GlcA 2-sulfate (2S), which has been described adjacent to GalNAc-6S, but has not been found next to nonsulfated GalNAc or GalNAc-4S. The epimerization to IdceA is found almost entirely adjacent to GalNAc-4S, but the presence of GalNAc-6S adjacent to IdceA has not been completely ruled out. The IdceA is frequently 2-sulfated, but has only been found adjacent to GalNAc-4S, consistent with the requirement of GalNAc-4S for epimerization of GlcA to IdceA (16–18). The amounts and distribution of epimerization and 2-sulfation in dermatan sulfate are good candidates for various functions, as exemplified by a repeat of three IdceA-2S–GalNAc-4S residues, which has been shown to be required for heparin cofactor II activity (12,13).

---

* Abbreviations: GalNAc, *N*-acetylgalactosamine; GlcA, glucuronate; IdceA, iduronate; Gal, galactose; Xyl, xylose; 2S, 2-sulfate; 4S, 4-sulfate; 6S, 6-sulfate; 4,6S, 4,6-disulfate; PAPS, 3'-phosphoadenylyl 5'-phosphosulfate; UDP, uridine diphosphate.

III.   DERMATAN/CHONDROITIN SULFATE BIOSYNTHESIS

The steps in the assembly of proteoglycans are: (1) synthesis of core protein, (2) xylosylation of specific serine moieties of the core protein in the endoplasmic reticulum and/or early Golgi, (3) sequential addition of two galactose (Gal) residues to the xylose (Xyl) in early Golgi, (4) sequential addition in later Golgi fractions of GlcA and GalNAc to complete a GalNAc-GlcA-Gal-Gal-Xyl pentasaccharide linkage region, (5) together with addition of the repeating disaccharide units consisting of alternating GlcA and GalNAc, (6) with modification of the growing polymer by sulfation of the GalNAc at the 4 or 6 position, (7) together with epimerization of varying amounts of the GlcA to IdceA in the case of dermatan sulfate, (8) followed by 2-sulfation of some IdceA or GlcA.

The polymerization to form glycosaminoglycans takes place on the nascent proteoglycan with UDP-GlcA and UDP-GalNAc as precursors (2). The nascent proteoglycan appears to remain attached to Golgi membranes during the entire process of assembly with channeling from individual membrane-bound enzymes to form the Gal-Gal-Xyl linkage and then to what appears to be membrane-bound enzyme complexes to complete the GalNAc-GlcA-Gal-Gal-Xyl linkage together with the glycosaminoglycan polymerization, sulfation, and epimerization (19).

Dermatan residues are formed by the C5 epimerization of GlcA to IdceA during or subsequent to polymerization of the glycosaminoglycan (16), and the only difference between proteochondroitin sulfate and proteodermatan sulfate is a result of the action of epimerase on some of the GlcA of the precursor proteochondroitin sulfate producing a mixture of dermatan (IdceA-containing) residues and chondroitin (GlcA-containing) residues. Although pure chondroitin sulfate is the only component of many proteoglycans, pure dermatan sulfate does not exist since there is always some chondroitin in the chain (20). The epimerization to IdceA is closely dependent upon 4-sulfation of adjacent GalNAc residues (18,21).

Sulfation of chondroitin takes place while the polymer is being formed (22) with the same Golgi subfractions that have polymerization activity (23). These subfractionation studies and experiments on the effects of the ionophore monensin on dermatan sulfate synthesis (24) have suggested that sulfation occurs in the *medial*, *trans*, or *trans*-Golgi network. Consequently 4-sulfating and 6-sulfating enzymes must be co-localized with the enzymes of polymerization. The chondroitin polymer is modified to form dermatan sulfate by transfer of sulfate from adenosine 3′-phosphoadenylyl 5′-phosphosulfate (PAPS) together with epimerization being found only where there is 4-sulfation (18), demonstrating that this enzyme as well is co-localized with the enzymes of polymerization and 4-sulfation. Sulfation of GalNAc residues near the linkage region (25), and at the terminal or preterminal GalNAc structure of chondroitin sulfate in relation to enzyme-substrate specificities has been examined in some detail (26,27).

Synthesis of the core protein with its transport to sites for glycosaminoglycan formation appear to be the sole controlling factor in formation of the proteoglycans under ordinary conditions. This has been demonstrated by the manyfold increases in formation of fully formed glycosaminoglycans that have been found when β-xylosides were added to many different cell culture systems, presenting an artificial substrate for steps 3 through 8 above. Consequently, cultured cells, and presumably cells in vivo, are ordinarily able to provide ample excess substrates and enzymes for a massive increase in production. Exceptions to this only appear to occur in situations in which there is a deficit in a particular enzyme or substrate brought about by one or another mutation. Thus, cells that lack full capacity to transport sulfate have diminished sulfation (28,29), and cells lacking a specific glycosyl transferase (30), specific sulfotransferase (31), or with a deficiency of an enzyme for transport (32) or formation (33) of a particular substrate, such as UDP-Gal or PAPS, show a limited capability to synthesize or to sulfate glycosaminoglycans.

IV. PRODUCTION OF UNDERSULFATED DERMATAN/ CHONDROITIN SULFATE

Undersulfation of proteoglycans can easily be produced in vitro with explants or cultures of some cells by restricting sulfate in the growth media (18,21,34–37) or in all cells by using chlorate (36,38,39) to block formation of PAPS. The former of these techniques is limited by the capability of some cells to produce their own sulfate from cysteine or methionine (40), while the latter technique will eliminate sulfation to various degrees depending upon the concentration of chlorate. Cells grown in the presence of chlorate, even at concentrations high enough to eliminate all sulfation, are surprisingly healthy, with little limitation in growth or subculturing. This has the advantage of examining the biosynthesis under conditions of limited sulfation even while serum is present in the culture medium. However, there is always the possibility that observed changes in cell function, metabolism, interactions, etc., could be due to effects of chlorate on cell growth or metabolism other than the direct blocking of sulfation.

Total matrix proteochondroitin sulfate and proteodermatan/chondroitin sulfate produced by human skin fibroblasts grown with sulfate concentrations of 0.3 mM have been shown to be close to 100% sulfated, with dermatan residues varying from 20 to 70% (18,21). It was also shown that undersulfation of chondroitin and dermatan/chondroitin resulted in a range of undersulfated glycosaminoglycan chains with a random or near random distribution of the unsulfated residues (18,21,35).

The advantage of using low sulfate concentrations for undersulfation is the lesser likelihood of disturbing other aspects of cell metabolism. However, some cells (28,40), including skin fibroblasts from some but not all individuals (21), are capable of making their own sulfate from cysteine or methionine so that sulfate in the growth media would not be needed to obtain sulfation. Even though no major changes in a 24-hr incubation of skin fibroblasts under these conditions were seen, there could well have been an effect upon the production of matrix over a longer time period.

We have previously reduced the sulfation of proteodermatan/chondroitin in skin fibroblast cultures to as low as 20% by reducing sulfate concentrations to 0.01 mM (18) and endothelial cells to less than 2% by use of 30 mM chlorate (40). However some small effects on sulfation were seen even at concentrations as high as 0.2 mM (18). Undersulfation of chondroitin and dermatan/chondroitin by incubations in low sulfate or with chlorate resulted in a range of undersulfated glycosaminoglycan chains with a random or near random distribution of the unsulfated residues (18,21,35,37). In no case was there any fully sulfated glycosaminoglycan if there were significant amounts of overall undersulfation, indicating that all chains were affected. Epimerization of dermatan was found to be limited to the same degree that 4-sulfation was limited, and GalNAc residues that were nonsulfated were always adjacent to GlcA, while GalNAc-4S was next to IdceA.

Normal serum sulfate concentrations in humans have been reported to range from approximately 0.2 to 0.4 mM (41–43), overlapping the range where undersulfation of dermatan/chondroitin sulfate can begin. This is in contrast to sulfate concentrations in other animals, such as mice and rats, which have serum levels as high as 1.2 mM (44). As might be expected, ingested drugs that are conjugated with sulfate for excretion (salicylates, acetominophen, paracetamol) have the effect of lowering serum sulfate (45), and lowering as much as 75% has been reported after intraperitoneal injection of salicylate into mice (44). Reduced incorporation of sulfate into proteoglycans has been seen with cultured cartilage explants from a number of animals (46), but only with human cartilage explants was there an effect within the physiological range of sulfate concentration (47). Diminution of sulfation by as much as one-third was seen when medium concentrations were lowered from 0.3 to 0.2 mM. It should be noted that cartilage cells require an extracellular source of sulfate in order to produce their large amount of proteoglycans, since chondrocytes appear to be incapable of obtaining sulfate by metabolism from cysteine or methionine. Therefore, cartilage should be the most sensitive tissue to sulfate depletion. Nevertheless, there has not been much attention given to the mechanism of why or how such undersulfation might affect cartilage structure and stability, and tissues other than cartilage have not been examined to any extent for decreases in sulfation due to sulfate depletion.

V. POTENTIAL EFFECTS OF UNDERSULFATION ON FUNCTION

An obvious effect of sulfate depletion might be a change in salt or water balance, filtration, physical changes, and connective tissue support due to decreases in the anionic nature of the large proteoglycans. In the case of skin, this would be versican. However, subtle effects would likely be missed with wound healing unless careful, detailed, blinded examinations of serum sulfate concentrations were monitored for comparison with wounds during the healing process. Animal experiments with and without drugs such as salicylates could be performed with little difficulty.

Effects of undersulfation on specific actions of cell surface proteoglycans might be of considerable importance. This would probably not apply to changes in sulfation of heparan sulfate since there are no clear mechanisms to lower sulfate levels in vivo to the degree that might affect its degree of sulfation. On the other hand, cell surface dermatan/chondroitin sulfate could well be affected, and examining this would seem to be the most logical direction in which to proceed. Thus, the specific epimerization, IdceA 2-sulfation, and GalNAc 4-sulfation could well be sensitive to blood sulfate levels, and examination of wound healing fluid for modifications in dermatan sulfate structure might be in order. Dermatan sulfate is the most prominent proteoglycan of wounds (see Chapter 1), and its release after injury has recently been shown to be a promoter of fibroblast growth factor-2 function (48). However, no detailed analysis for degree and localization of sulfation or epimerization has been reported.

The dermatan sulfate–containing proteoglycan, decorin, is a good candidate for producing changes in structure/function by undersulfation, since it is involved in collagen fibril orientation. The shape of vertebrates is largely fashioned out of extracellular matrix and depends upon getting collagen fibrils of the right size into the right places and maintaining them there. It has been apparent for many years that a proteodermatan sulfate is involved in collagen fibril orientation (49), and the term ''decorin'' was later applied because it ''decorated'' collagen fibers. Regular, frequent, and specifically located proteoglycan attachments or bridges between collagen fibrils were first seen by electron microscopy in a number of tissues (11,50–52) by use of Cupromeronic blue™, a specific electron histochemical stain developed for proteoglycans (53), and uranyl acetate to counterstain the collagen fibrils. It was proposed that decorin in tissues such as skin, cornea, tendon, and cartilage attaches to and forms bridges between adjacent collagen fibrils by means of an association of the single glycosaminoglycan chain on each decorin molecule. The center-to-center distance between the fibrils appears to be a function of the length of the glycosaminoglycan chains. In addition to tissues, the Cupromeronic blue staining technique has been applied to cultured skin fibroblasts, which make a matrix with a similar array of collagen bridged by proteoglycan (54). Thus, these proteoglycans appear to play an important role in orienting, organizing, and maintaining an ordered fibrillar matrix.

It was determined that the small proteodermatan/chondroitin sulfate in skin, tendon, and cornea was decorin and that it occupied up to four binding sites in each D period of the α 1 chain of type I collagen fibrils through the attachment of a horseshoe-shaped decorin core protein (55,56). Stereological evidence was used to support the suggestion that the bridges between the collagen fibrils contained the two glycosaminoglycan chains consisting of the single chain from each decorin molecule. Upon examination of the tertiary structures of glycosaminoglycans, it became apparent that only an antiparallel association could occur (57) and that this was consistent with the conformation of dermatan-4S but not chondroitin-4S. Thus, dermatan-4S residues have their sulfate charges concentrated in a position reducing electrostatic repulsion, while the chondroitin-4S residues have their sulfate charges in a position which results in repulsion. Recently, the role of decorin in skin collagen fibril morphology has been confirmed directly by electron microscopic examination of skin from a spontaneously aborted decorin-deficient human fetus (54) and skin from decorin null mice (58,59). This clearly demonstrated a loss of the glycosaminoglycan bridging between collagen fibrils which was accompanied by marked skin fragility. Other tissues, including cartilage, were not notably weakened.

Since disruption in the maintenance of collagen fibril placement might be expected to modify shape and destabilize the extracellular matrix, any defect in dermatan formation resulting in a decrease of fibril-to-fibril stability might affect connective tissue to a considerable degree. Degradation or destabilization of matrix due to lower sulfation may be highly relevant in wound healing, since the lower range of normal sulfate concentration in human serum is near the concentration that results in undersulfation in cultured cells. Thus, modification in sulfate levels, such as occurs when sulfate is depleted by conjugation with aspirin or acetaminophen, might be of considerable significance.

VI. POTENTIAL EFFECTS OF UNDERSULFATION ON DEGRADATION AND TURNOVER

The turnover of proteoglycans in connective tissue is primarily a function of metalloproteases (60) followed by endocytosis of intact or large pieces of glycosaminoglycan (19,61,62) which are then degraded mainly by lysosomal exoenzymes (glycosidases and sulfatases). However, glycosaminoglycan endohydrolases of the testicular hyaluronidase-type have been found in lysosomes and in the matrix of some mammalian tissues, including skin (63), skin wound (64), synovial fluid (65), synovial cell culture (66), and serum (62,65,67–69). It is not clear whether the matrix enzymes are all lysosomal with leakage into connective tissue secondary to cell modification/destruction, or whether they are normally excreted in small quantity into tissues such as skin. This latter may occur, since small pieces of glycosaminoglycan have been found in urine, presumably the product of some extracellular degradation of matrix glycosaminoglycans. However, examination of matrix to detect small amounts of extracellular glycosaminoglycan endohydrolase has not been reported in any detail.

All of the mammalian glycosaminoglycan endohydrolases of the testicular hyaluronidase-type appear to have the same substrate specificities (61). These enzymes are highly active on hyaluronan and nonsulfated chondroitin, yielding tetrasaccharide and larger oligosaccharides. They also have some activity on chondroitin sulfate, but much less than on nonsulfated chondroitin. None of these enzymes has any activity on the dermatan linkage of GalNAc-IdceA. Therefore, dermatan sulfate residues in connective tissue proteodermatan/chondroitin sulfate will be completely resistant to any connective tissue chondroitin endohydrolases, and chondroitin sulfate residues will be partially resistant. However, any modification which would diminish the percentage of dermatan and provide nonsulfated chondroitin would also provide a large increase in susceptibility to these enzymes. Most hyaluronidases are active at acid pH with little or no activity at neutral pH, and activity has not generally been found in ordinary tissue culture. However, hyaluronan depolymerization has been described in cultured human skin fibroblasts grown at near-neutral pH (70), yielding large pieces of glycosaminoglycan. Similar examination for chondroitin depolymerization was not reported. At least some other hyaluronidases are not inactivated at neutral pH, and activity has been found when tissue culture medium has been concentrated and then assayed at acidic pH (71).

The presence of extracellular hyaluronidase-type glycosaminoglycan endohydrolase in skin suggests that there might be minor degradation of chondroitin sulfate, but much more degradation whenever there would be undersulfation. This could have a significant effect on versican chondroitin sulfate turnover with an even more significant effect on collagen orientation. Since undersulfation of dermatan is accompanied by underepimerization of the same disaccharide residues, this would make the glycosaminoglycan much more susceptible to tissue endohydrolases should these enzymes be capable of reaching the sites of the proteoglycans. Any changes in turnover due to undersulfation would in turn be expected to modify wound healing, most likely through destabilization of collagen placement by affecting the structure of the dermatan with loss of antiparallel association. Increased susceptibility to animal glycosaminoglycan-degrading endoenzymes requiring the presence of GlcA would destabilize collagen placement still further.

VII. CONSIDERATIONS

There have been no significant studies regarding the relationship of sulfate metabolism or specific glycosaminoglycan sulfate fine structure to wound healing. However, it is clear that dermatan/chondroitin sulfate proteoglycans are important factors in healing, and that their structures can be modified greatly under conditions of low sulfate availability. Moreover, effects of undersulfation on dermatan/chondroitin sulfate proteoglycans produced by human skin fibroblasts in culture have been shown to be highly variable (21). Thus fibroblasts from some individuals are capable of synthesizing as much sulfate as necessary from cysteine and/or methionine, while fibroblasts from others are not. Sulfate in humans is derived directly by ingestion of sulfate-containing substances, but metabolism (mainly in the liver) of dietary sulfhydryl-containing amino acids is the main source. A decrease in the capacity of liver to produce sulfate, or any protein deficiency, could easily lead to undersulfation if dietary sulfate were low. Should this occur, one might find that the simple expedient of providing supplementary sulfate could protect against inadequate wound healing possibly due to inadequate sulfation. This could be accomplished by increased sulfate intake or even by local administration. It would be of particular importance for those individuals whose skin lacked the capacity for forming sulfate from the sulfhydryl-containing amino acids.

REFERENCES

1. Kjellen L, Lindahl U. Proteoglycans: structures and interactions. Annu Rev Biochem 1991; 60:443–475.
2. Silbert JE, Bernfield M, Kokenyesi R. Proteoglycans: a special class of glycoproteins. In: Montreuil J, Vliegenthart JFG, Schachter H, eds. Glycoproteins II. Amsterdam: Elsevier, 1997: 1–31.
3. Bernfield M, Sanderson RD. Syndecan, a developmentally regulated cell surface proteoglycan that binds extracellular matrix and growth factors. Philos Trans R. Soc Lond (Biol) 1990; 327:171–186.
4. Marcum JA, Rosenberg RD. Anticoagulantly active heparan sulfate proteoglycan and the vascular endothelium. Semin Thromb Hemost 1987; 13:464–474.
5. Bashkin P, Doctrow S, Klagsbrun M, Svahn CM, Folkman J, Vlodavsky I. Basic fibroblast growth factor binds to subendothelial extracellular matrix and is released by heparitinase and heparin-like molecules. Biochemistry 1989; 28:1737–1743.
6. Laterra J, Silbert JE, Culp LA. Cell surface heparan sulfate mediates adhesive responses to glycosaminoglycan-binding matrices, including fibronectin. J Cell Biol 1983; 96:112–123.
7. Gill PJ, Silbert CK, Silbert JE. Effects of heparan sulfate removal on attachment and reattachment of fibroblasts and endothelial cells. Biochemistry 1986; 25:405–410.
8. Gallagher JT. The extended family of proteoglycans: social residents of the pericellular zone. Curr Opin Cell Biol 1989; 1:1201–1218.
9. Ruoslahti E. Proteoglycans in cell regulation. J Biol Chem 1989; 264:13369–13372.
10. Toole BP. Glycosaminoglycans in morphogenesis. In: Hay ED, ed. Cell Biology of Extracellular Matrix. New York: Plenum, 1981:259–294.
11. Scott JE. Extracellular matrix, supramolecular organization and shape. J Anat 1995; 187:259–269.

12. Maimone MM, Tollefsen DM. Structure of a dermatan sulfate hexasaccharide that binds to heparin cofactor II with high affinity. J Biol Chem 1990; 265:18263–18271.

13. Tollefsen DM. Insight into the mechanism of action of heparin cofactor II. Thromb Haemost 1995; 74:1209–1214.

14. Fransson LA, Havsmark B, Silberberg I. A method for the sequence analysis of dermatan sulphate. Biochem J 1990; 269:381–388.

15. Plaas AHK, Wong-Palms S, Roughley PJ, Midura RJ, Hascall VC. Chemical and immunological assay of the nonreducing terminal residues of chondroitin sulfate from human aggrecan. J Biol Chem 1997; 272:20603–20610.

16. Malmstrom A, Fransson LA, Hook M, Lindahl U. Biosynthesis of dermatan sulfate: formation of L-iduronic acid residues. J Biol Chem 1975; 250:3419–3425.

17. Malmstrom A. Biosynthesis of dermatan sulfate. II. Substrate specificity of the C-5 uronosyl epimerase. J Biol Chem 1981; 259:161–165.

18. Silbert JE, Palmer ME, Humphries DE, Silbert CK. Formation of dermatan sulfate by cultured human skin fibroblasts: effects of sulfate concentration on proportions of dermatan/chondroitin. J Biol Chem 1986; 261:13397–13400.

19. Silbert JE, Sugumaran G. Intracellular membranes in the synthesis, transport, and metabolism of proteoglycans. Biochim Biophys Acta 1995; 1241:371–384.

20. Fransson LA, Roden L. Structure of dermatan sulfate. II. Characterization of products obtained by hyaluronidase digestion of dermatan sulfate. J Biol Chem 1967; 242:4170–4175.

21. Silbert CK, Humphries DE, Palmer ME, Silbert JE. Effects of sulfate deprivation on the production of chondroitin/dermatan sulfate by cultures of skin fibroblasts from normal and diabetic individuals. Arch Biochem Biophys 1991; 285:137–141.

22. Sugumaran G, Silbert JE. Relationship of sulfation to ongoing chondroitin polymerization during biosynthesis of chondroitin 4-sulfate by microsomal preparations from cultured mouse mastocytoma cells. J Biol Chem 1990; 265:18284–18288.

23. Sugumaran G, Silbert JE. Subfractionation of chick embryo epiphyseal cartilage Golgi: localization of enzymes involved in the synthesis of the polysaccharide portion of proteochondroitin sulfate. J Biol Chem 1991; 266:9565–9569.

24. Hoppe U, Glossl J, Kresse H. Influence of monensin on biosynthesis, processing and secretion of proteodermatan sulfate by skin fibroblasts. Eur J Biochem 1985; 152:91–97.

25. Kitagawa H, Oyama M, Masayama K, Yamaguchi Y, Sugahara K. Structural variations in the glycosaminoglycan-protein linkage region of recombinant decorin expressed in Chinese hamster ovary cells. Glycobiology 1997; 7:1175–1180.

26. Silbert JE. Biosynthesis of chondroitin sulfate: chain termination. J Biol Chem 1978; 253:6888–6892.

27. Cogburn JN, Silbert JE. The effect of penultimate N-acetylgalactosamine 4-sulfate on chondroitin chain elongation. Carbohyd Res 1986;151:207–212.

28. Esko JD, Elgavish A, Prasthofer T, Taylor WH, Weinke JL. Sulfate transport-deficient mutants of Chinese hamster ovary cells: sulfation of glycosaminoglycans dependent on cysteine. J Biol Chem 1986; 261:15725–15733.

29. Rossi A, Bonaventure J, Delezzolde A-L, Cetta G, Superti-Furga A. Undersulfation of proteoglycans synthesized by chondrocytes from a patient with achondrogenesis

type 1B homozygous for an L483P substitution in the diastrophic dysplasia sulfate transporter. J Biol Chem 1996; 271:18456–18464.

30. Lidholt K, Weinke JL, Kiser CS, Lugemwa FN, Bame KJ, Cheifetz S, Massague J, Lindahl U, Esko JD. A single mutation affects both *N*-acetylglucosaminyltransferase and glucuronosyltransferase activities in a Chinese hamster ovary cell mutant defective in heparan sulfate biosynthesis. Proc Natl Acad Sci USA 1992;89:2267–2271.

31. Bai X, Esko JD. An animal cell mutant defective in heparan sulfate hexuronic acid 2-*O*-sulfation. J Biol Chem 1996; 271:17711–17717.

32. Toma L, Pinhal MAS, Dietrich CP, Nader HB, Hirschberg CB. Transport of UDP-galactose into the Golgi lumen regulates the biosynthesis of proteoglycans. J Biol Chem 1996; 271:3897–3901.

33. Lyle S, Stanczak JD, Westley J, Schwartz NB. Sulfate-activating enzymes in normal and brachymorphic mice: evidence for a channeling defect. Biochemistry 1995; 34:940–945.

34. Sobue M, Takeuchi J, Ito K, Kimata K, Suzuki S. Effect of environmental sulfate concentration on the synthesis of low and high sulfated chondroitin sulfates by chick embryo cartilage. J Biol Chem 1978; 253:6190–6196.

35. Humphries DE, Silbert CK, Silbert JE. Glycosaminoglycan production by bovine aortic endothelial cells cultured in sulfate-depleted medium. J Biol Chem 1986; 261:9122–9127.

36. Humphries DE, Sugumaran G, Silbert JE. Techniques to decrease proteoglycan sulfation in cultured cells. Methods Enzymol 1989; 179:428–434.

37. Silbert JE, Sugumaran G, Cogburn JN. Sulfation of proteochondroitin and 4-methylumbelliferyl β-D-xyloside-chondroitin formed by mouse mastocytoma cells cultured in sulfate-deficient medium. Biochem J 1993; 296:119–126.

38. Humphries DE, Silbert JE. Chlorate: a reversible inhibitor of proteoglycan sulfation. Biochem Biophys Res Commun 1988; 154:365–371.

39. Greve H, Cully Z, Blumberg P, Kresse H. Influence of chlorate on proteoglycan biosynthesis by cultured human fibroblasts. J Biol Chem 1988; 263:12886–12892.

40. Humphries DE, Silbert CK, Silbert JE. Sulphation by cultured cells: cysteine, cysteinesulphinic acid, and sulphite as sources for proteoglycan sulphate. Biochem J 1988; 252:305–308.

41. Ziemniak JA, Allison N, Boppana VK, Dubb J, Stote R. The effect of acetaminophen on the disposition of fenoldopam: competition for sulfation. Clin Pharmacol 1988; 3:275–281.

42. Morris ME, Benincosa LJ. Sulfate homeostasis. II Influence of chronic aspirin administration on inorganic sulfate in humans. Pharm Res 1990; 7:719–722.

43. Edwards DJ, Altman HJ, Galinsky RE. Plasma concentrations of inorganic sulfate in Alzheimer's disease. Neurology 1993; 43:1637–1838.

44. de Vries BJ, van den Berg WB, van de Putte LBA. Salicylate-induced depletion of endogenous inorganic sulfate: the potential role in the suppression of sulfated glycosaminoglycan synthesis in murine articular cartilage. Arthritis Rheum 1985; 28:922–929.

45. van der Kraan PM, de Vries BJ, Vitters EL, van den Berg WB, van de Putte LBA.

Inhibition of glycosaminoglycan synthesis in anatomically intact rat patellar cartilage by paracetamol-induced serum sulfate depletion. Biochem Pharmacol 1988; 37: 3683–3690.

46. van der Kraan PM, de Vries BJ, Vitters EL, van den Berg WB, van de Putte LBA. The effect of low sulfate concentrations on the glycosaminoglycan synthesis in anatomically intact articular cartilage in the mouse. J Orth Res 1989; 7:645–653.

47. van der Kraan PM, Vitters EL, de Vries BJ, van den Berg WB. High susceptibility of human articular cartilage glycosaminoglycan synthesis to changes in inorganic sulfate availability. J Orthop Res 1990; 8:565–571.

48. Penc SF, Pomahac B, Winkler T, Dorschner RA, Eriksson E, Herndon M, Gallo RL. Dermatan sulfate released after injury is a potent promoter of fibroblast growth factor-2 function. J Biol Chem 1998; 273:28116–28121.

49. Toole BP, Lowther DA. Dermatan sulfate-protein: isolation from and interaction with collagen. Arch Biochem Biophys 1968; 128:567–578.

50. Orford CR, Gardner DL. Proteoglycan association with collagen d band in hyaline articular cartilage. Connect Tissue Res 1984; 12:345–348.

51. Scott JE, Haigh M. Proteoglycan-collagen interactions in intervertebral disc: a chondroitin sulphate proteoglycan associates with collagen fibrils in rabbit annulus fibrosus at the d-e bands. Biosci Rep 1986; 6:879–888.

52. Scott JE. Supramolecular organization of extracellular matrix glycosaminoglycans, in vitro and in the tissues. FASEB J 1992; 6:2639–2645.

53. Scott JE, Orford CR. Dermatan sulphate-rich proteoglycan associates with rat tail-tendon collagen at the d band in the gap region. Biochem J 1981; 197:213–216.

54. Scott JE, Dyne K, Thomlinson AM, Ritchie M, Bateman J, Cetta G, Valli M. Human cells unable to express decoron produced disorganized extracellular matrix lacking "shape modules" (interfibrillar proteoglycan bridges). Exp Cell Res 1998; 243:59–66.

55. Scott JE. Proteodermatan and proteokeratan sulfate (decorin, lumican/fibromodulin) proteins are horseshoe shaped: implications for their interactions with collagen. Biochemistry 1996; 35:8795–8799.

56. Weber IT, Harrison RW, Iozzo RV. Model structure of decorin and implications for collagen fibrillogenesis. J Biol Chem 1996; 271:31767–31770.

57. Scott JE, Heatley F, Wood B. Comparison of secondary structures in water of chondroitin-4-sulfate and dermatan sulfate: implications in the formation of tertiary structures. Biochemistry 1995; 34:15467–15474.

58. Danielson KG, Baribault H, Holmes DF, Graham H, Kadler KE, Iozzo RV. Targeted disruption of decorin leads to abnormal collagen fibril morphology and skin fragility. J Cell Biol 1997; 136:729–743.

59. Keene DR, Ridgway CC, Iozzo RV. Type VI microfilaments interact with a specific region of banded collagen fibrils in skin. J Histochem Cytochem 1998; 46:215–220.

60. Woessner JF. Matrix metalloproteinases and their inhibitors in connective tissue remodeling. FASEB J 1991; 5:2145–2154.

61. Silbert JE. Advances in the biochemistry of proteoglycans. In: Uitto J, Perejda AF, eds. Diseases of Connective Tissue: The Molecular Pathology of the Extracellular Matrix. New York: Marcel Dekker, 1987:83–98.

62. Roden L, Campbell P, Fraser JRE, Laurent TC, Pertoft H, Thompson JN. Enzymic

pathways of hyaluronan catabolism. In: The Biology of Hyaluronan. Ciba Found Sym 1989; 143:60–86.

63. Cashman DC, Laryea JU, Weissmann B. The hyaluronidase of rat skin. Arch Biochem Biophys 1969; 135:387–395.

64. Bertolami CN, Donoff RB. Identification, characterization, and partial purification of mammalian skin wound hyaluronidase. J Invest Derm 1982; 79:417–421.

65. Bollet AJ, Bonner WM Jr, Nance JL. The presence of hyaluronidase in various mammalian tissues. J Biol Chem 1963; 238:3522–3527.

66. Orkin RW, Toole BP. Isolation and characterization of hyaluronidase from cultures of chick embryo skin- and muscle-derived fibroblasts. J Biol Chem 1980; 255:1036–1042.

67. Aronson NN Jr, Davidson EA. Lysosomal hyaluronidase from rat liver. J Biol Chem 1967; 242:437–440, 441–444.

68. Afify AM, Stern M, Guntenhoener M, Stern R. Purification and characterization of human serum hyaluronidase. Arch Biochem Biophys 1993; 305:434–441.

69. Zhu L, Hope TJ, Hall J, Davies A, Stern M, Muller-Eberhard U, Stern R, Parslow TG. Molecular cloning of a mammalian hyaluronidase reveals identity with hemopexin, a serum heme-binding protein. J Biol Chem 1994; 269:32092–32097.

70. Nakamura T, Takagaki K, Kubo K, Morikawa A, Tamura S, Endo M. Extracellular depolymerization of hyaluronic acid in cultured human skin fibroblasts. Biochem Biophys Res Commun 1990; 172:70–76.

71. Orkin RW, Toole BP. Chick embryo fibroblasts produce two forms of hyaluronidase. J Cell Biol 1980; 85:248–257.

3
Syndecan Biology in Wound Repair

Richard L. Gallo
*University of California, San Diego, and San Diego VA Medical Center,
San Diego, California*

Merton Bernfield
*The Children's Hospital and Harvard Medical School,
Boston, Massachusetts*

Varpu Kainulainen
Turku Centre for Biotechnology, Turku, Finland

I. INTRODUCTION

The repair of injury is orchestrated by a wide variety of soluble effectors, including growth factors, cytokines, chemokines, proteases, antiproteases, and insoluble extracellular matrix components. The presence of visible scar, or disorganized dermal architecture and fibrosis, is influenced by many of these soluble and insoluble effectors of wound repair. This chapter discusses evidence that demonstrates proteoglycans, in particular syndecans, may control the wound repair process by binding many of these effectors and influencing their function.

II. CELL SURFACE HEPARAN SULFATE BINDS EFFECTORS OF TISSUE REPAIR

The syndecans are cell surface proteoglycans (PGs) that are synthesized with covalently attached heparan sulfate (HS) glycosaminoglycan (GAG) chains. Much of the heparan sulfate on epithelial cells is associated with syndecans. To understand how syndecans may function it is important to first understand the actions of heparan sulfate itself.

37

Heparan sulfate binds growth factors such as fibroblast growth factor-2 (FGF-2), involved in fibroblast and endothelial cell proliferation and connective tissue formation; heparin-binding epidermal growth factor (HB-EGF), a powerful epithelial and smooth muscle cell mitogen; platelet-derived growth factor (PDGF), involved in fibroblast migration and proliferation; transforming growth factor-β (TGF-β), a major determinant of extracellular matrix (ECM) production and remodeling and an inhibitor of epithelial cell proliferation; and vascular endothelial growth factor (VEGF), also known as vascular permeability factor (VPF), which increases endothelial permeability as well as capillary endothelial cell growth (1). Heparan sulfate chains bind to the powerful neutrophil-derived proteases (viz., elastase, cathepsin G) and can protect them against inhibition by α1-antiprotease and α1-antichymotrypsin, respectively. Extracellular superoxide dismutase, a major protectant against oxidative injury, binds to heparan sulfate with high affinity. A variety of growth factor–binding proteins (BPs) also bind to heparan sulfate chains, including insulin-like growth factor (IGF)–BPs 3 and 5, as well as TGE-β–BP. Fibrosis involves the accumulation of a variety of insoluble extracellular matrix components, including the fibrillar collagens (types I, III, and V), fibronectin, tenascin, thrombospondin, and vitronectin (2). Since heparan sulfate acts on each of these effectors involved in the repair of injury (Fig. 1) it is reasonable to speculate that heparan sulfate could influence scarring.

Heparan sulfate chains are linked to specific core proteins as proteoglycans. Heparan sulfate PGs are found within intracellular vesicles, at cell surfaces, and in the ECM. Heparan sulfate is qualitatively similar in structure to the pharmaceutical product, heparin, and is the most acidic molecule made by animal cells. Heparan sulfate chains bind protein ligands at high affinity. The high binding affinities (Kd ranging from 1–100 nM) result from the conformational flexibility and strong anionic charge of the HS chains. Some heparan sulfate chains are comprised of highly sulfated regions (heparin-like domains) alternating with relatively unmodified domains, and this macroscopic structure appears to vary with cell type (3).

Cell surface heparan sulfate proteoglycans, like syndecans, provide cells with a mechanism to snare a wide variety of physiological effectors without requiring that evolution generate multiple novel binding proteins. The interaction of FGF-2 with cell surface heparan sulfate is a well studied example: This growth factor binds at nM affinities to heparan sulfate chains, which are 20- to 50-fold more abundant at the cell surface than the signal transducing FGF receptors. Once formed, the FGF-heparan sulfate complex forms a higher-affinity ternary complex with the FGF receptor which, when occupied, initiates a signaling cascade within the cell (4,5). Analogous co-receptor interactions occur with other extracellular effectors, e.g., fibronectin initiates stress fiber formation only when both its heparan sulfate- and integrin-binding domains are engaged (6).

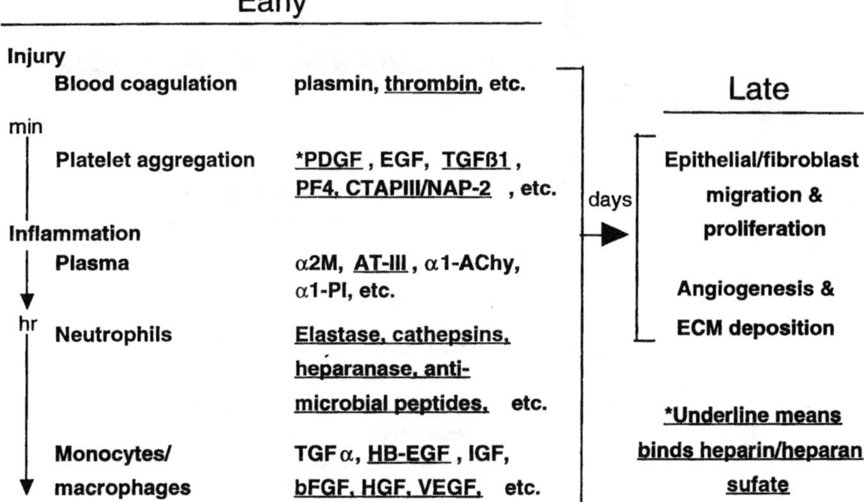

Figure 1   Effectors involved in repair of injury. During the process of wound repair multiple proteins are regulated by binding to heparan sulfate. Underlined items in this partial list of wound repair components illustrates heparan sulfate–binding effectors.

III. BASICS OF PROTEOGLYCAN STRUCTURE

In the past, terms such as "ground substance" or "mucopolysaccharide" had been used to describe proteoglycans because of their appearance histologically and their thick and mucinous nature when isolated. Due to these physical properties, proteoglycans were historically difficult to study and poorly understood. Over the last decade, however, our understanding of these complex molecules has increased. Among the most important advances in our knowledge of proteoglycans has been the identification of specific core proteins and recognition of sequence specificity in glycoaminoglycans. Information derived from this has helped us understand proteoglycan structure.

Proteoglycans are known by specific gene families based on sequence information derived from proteoglycan core proteins and direct molecular cloning techniques. The prototypical proteoglycan consists of a single core protein linked to one or more linear glycosaminoglycans (Fig. 2). Each core protein has the capacity to accept a variety of GAG chains. The general terms used to describe sulfated GAGs are heparan sulfate, keratan sulfate, or chondroitin sulfate A, B, and C. Chondroitin sulfate B is also known as dermatan sulfate. Therefore, the

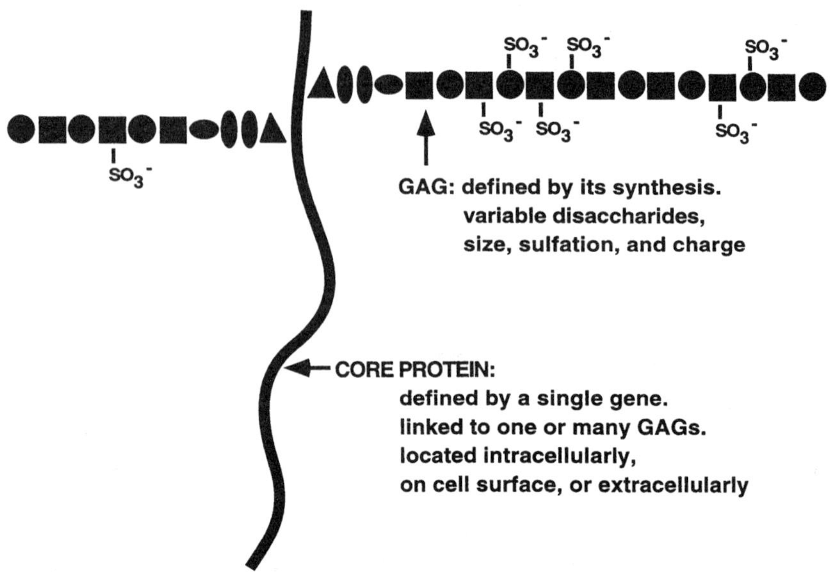

Figure 2 Schematic representation of proteoglycan structure. Proteoglycans are composed of central ''core'' protein, illustrated here as a solid line, to which one or more glycosaminoglycan chains are attached. The glycosaminoglycan (GAG) is attached to the core protein by a xylose (triangle) followed by two galactose residues (vertical oval) and a glucuronic acid (horizontal oval). The complete GAG is then assembled with variable repeating disaccharide units with variable sulfation patterns (squares and circles).

nomenclature for proteoglycans is complicated in that individual molecules must be defined based on the core protein and the associated GAG. For example, syndecans may have heparan sulfate or chondroitin sulfate GAGs. The nature of the GAGs will change function. Similarly, heparan sulfate may be on many different core proteins. Different core proteins can convey different functions to the GAG.

For purposes of organization, it is useful to group proteoglycans based on their site of expression by the cell. Specific proteoglycan core proteins have been identified within the cell, attached to the cell surface, and bound within the extracellular matrix (Table 1).

The diversity of proteoglycans suggests many biological activities may be associated with different core proteins or attached glycoaminoglycans. A specific example is the clinical disorder Simpson-Golabi-Behmel. This disorder is due to a deficiency in glypican-3, resulting in numerous visceral and skeletal abnormalities and decorin-deficent mice, which have abnormal collagen organization and

Table 1 Core Proteins of Proteoglycans

Core protein	Location	Reference
Intracellular		
Serglycin	Mast cells, basophils	Stevens (118)
Cell surface		
Syndecan-1	Keratinocytes, other epithelia	Saunders et al. (8)
Syndecan-2	Fibroblasts, endothelia	Marynen et al. (7)
		Mali et al. (10)
Syndecan-3	Neural cells	Gould et al. (13)
		Carey et al. (11)
Syndecan-4	Ubiquitous, lymphoid	Kojima et al. (14)
		David et al. (12)
NG-2	Neural, melanoma	Nishiyama and Stallcup (119)
Glypican		David et al. (120)
Cerebroglycan		Stipp et al. (121)
OCI-5		Filmus et al. (122)
K Glypican	Kidney, brain	Watanabe et al. (123)
Glypican–5	Brain, bone	Veugelers et al. (124)
Epican	Keratinocytes	Haggerty et al. (125)
Betaglycan	Fibroblasts, epithelia	Wang et al. (126)
Extracellular matrix		
Aggracan	Cartilage	Doege et al. (127)
		Daege et al. (128)
Versican	Fibroblasts	Zimmermann et al. (129)
		LeBaron et al. (130)
		Kahari et al. (131)
Brevican	Brain	Yamada et al. (132)
Neurocan	Brain	Perides et al. (133)
		Rauch et al. (134)
Decorin	Fibroblasts, others	Brennan et al. (135)
Biglycan	Bone	Fisher et al. (136)
Epiphycan	Cartilage	Johnson et al. (137)
Fibromodulin	Fibroblasts	Oldberg et al. (138)
Lumican	Cornea	Blochberger et al. (139)
OIF	Cartilage	Shinomura et al. (140)
Agrin	Brain	Tsen et al. (141)
Perlecan	Basement membranes	Noonan et al. (142)
		Murdoch et al. (143)
Bamacan	Basement membranes	Couchman et al. (144)

skin fragility. It is unclear, however, if the physiological manifestations of these specific proteoglycan deficiencies are due to the lack of core protein or associated GAG, or both.

The syndecan family of proteoglycans has been the most extensively studied with relation to wound repair and fibrosis. These proteoglycans illustrate the functional relevance of both proteoglycan core protein and associated glycosaminoglycan and can serve as a prototype to understand proteoglycan function in general.

IV. SYNDECAN FAMILY OF HEPARAN SULFATE PROTEOGLYCANS

Altogether four syndecan heparan sulfate proteoglycan genes have been cloned from mammals (7–17). Their chromosomal localization, exon organization, and sequence relationships with a *Drosophila* syndecan (18), a *C. elegans* syndecan and *Xenopus* syndecan (19) indicate that the mammalian syndecan family arose by gene duplication from a single ancestral gene (Fig. 3). All syndecans are type I transmembrane proteins, with an N-terminal signal peptide, an ectodomain that contains several Ser-Gly consensus sequences for GAG attachment sites, a single hydrophobic transmembrane domain, and a short C-terminal cytoplasmic domain. Syndecan-1 and -3, and syndecan-2 and -4 can be considered to form subfamilies based on sequence similarities, GAG attachment sites, and core protein size (see Fig. 3). In syndecans-1 and -3 the GAG sites occur in two clusters, one near the N-terminus and the other near the plasma membrane. A variable proportion of these attachment sites may be glycanated. The structural elements of the core protein determine if a site will be glycanated, and if so, whether with heparan or chondroitin sulfate (20). The majority of GAG chains added to syndecans are heparan sulfate, although syndecan-1 (21) and syndecan-4 (22) have been shown to bear chondroitin sulfate as well. Other than the GAG attachment sites, syndecan extracellular domain sequences are highly variable. This is apparent when the sequence of a specific syndecan is compared across species.

In contrast to the extracellular domain, transmembrane and cytoplasmic domains of different syndecans are highly conserved (see Fig. 3). The cytoplasmic domains are short, but highly conserved. All syndecan core proteins have an identical tetrapeptide sequence EFYA at the C-terminus and three invariant tyrosines and one invariant serine in the cytoplasmic domain. Syntenin, a PDZ protein, binds the FYA sequence and affects membrane-cytoskeleton organization (23). Syntenin is a candidate for linking syndecan-supported recognition processes to the cytoskeleton and cytoplasmic signal-effector systems. The presence of four phosphorylatable residues in the cytoplasmic tail of all the syndecans suggests that the tail could be a kinase substrate in vivo. Phosphorylation of the cytoplasmic tails has been detected in the serine residue of all syndecans (24–

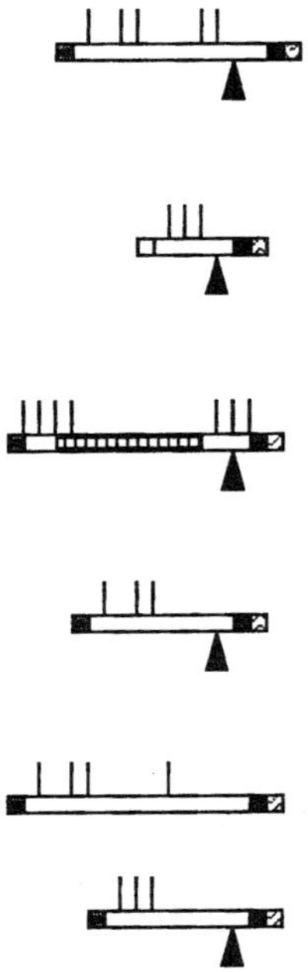

Schematic diagram	Name (synonyms)	Species	Size of core protein (aa)	Size of mRNA (kb)	Type of GAG	Reference
	Syndecan-1 (Syndecan, B-B4, CD138)	mouse	311	2.6, 3.4	HS, CS	Saunders et al., 1989
		human	310	2.6, 3.4		Mali et al., 1990
		hamster	309	2.4, 3.2		Kiefer et al., 1990
		rat	313	2.6, 3.4		Kojima et al., 1992
	Syndecan-2 (Fibroblycan)	human	201	2.6, 3.4	HS	Marynen et al., 1989
		rat	211	1.1, 2.2, 3.4		Pierce et al., 1992
	Syndecan-3 (N-Syndecan)	rat	442	2.6	HS, CS	Carey et al., 1992 & 1997
		chicken		7.0		Gould et al., 1992
	Syndecan-4 (Ryudocan, Amphiglycan)	human	198	2.6	HS	David et al., 1992
		rat	202	2.6		Kojima et al., 1992
		chicken	197	0.9, 1.3, 2.9		Baciu et al., 1994
		mouse	198	2.7		Tsuzuki et al., 1997
	D. melanogaster syndecan		367	2.3, 3.9	HS	Spring et al., 1994
	Xenopus syndecan		191	2, 4	HS	Rosenblum et al., 1995

Figure 3 Syndecan family of cell surface heparan sulfate proteoglycans. Four distinct syndecans are known in mammals, two in chicken, and one in *Drosophila* and *Xenopus*. The schematic diagram illustrates the similarity in core proteins among the syndecans. GAG attachment sites are shown by solid lines and predicted protease cleavage sites in the extracellular domain are shown with arrows.

28) and in tyrosine residues of syndecan-1 (26). Syndecan-4 phosphorylation is enhanced by treatment with PMA and decreased by FGF-2, and the phosphorylation site is localized to Ser^{183} that is conserved in all syndecans (28). Thus, this finding may be relevant for all syndecan family members. In addition, recent data show that the cortacin-Src kinase signaling pathway is involved in syndecan-3–dependent neurite outgrowth by heparin-binding growth-associated molecule (HB-GAM). Furthermore, Src family tyrosine kinases and their substrates can bind a region (RMKKKDEGSY) in the syndecan-3 cytoplasmic domain that is conserved in all syndecans (29). Thus, all syndecans may interact with the Src family kinases through their conserved cytoplasmic domains.

Interrupting the conserved domains within the cytoplasmic tail of the syndecans are variable regions that show less similarity between syndecans-1, -2, -3, and -4. Interestingly, these variable regions are highly conserved between different species among each specific syndecans. For example, a sequence unique to the syndecan-4 cytoplasmic domain binds both protein kinase C alpha (PKCα) (30) and phosphatidylinositol 4,5-bisphosphate (PIP_2) (31). This binding promotes syndecan-4 cytoplasmic tail oligomerization (32) and potentiates protein kinase C activation (33). These studies further suggest a specific role for syndecan-4 at focal contacts. Overall, structural similarities in cytoplasmic domains, and diversity of the ectodomains, suggests that syndecans were evolved to carry out similar, but not identical functions.

V.　GENOMIC ORGANIZATION AND REGULATORY ELEMENTS OF SYNDECANS

The syndecan genes are dispersed throughout the mouse and human genomes, but each syndecan gene is linked to four members of the myc oncogene family of transcription factors (34). Syndecan-1 is next to Nmyc, syndecan-2 close to myc, syndecan-3 near Lmyc, and syndecan-4 on the same chromosome as Bmyc (34). The physical relationship between the members of these two gene families appears to be ancient and conserved after two genome duplications thought to have occurred during vertebrate evolution. The syndecan-1 gene maps to human chromosome 2p23 (35), syntenic region in the mouse is on chromosome 12 (36); syndecan-2 gene on chromosome 8q23 (7), in mouse 15 (34); syndecan-3 on chromosome 1p32-p36 (34), in mouse 4 (34); and syndecan-4 on 20q12-q13 (37), in mouse 2 (34).

The genomic organization of the mammalian syndecans (38,39) is similar to that of the *Drosophila* and *C. elegans* syndecans. They show a strikingly similar exon–intron organization, which supports the idea that syndecans arose by gene duplication from a single ancestral gene. Each exon encodes discrete functional domains in syndecans: exon 1 encodes the 5′-untranslated region and signal peptide, exon 2 encodes the N-terminal cluster of GAG attachment sites, exon

3 encodes the ectodomain spacer region, exon 4 encodes the transmembrane cluster of GAG attachment sites and 10bp of the transmembrane domain, and exon 5 encodes the rest of the transmembrane domain, the cytoplasmic domain and 3'-untranslated region. The most variable exon in length and sequence is exon 3, which encodes an ectodomain region without the conserved GAG attachment sites. The most conserved exons are 4 and 5, coding transmembrane and cytoplasmic domains, respectively.

Upstream sequences of the syndecan-1 gene have promotor activity and contain TATA and CAAT boxes as well as a variety of other potential binding sites for transcription factors, including Sp-1, NF-κB, MyoD (E-box) and Antennapedia (38). Wilms' tumor protein WT1, which is required for kidney development, is a transcriptional activator of the syndecan-1 gene and has multiple binding sites in the promotor (40). Constitutive high level of syndecan-1 expression in epithelial cells is due to proximal Sp-1 binding sites (41), which is typical for many constitutively expressed genes. Syndecan-1 gene has also a secondary far-upstream enhancer that is activated in migrating keratinocytes during wound re-epithelialization (42). Syndecan-1 expression is down-regulated during myoblast terminal differentiation, however, by a myogenin- and E-box independent pathway. Its expression in myoblasts is controlled by a proximal region of promotor that is influenced by FGF-2, TGF-β and retinoic acid (43).

An analysis of syndecan mRNA levels in various mouse cells and tissues showed that virtually all tissues and cells express at least one syndecan, and most cells and tissues express multiple family members (44). However, each syndecan family member is expressed in a distinct cell-, tissue-, and development-specific pattern, suggesting distinct functions of each syndecan. For example, brain contains almost exclusively syndecan-3 mRNA, kidney mostly syndecan-4, and liver high levels of syndecans-1, -2, and -4, but no syndecan-3 (44).

VI. DEVELOPMENTAL REGULATION OF SYNDECANS

Spatial and temporal changes of syndecan expression occur during early embryogenesis (1,45,46). Syndecan-1 is first detected at the 4-cell stage. Between the 4-cell stage and late morula stages, syndecan-1 is present intracellularly and on the cell surfaces of the blastomeres. At the blastocyst stage, syndecan-1 is detected at cell–cell contacts throughout the embryo, and later at the interface of the primitive ectoderm and endoderm, the initial site of matrix accumulation. During gastrulation, syndecan-1 is expressed at the basolateral surfaces of ectoderm cells and on its derivatives, definitive endoderm and undifferentiated mesenchyme. Syndecan-1 is then lost from the neural plate in an asymmetrical pattern from the mesenchyme. This asymmetry exhibits only in embryonic mesenchyme; syndecan-1 expression is uniform in the extraembryonic mesechyme and is strongly expressed by the cells undergoing trophoblast giant cell differentiation, suggesting a role in placental development.

The morphogenesis is modified by reciprocal interactions between epithelial derivatives (ectoderm and endoderm) and mesenchyme. Embryonic syndecan-1 expression has been suggested to have a role in this interplay during the development of several organs, including tooth (47), kidney (48), limb (49), lung (50), and the optic, vibrissal, nasal, and otic analog (51). Syndecan-1 expression during the development of these organs shares some common features. In general, the epithelium changing its shape (e.g., forming a bud) transiently loses its cell surface syndecan-1 expression while the condensing and proliferating mesenchyme around the epithelium begins to express syndecan-1. With further development, the morphologically stable epithelium reexpresses syndecan-1 while the terminally differentiated mesechymal cells lose it (e.g., when limb bud mesechymal cells form chondroblasts).

Similar findings have been shown with syndecan-3. During limb development, syndecan-3 is transiently expressed in condensing mesenchyme (13,52), and this expression is closely associated with tenascin-C expression, an ECM protein that binds syndecans (53). In the embryo tibia, syndecan-3 is expressed in proliferating, immature chondrocytes, while differentiated chondrocytes lack the expression (54), suggesting a regulatory role of proliferation during bone development. Furthermore, limb cartilage differentiation can be inhibited with syndecan-3 antibodies in vitro (55). Thus, syndecan-1 and-3 expression in epithelia correlates with epithelial maturation and in mesenchyme with cell proliferation and migration, consistent with their proposed functions as matrix receptors and growth factor co-receptors. Interestingly, syndecan-3 might also have a role in oligodendrocyte differentiation, since its expression is highly up-regulated during that time of postnatal central nervous system development (56).

VII. SYNDECANS IN MALIGNANT TRANSFORMATION

Consistent with its proposed role as a modulator of growth factor actions and as an ECM receptor, syndecan-1 exhibits a regulated pattern of expression during cell differentiation and malignant transformation. In mature tissues, syndecan-1 is most abundant in stratified epithelia where it is localized over the entire surface of suprabasal keratinocytes, whereas basal and the most superficial layers are stained only weakly (8,57,58). Increased proliferation of keratinocytes without malignant growth during wound repair is associated with increased syndecan-1 expression (59). However, development of dysplasia, a premalignant neoplasia, is associated with the loss of syndecan-1 (60).

The formation of carcinomas is associated with marked reduction in syndecan-1 expression in several human carcinomas (61,62) and in animal models

(60,63). However, syndecan-1 expression is not totally lost from malignant tumors, but is retained in tumors showing high degree of differentiation (61–63). In squamous cell carcinomas (SCCs), retained syndecan-1 is localized around the keratin pearls, but is lost on the actively proliferating cells in tumor mass (64). This pattern of expression suggests that syndecan-1 may have a role in keratinocyte differentiation during neoplastic growth. In addition, the loss of syndecan-1 expression in SCC of the head and neck is associated with the poor clinical outcome (64). In SCCs syndecan-1 and E-cadherin show similar expression; both are expressed in well-differentiated cells, while lacking from poorly differentiated ones. Furthermore, they show coordinated expression in mammary epithelial cells genetically manipulated with E-cadherin (65). Both molecules have been suggested to have a role in the polarization and maintenance of cytoskeleton and cell morphology.

The possible role of syndecan-1 in malignant transformation and maintaining the epithelial morphology has been studied in vitro using mouse mammary tumor cells (S115). These cells respond to steroid hormones by changing their morphology to fusiform type, increasing growth rate and anchorage-independent growth. When transfected with syndecan-1 cDNA they exhibit benign characteristics also in the presence of steroids (66). This effect is mediated ectodomain since S155 cells transfected with a mutant syndecan-1 lacking cytoplasmic and transmembrane domains also show benign characteristics (67). Also, overexpression of syndecan-1 in transformed human renal epithelial cells causes cells to become more anchorage dependent and less motile (68). Thus, syndecan-1 expression seems to be required for maintenance of a differentiated epithelial phenotype. A similar conclusion was reached from experiments in which endogenous syndecan-1 expression was suppressed in epithelial cells by transfection with antisense cDNA (69). These cells showed a striking change in morphology, from a cuboidal shape to fusiform cells that lose E-cadherin expression and gain the ability to migrate in collagen gels, and grow anchorage independently.

VIII. REGULATION OF SYNDECANS DURING TISSUE INJURY

Both cell surface expression and shedding of syndecan-1 and -4 are induced in response to injury. For example, syndecan-1 is induced in aortic neointima in response to a balloon catheter induced by vascular wall injury (70). The best-studied example, however, is cutaneous wound repair. Syndecan-1 is transiently induced in proliferating keratinocytes at the wound edge and in the endothelial cells of the wound bed (59), while syndecan-4 is induced on the fibroblasts that form granulation tissue (71). This induction in mesenchymal cells has been shown to be, in part, due to action of neutrophil-derived antimicrobial peptide PR-39

(72). However, syndecan-1 is lost from the keratinocytes that migrate into the wound (59), and the induced endothelial cell expression of syndecan-1 is suppressed upon repair of the wound. Also, induced keratinocyte expression is normalized upon reepithelialization of the wound (59).

IX. REGULATION OF CELL SURFACE SYNDECAN RELEASE

A common mechanism of HSPG turnover involves endocytosis and degradation in lysosomes, and a significant fraction of syndecans are removed by this mechanism (73). However, an additional mechanism for removal of syndecans from the cell surfaces is the release of the entire ectodomain into extracellular space in a process called shedding (74,75). This release is mediated by a proteolytic activity of unknown identity. However, syndecan shedding can be inhibited by treatment of the cells with metalloproteinase inhibitors suggesting that a metalloproteinase is involved. The precise site of cleavage within the ectodomain is not identified. The dibasic sequence adjacent to the plasma membrane attachment site has been considered to be the prime candidate, but shedding of the *Drosophila* syndecan that lacks these basic residues (18) suggests that this supposition is not true.

Enhanced syndecan shedding by phorbol esters (76) resembles that of other membrane proteins, including growth factors, cytokine receptors, cell adhesion molecules, and some enzymes, suggesting a common regulated mechanism for the proteolytic cleavage. Importantly, syndecan-1 and -4 shedding is enhanced by the proteases (thrombin, plasmin) and growth factors (EGF-family members) involved in tissue injury (76). Furthermore, there is evidence that syndecan shedding also occurs in vivo. For example, soluble syndecan-1 and -4 are found from acute cutaneous wound fluids and tracheal aspirates (76) and syndecan-3 from an aqueous extraction of neonatal rat brain (56). Elevated levels of soluble syndecan-1 correlates with tumor mass and decreased matrix metalloproteinase-9 activity is found in the serum of multiple myeloma patients (77). These soluble syndecans are not stained on immunoblots with antibodies directed against cytoplasmic domains, consistent with the loss of a cytoplasmic domain by proteolysis.

X. FUNCTIONS OF SYNDECANS

As discussed earlier, many extracellular proteins bind heparan sulfate. Therefore, syndecan-1 binds cells via its heparan sulfate chains to a variety of extracellular matrix components, including types I, III, and V fibrillar collagen (78), fibronectin (79), thrombospondin (80) and tenascin (81). Syndecan-1 expression is also consistent with its role as matrix receptor. It polarizes to the basolateral surface of cultured epithelial cells (82) and in simple epithelia (57), and localizes in early embryogenesis to the site of matrix accumulation (45). In addition, syndecan-1 and -3 co-localize with tenascin during tooth (83) and limb (53) development, respectively. Furthermore, syndecan-1 binds B-cells to type I collagen (84), and it is expressed on these cells while in contact with matrix, e.g., on pre-B cells in bone marrow and on differentiated plasma cells in lymphoid tissues (85). Syndecan-1 expression inhibits cell invasion into type I collagen (86) and mediates cell–cell adhesion via its heparan sulfate chains (87).

Despite ligand binding to heparan sulfate chains, the syndecan core proteins also have important roles in cell adhesion. Syndecan-1 expressed in Schwann cells coaligns with actin filaments in response to antibody ligation, which is dependent on the third conserved tyrosine in the syndecan-1 cytoplasmic domain (88). Syndecan-1 also mediates cell spreading on core protein-specific antibody that is not dependent on heparan sulfate or the cytoplasmic domain and can be inhibited by agents that block actin and microtubule polymerization (89). These data suggest that the core protein of syndecan-1 mediates spreading through the formation of a multimolecular signaling complex at the cell surface that signals cytoskeletal reorganization. Indeed, binding of fibroblasts and endothelial cells to the extracellular part of the syndecan-4 core protein suggests an association between the core and other cell surface molecules (90).

Engagement of proteoglycans with other cell surface receptors may be a common adhesion and growth factor signaling mechanism. For example, the interaction between cell surface heparan sulfate proteoglycans and fibronectin stimulates focal adhesion formation but only in cooperation with integrins (6,91). Syndecan-4 becomes inserted into the focal adhesions of a number of cell types, such as fibroblasts, smooth muscle cells, and endothelial cells (91), when protein kinase C (PKC) is activated (92). Recently, it has been shown that a unique sequence in the central part of the cytoplasmic domain of syndecan-4 can directly activate PKCα and potentiate its activity by phospholipid mediators when the cytoplasmic domain is oligomerized (30,33). This was the first report of direct transmembrane signaling through cell surface proteoglycans.

Syndecan-1, -3, and -4 have been shown to specifically bind FGF-2 (93–96), syndecan-3 binds heparin-binding growth-associated molecule (97) and syndecan-4 binds midkine, a heparin-binding growth/differentiation factor related to HB-GAM (96). As discussed earlier in this chapter these binding interactions are through the heparan sulfate GAG chains on syndecan. The importance of cell surface heparan sulfate proteoglycans in the action of heparin-binding growth factor signaling came from the studies that showed that cells deficient in heparan sulfate, or cells treated with chlorate to block heparan sulfate sulfation, or mutated in an enzyme needed for heparan sulfate biosynthesis, caused failure of FGFs to activate FGF receptor (98–101). Thus, heparan sulfate proteoglycans were determined to function as co-receptors for FGF-2 (Fig. 4) (102,103). An augmenting effect of heparan sulfate on signaling has so far been demonstrated for FGF-1, -2, -4, -5, -8, and -9 (5). However, to determine the role of syndecans and other proteoglycans in FGF-receptor signaling has been challenging. First, it was found that FGF-2–induced cell proliferation was strongly inhibited in 3T3 cells overexpressing syndecan-1, both on the cell surface and in the culture medium (104), and that soluble syndecan-1 and -2 inhibited FGF-2 receptor binding in cell free assays (105). However, when syndecans-1, -2, -4 or glypican were transfected in 3T3 cells, which normally express low levels of cell surface heparan sulfate proteoglycans, the FGF-2 receptor signaling was stimulated (106). The soluble syndecan-4 ectodomain had no effect on FGF-2 binding to the receptor. On the contrary, soluble basement membrane proteoglycan perlecan was found to promote FGF-receptor binding, mitogenesis, and angiogenesis (107). Furthermore, in wound fluids, dermatan sulfate proteoglycans are a major and potent promoter of FGF-2 activity (108). Thus, other proteoglycans are functional. Furthermore the location of the proteoglycan at either the cell surface or in solution has important functional consequences (109–111).

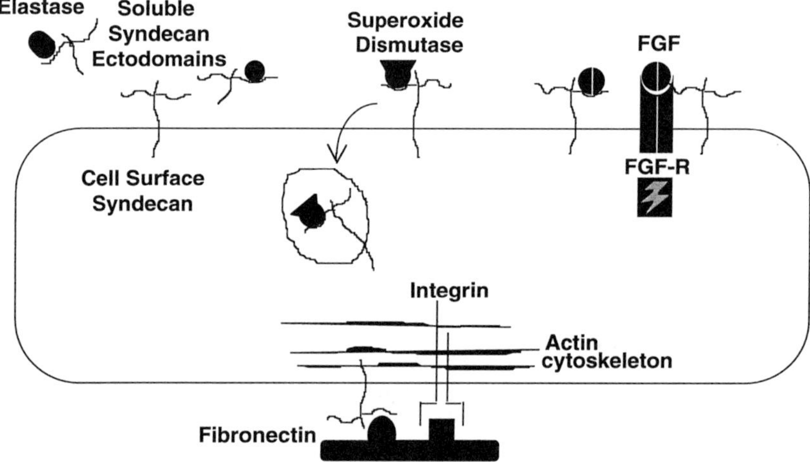

Figure 4   A model for syndecan function. Syndecan (†) can act in many ways at either the cell surface or in a soluble form in the extracellular space. Enzymes, such as elastase (●), can bind the GAG on syndecan and change activity. Other molecules, such as superoxide dismutase (▼), bind syndecan and are internalized. Growth factors, such as members of the FGF family (◖), must bind GAG to activate their receptor (FGF-R). Syndecans can also act with cell adhesion molecules, such as the integrins, to bind the cell to components of the extracellular matrix.

Proteoglycan interactions with heparin-binding growth factors and their receptors provide an attractive mechanism to regulate growth factor actions. Adjustments to cellular responses to growth factors could result from changes of syndecan expression, shedding, and in the fine structure of GAG chains attached to syndecans. This could be especially important during development and tissue injury, when rapid changes in cellular responses are required. In the developing neuroepithelium, heparan sulfate structure undergoes a rapid change in growth factor–binding specificity concomitant with the temporal expression of FGFs (112). Also, during malignant transformation, FGF-2 binding to heparan sulfate around microvessels is lost with breast carcinomas (113). Indeed, rapid changes in syndecan expression and shedding have been observed during development, malignant transformation, and wound repair.

Syndecans also bind extracellular ligands that are not growth factors or do not mediate cell adhesion. These include lipoprotein metabolism enzymes (e.g., lipoprotein lipase, low density lipoprotein) and serine proteases and their inhibitors (serpins). Like other known binding properties of extracellular ligands, these interactions are mediated by heparan sulfate chains.

The metabolism of lipoproteins is partially regulated by heparan sulfate proteoglycans through their interactions with lipoproteinlipase (LPL), lipoproteins, and apolipoproteins B and E (apoB and apoE). LPL hydrolyses triglycerides in very low density lipoproteins and chylomicrons, thus controlling the delivery of fatty acids to tissues. The primary site of LPL is in the luminal surface of capillary endothelial cells where the enzyme is anchored to heparan sulfate proteoglycans, mainly syndecan-1 (114). Surprisingly, LPL is synthesized in myocytes and adipocytes. Presumably, LPL bound to heparan sulfate proteoglycans is internalized and translocated to the apical site. Indeed, syndecan-1 can mediate binding and internalization of lipoproteins, thus functioning as lipoprotein receptor (115).

Another class of enzymes regulated by heparin/heparan sulfate is serine proteases and their inhibitors (serpins). Antithrombin III (ATIII), a serpin that inhibits thrombin and other coagulation proteases, binds a heparin-like sequence in heparan sulfate, which dramatically accelerates enzyme-ATIII complex formation (for review see Rosenberg et al. [116]). Thus, heparin has long been clinically used as an anticoagulant. ATIII binding to syndecans on the luminal surface of endothelial cells can contribute to the establishment of a nonthrombogenic lining of blood vessels (117). Because only a small proportion of syndecans polarize to the luminal surface, other HSPGs may also be involved in producing a nonthrobogenic endothelial luminal surface.

Syndecans can function as receptors, co-receptors, and soluble effectors for many types of heparin-binding molecules (see Fig. 4). Because soluble and cell surface syndecans compete for the same ligands, the soluble syndecan ectodomain may also function as an inhibitor. In the wound environment, each of these functions is likely to influence the balance of events that leads to excessive fibrosis or effective tissue remodeling. To better understand how syndecans can act in vivo, the syndecan-1 gene was disrupted by homologous recombination in mouse embryonic stem cells. Surprisingly, syndecan-1 null mice are viable, develop normally, are fertile, and are indistinguishable from wild type littermates by histological evaluation (M. Bernfield, unpublished observations, 1999). The sole abnormality detected in the synd-1 −/− mouse is defective repair of skin and corneal wounds. At both sites, lack of syndecan-1 prevents keratinocytes migrating into the wound from restoring their stable cell-cell and cell-matrix contacts at a normal rate. The result is a marked delay in reconstitution of the normal epithelium. The essential function of syndecan-1 appears to be for normal epithelial behavior during wound repair.

To further evaluate the functions of syndecan-1 during skin wound repair, wounds were studied in mice overexpressing syndecan-1 in the skin under the influence of the CMV promoter/enhancer (M. Bernfield, unpublished observations, 1999). Compared with wild-type mice, wound closure, reepithelialization, granulation tissue formation, and remodeling were delayed approximately five days in mice that overexpress syndecan-1. Wounding in both wild-type and in overexpressing mouse skin caused shedding of the soluble syndecan-1 ectodomain into wound fluids, but the shedding was markedly enhanced and prolonged in wounds from overexpressing mice. Wounds in overexpressing mice showed markedly reduced cell proliferation rates of keratinocytes at wound edges and cells within granulation tissue. Furthermore, fluids from these wounds contained increased elastolytic activity. The reduced cell proliferation rates and enhanced proteolytic activity were due to excess soluble syndecan-1 ectodomain in the wound. Thus, it appears that soluble syndecan-1 also acts as a dominant negative inhibitor of cell proliferation during wound repair. Taken together, these observations of the physiological effects of genetic manipulation of syndecan-1 gene expression confirm the in vitro findings that a delicate balance of syndecan expression is required for the function of many cellular events. Future work will define which of these events can be taken advantage of to influence clinical outcome and define the specific functions of syndecans and other proteoglycans in the skin.

REFERENCES

1. Bernfield M, Kokenyesi R, Kato M, Hinkes MT, Spring J, Gallo RL, Lose EJ. Biology of the syndecans: a family of transmembrane heparan sulfate proteoglycans. Annu Rev Cell Biol 1992; 8:365–398.
2. Conrad HE: *Heparin-Binding Proteins*. San Diego: Academic Press, 1998.
3. Kato M, Wang H, Bernfield M, Gallagher JT, Turnbull JE. Cell surface syndecan-

1 on distinct cell types differs in fine structure and ligand binding of its heparan sulfate chains. J Biol Chem 1994; 269:1881–1980.

4. Gallagher JT, Turnbull JE. Heparan sulphate in the binding and activation of basic fibroblast growth factor. Glycobiology 1992; 2:523–528.

5. Rapraeger AC. In the clutches of proteoglycans: how does heparan sulfate regulate FGF binding? Chem Biol 1995; 2:645–649.

6. Woods A, McCarthy JB, Furcht LT, Couchman JR. A synthetic peptide from the COOH-terminal heparin-binding domain of fibronectin promotes focal adhesion formation. Mol Biol Cell 1993; 4:605–613.

7. Marynen P, Cassiman J-J, Van den Berghe H, David G. Partial primary structure of the 48- and 90-kilodalton core proteins of cell surface-associated heparan sulfate proteoglycans of lung fibroblasts—prediction of an integral membrane domain and evidence for multiple distinct core proteins at the cell surface of human lung fibroblasts. J Biol Chem 1989; 264:7017–7024.

8. Saunders S, Jalkanen M, O'Farrell S, Bernfield M. Molecular cloning of syndecan, an integral membrane proteoglycan. J Cell Biol 1989; 108:1547–1556.

9. Kiefer MC, Stephans JC, Crawford K, Okino K, Barr PJ. Ligand-affinity cloning and structure of a cell surface heparan sulfate proteoglycan that binds basic fibroblast growth factor. Proc Natl Acad Sci USA 1990; 87:6985–6989.

10. Mali M, Jaakkola P, Arvilommi A-M, Jalkanen M. Sequence of human syndecan indicates a novel gene family of integral membrane proteoglycans. J Biol Chem 1990; 265:6884–6889.

11. Carey DJ, Evans DM, Stahl RC, Asundi VK, Conner KJ, Garbes P, Cizmeci-Smith G. Molecular cloning and characterization of N-syndecan, a novel transmembrane heparan sulfate proteoglycan. J Cell Biol 1992; 117:191–201.

12. David G, van der Schueren B, Marynen P, Cassiman J-J, Van den Berghe H. Molecular cloning of amphiglycan, a novel integral membrane heparan sulfate proteoglycan expressed by epithelial and fibroblastic cells. J Cell Biol 1992; 118:961–969.

13. Gould SE, Upholt WB, Kosher RA. Syndecan-3: a new member of the syndecan family of membrane-intercalated proteoglycans that is expressed in high amounts at the onset of chick limb cartilage differentiation. Proc Natl Acad Sci 1992; 89:3271–3275.

14. Kojima T, Shworak NW, Rosenberg RD. Molecular cloning and expression of two distinct cDNA-encoding heparan sulfate proteoglycan core proteins from a rat endothelial cell line. J Biol Chem 1992; 267:4870–4877.

15. Baciu PC, Acaster C, Goetinck PF. Molecular cloning and genomic organization of chicken syndecan-4. J Biol Chem 1994; 261:696–703.

16. Carey DJ. Syndecans: multifunctional cell-surface co-receptors. Biochem J 1997; 327:1–16.

17. Tsuzuki S, Kojima T, Katsumi A, Yamazaki T, Sugiura I, Saito H. Molecular cloning, genomic organization, promoter activity, and tissue-specific expression of the mouse ryudocan gene. J Biochem 1997; 122:17–24.

18. Spring J, Paine-Saunders SE, Hynes RO, Bernfield M. *Drosophila* syndecan: conservation of a cell surface heparan sulfate proteoglycan. Proc Natl Acad Sci USA 1994; 91:3334–3338.

19. Rosenblum ND, Botelho BB, Bernfield M. Expression of a *Xenopus* counterpart of mammalian syndecan 2 during embryogenesis. Biochem J 1995; 309I:69–76.

20. Kokenyesi R. Core protein structure and sequence determine the site and presence of heparan sulfate and chondroitin sulfate on syndecan-1. J Biol Chem 1994; 269:12304–12309.

21. Rapraeger A, Jalkanen M, Endo E, Koda JE, Bernfield M. Cell surface proteoglycan from mouse mammary epithelial cells bears chondroitin sulfate and heparan sulfate glycosaminoglycans. J Biol Chem 1985; 260:11046–11052.

22. Shworak NW, Shirakawa M, Mulligan RC, Rosenberg RD. Characterization of ryudocan glycosaminoglycan acceptor sites. J Biol Chem 1994; 269:21204–21214.

23. Grootjans JJ, Zimmermann P, Reekmans G, Smets A, Degeest G, Durr J, David G. Syntenin, a PDZ protein that binds syndecan cytoplasmic domains. Proc Natl Acad Sci USA 1997; 94:13683–13688.

24. Prasthofer T, Ek B, Ekman P, Owens R, Hook M, Johansson S. Protein kinase C phosphorylates two of the four known syndecan cytoplasmic domains in vitro. Biochem Mol Biol Intl 1995; 36:793–802.

25. Itano N, Oguri K, Nagayasu Y, Kusano Y, Nakanishi H, David G, Okayama M. Phosphorylation of a membrane-intercalated proteoglycan, syndecan-2, expressed in a stroma-inducing clone from a mouse Lewis lung carcinoma. Biochem J 1996; 315:925–930.

26. Reiland J, Ott VL, Lebakken CS, Yeaman C, McCarthy J, Rapraeger AC. Pervanadate activation of intracellular kinases leads to tyrosine phosphorylation and shedding of syndecan-1. Biochem J 1996; 319:39–47.

27. Oh ES, Couchman JR, Woods A. Serine phosphorylation of syndecan-2 proteoglycan cytoplasmic domain. Arch Biochem Biophys 1997; 344:67–74.

28. Horowitz A, Simmons M. Regulation of syndecan-4 phosphorylation in vivo. J Biol Chem 1998; 273:10914–10918.

29. Kinnuenen T, Kaksonen M, Saarinen J, Kalkkienen N, Peng HB, Rauvala H. Cortactin-Src kinase signaling pathway is involved in N-syndecan-dependent neurite outgrowth. J Biol Chem 1998; 273:10702–10708.

30. Oh ES, Woods A, Couchman JR. Syndecan-4 proteoglycan regulates the distribution and activity of protein kinase C. J Biol Chem 1997; 272:8133–8136.

31. Oh ES, Woods A, Lim S-T, Theibert AW, Couchman JR. Syndecan-4 proteoglycan cytoplasmic domain and phospatidylinositol 4,5-bisphosphate coordinately regulate protein kinase C activity. J Biol Chem 1998; 273:10624–10629.

32. Lee D, Oh ES, Woods A, Couchman JR, Lee W. Solution structure of a syndecan-4 cytoplasmic domain and its interaction with phospatidylinositol 4,5-bisphosphate. J Biol Chem 1998; 273:13022–13029.

33. Oh ES, Woods A, Couchman JR. Multimerization of the cytoplasmic domain of syndecan-4 is required for its ability to activate protein kinase C. J Biol Chem 1997; 272:11805–11811.

34. Spring J, Goldberger OA, Jenkins NA, Gilbert DJ, Copeland NG, Bernfield M. Mapping of the syndecan genes in the mouse: linkage with members of the Myc gene family. Genomics 1994; 21:597–601.

35. Ala-Kapee M, Nevanlinna H, Mali M, Jalkanen M, Schröder J. Localization of

gene for human syndecan, an integral membrane proteoglycan and a matrix receptor to chromosome 2. Somatic Cell Mol Genet 1990; 16:501–505.

36. Oettinger HF, Streeter H, Lose E, Copeland NG, Gilbert DJ, Justice MJ, Jenkins NA, Mohandas T, Bernfield M. Chromosome mapping of the murine syndecan gene. Genomics 1991; 11:334–338.

37. Kojima T, Inazawa J, Takamatsu J, Rosenberg RD, Saito H. Human ryudocan core protein: molecular cloning and characterization of the cDNA, and chromosomal localization of the gene. Biochem Biophys Res Commun 1993; 190:814–822.

38. Hinkes MT, Goldberger OA, Neumann PE, Kokenyesi R, Bernfield M. Organization and promoter activity of the mouse syndecan-1 gene. J Biol Chem 1993; 268: 11440–11448.

39. Vihinen T, Auvinen P, Alanen-Kurki L, Jalkanen M. Structural organization and genomic sequence of mouse syndecan-1 gene. J Biol Chem 1993; 268:17261–17269.

40. Cook DM, Hinkes M, Bernfield M, Rauscher III FJ. Transcriptional activation of the syndecan-1 promotor by the Wilms' tumor protein WT1. Oncogene 1996; 13: 1789–1799.

41. Vihinen T, Maatta A, Jaakkola P, Auvinen P, Jalkanen M. Functional characterization of mouse syndecan-1 promotor. J Biol Chem 1996; 271:12532–12541.

42. Jaakkola P, Kontusaari S, Kauppi T, Maatta A, Jalkanen M. Wound reepithelization activates a growth factor responsive enhancer in migrating keratinocytes. FASEB J 1998; 12:959–969.

43. Larrain J, Cizmeci-Smith G, Troncoso V, Stahl RC, Carey D, Brandan E. Syndecan-1 expression is down-regulated during myoblast terminal differentiation. Modulation by growth factors and retinoic acid. J Biol Chem 1997; 272:18418–18424.

44. Kim CW, Goldberger OA, Gallo RL, Bernfield M. Members of the syndecan family of heparan sulfate proteoglycans are expressed in distint cell-, tissue-, and development-specific patterns. Mol Biol Cell 1994; 5:797–805.

45. Sutherland AE, Sanderson RD, Mayes M, Siebert M, Calarco PG, Bernfield M, Damsky CH. Expression of syndecan, a putative low affinity fibroblast growth factor receptor, in the early mouse embryo. Development 1991; 113:339–351.

46. Bernfield M, Hinkes MT, Gallo RL. Developmental expression of the syndecans: possible function and regulation. Development 1993; (suppl):205–212.

47. Thesleff I, Jalkanen M, Vainio S, Bernfield M. Cell surface proteoglycan expression correlates with epithelial-mesenchymal interaction during tooth morphogenesis. Dev Biol 1988; 129:565–572.

48. Vainio S, Jalkanen M, Thesleff I. Syndecan and tenascin expression is induced by epithelial-mesenchymal interactions in embryonic tooth mesenchyme. J Cell Biol 1989; 108:1945–1954.

49. Solursh M, Reiter RS, Jensen KL, Kato M, Bernfield M. Transient expression of a cell surface heparan sulfate proteoglycan (syndecan) during limb development. Dev Biol 1990; 140:83–92.

50. Brauker JH, Trautman MS, Bernfield M. Syndecan, a cell surface proteoglycan, exhibits molecular polymorphism during lung development. Dev Biol 1991; 147: 285–292.

51. Trautman MS, Kimelman J, Bernfield M. Developmental expression of syndecan,

an integral membrane proteoglycan, correlates with cell differentiation. Development 1991; 111:213–220.

52. Gould SE, Upholt WB, Kosher RA. Characterization of chicken syndecan-3 as a heparan sulfate proteoglycan and its expression during embryogenesis. Dev Biol 1995; 168:438–451.

53. Koyama E, Leatherman JL, Shimazu A, Hah HD, Pacifici M. Syndecan-3 tenascin-C, and the development of catilaginous skeletal elements and joints in chick limbs. Dev Dyn 1995; 203:152–162.

54. Shimazu A, Nah HD, Kirsch T, Koyama E, Leatherman JL, Golden EB, Kosher RA, Pacifici M. Syndecan-3 and the control of chondrocyte proliferation during endochondral ossification. Exp Cell Res 1996; 229:126–136.

55. Seghatoleslami MR, Kosher RA. Inhibition of in vitro limb cartilage differentiation by syndecan-3 antibodies. Dev Dyn 1996; 207:114–119.

56. Carey DJ, Conner K, Asundi VK, O'Mahony DJ, Stahl RC, Showalter L, Cizmeci-Smith G, Hartman J, Rothblum LI. cDNA cloning, genomic organization, and in vivo expression of rat N-syndecan. J Biol Chem 1997; 272:2873–2879.

57. Hayashi K, Hayashi M, Jalkanen M, Firestone J, Trelstad RL, Bernfield M. Immunocytochemistry of cell surface heparan sulfate proteoglycan in mouse tissues. A light and electron microscopic study. J Histochem Cytochem 1987; 35:1079–1088.

58. Sanderson RD, Hinkes MT, Bernfield M. Syndecan, a cell surface proteoglycan, changes in size and abundance when keratinocytes stratify. J Invest Dermatol 1992; 99:1–7.

59. Elenius K, Vainio S, Laato M, Salmivirta M, Thesleff I, Jalkanen M. Induced expression of syndecan in healing wounds. J Cell Biol 1991; 114:585–595.

60. Inki P, Stenback F, Talve L, Jalkanen M. Immunohistochemical localization of syndecan in mouse skin tumors induced by UV irradiation. Am J Pathol 1991; 139: 1333–1340.

61. Inki P, Larjava H, Haapasalmi K, Miettinen HM, Grenman R, Jalkanen M. Expression of syndecan-1 induced by differentiation and suppressed by malignant transformation of human keratinocytes. Eur J Cell Biol 1994; 63:43–51.

62. Inki P, Stenback F, Grenman S, Jalkanen M. Immunohistochemical localization of syndecan-1 in normal and pathological human uterine cervix. J Pathol 1994; 172: 349–355.

63. Inki P, Kujari H, Jalkanen M. Syndecan in carcinomas produced from transformed epithelial cells in nude mice. Lab Invest 1992; 66:314–323.

64. Inki P, Joensuu H, Grenman R, Klemi P, Jalkanen M. Association between syndecan-1 expression and clinical outcome in squamous cell carcinoma of the head and neck. Br J Cancer 1994; 70:319–323.

65. Leppa S, Vleminckx K, Van Roy F, Jalkanen M. Syndecan-1 expression in mammary epithelial tumor cells is E-cadherin-dependent. J Cell Sci 1996; 109:1393–1403.

66. Leppa S, Mali M, Miettinen H, Jalkanen M. Syndecan expression regulates cell morphology and growth of mouse mammary epithelial tumor cells. Proc Natl Acad Sci USA 1992; 89:932–936.

67. Mali M, Andtfolk H, Miettinen HM, Jalkanen M. Suppression of tumor cell growth by syndecan-1 ectodomain. J Biol Chem 1994; 269:27795–27798.

68. Numa F, Hirabayashi K, Tsunaga N, Kato H, O'Rourke K, Shao H, Stechmann-Lebakken C, Varani J, Rapraeger A, Dixit VM. Elevated levels of syndecan-1 expression confer potent serum-dependent growth in human 293T cells. Cancer Res 1995; 55:4676–4680.

69. Kato M, Saunders S, Nguyen H, Bernfield M. Loss of cell surface syndecan-1 causes epithelia to transform into anchorage-independent mesenchyme-like cells. Mol Biol Cell 1995; 6:559–576.

70. Wang H, Moore S, Alavi MZ. Expression of syndecan-1 in rabbit neointima following de-endothelialization by a balloon catheter. Artherosclerosis 1997; 131:141–147.

71. Gallo RL, Kim C, Kokenyesi R, Adzick NS, Bernfield M. Syndecans-1 and -4 are induced during wound repair of neonatal but not fetal skin. J Invest Dermatol 1996; 107:667–683.

72. Gallo RL, Ono M, Povsic T, Page C, Eriksson E, Klagsbrun M, Bernfield M. Syndecans, cell surface heparan sulfate proteoglycans, are induced by a proline-rich antimicrobial peptide from wounds. Proc Natl Acad Sci USA 1994; 91:11035–11039.

73. Yanagishita M, Hascall VC. Cell surface heparan sulfate proteoglycans. J Biol Chem 1992; 267:9451–9454.

74. Jalkanen M, Rapraeger A, Saunders S, Bernfield M. Cell surface proteoglycan of mouse mammary epithelial cells is shed by cleavage of its matrix-binding ectodomain from its membrane-associated domain. J Cell Biol 1987; 105:3087–3096.

75. Weitzhandler M, Streeter HB, Henzel WJ, Bernfield M. The cell surface proteoglycan of mouse mammary epithelial cells—the extracellular domain contains the N terminus and a peptide sequence present in a conditioned medium proteoglycan. J Biol Chem 1988; 263:6949–6952.

76. Subramanian SV, Fitzgerald ML, Bernfield M. Regulated shedding of syndecan-1 and -4 ectodomains by thrombin and growth factor activation. J Biol Chem 1997; 272:14713–14720.

77. Dhodapkar MV, Kelly T, Theus A, Athota AB, Barlogie B, Sanderson RD. Elevated levels of shed syndecan-1 correlates with tumor mass and decreased matrix metalloproteinase-9 activity in the serum of patients with multiple myeloma. Br J Haematol 1997; 99:368–371.

78. Koda JE, Bernfield M. Heparan sulfate proteoglycans from mouse mammary epithelial cells: basal extracellular proteoglycan binds specifically to native type I collagen fibrils. J Biol Chem 1984; 259:11763–11770.

79. Saunders S, Bernfield M. Cell surface proteoglycan binds mouse mammary epithelial cells to fibronectin and behaves as a receptor on epithelial for interstitial matrix. J Cell Biol 1988; 106:423–430.

80. Sun X, Mosher DF, Rapraeger A. Heparan sulfate-mediated binding of epithelial cell surface proteoglycan to thrombospondin. J Biol Chem 1989; 264:2885–2889.

81. Salmivirta M, Elenius K, Vainio S, Hofer U, Chiquet-Ehrismann R, Thesleff I, Jalkanen M. Syndecan from embryonic tooth mesenchyme binds tenascin. J Biol Chem 1991; 266:7733–7739.

82. Rapraeger A, Jalkanen M, Bernfield M. Cell surface proteoglycan associates with the cytoskeleton at the basolateral cell surface of mouse mammary epithelial cells. J Cell Biol 1986; 103:2683–2696.

83. Vainio S, Lehtonen E, Jalkanen M, Bernfield M, Saxen L. Epithelial-mesenchymal interactions regulate the stage-specific expression of a cell surface proteoglycan, syndecan, in the developing kidney. Dev Biol 1989a; 134:382–391.

84. Sanderson RD, Sneed T, Young L, Sullivan G, Lander A. Adhesion of B lymphoid (MPC-11) cells to type I collagen is mediated by the integral membrane proteoglycan, syndecan. J Immunol 1992; 148:3902–3911.

85. Sanderson RD, Lalor P, Bernfield M. B lymphocytes express and lose syndecan at specific stages of differentiation. Cell Reg 1989; 1:27–35.

86. Liebersbach BF, Sanderson RD. Expression of syndecan-1 inhibits cell invasion into type I collagen. J Biol Chem 1994; 269:20013–20019.

87. Stanley MJ, Liebersbach BF, Liu W, Anhalt DJ, Sanderson RD. Heparan sulfate-mediated cell aggregation. Syndecans-1 and -4 mediate intercellular adhesion following their transfection into human B lymphoid cells. J Biol Chem 1995; 270: 5077–5083.

88. Carey DJ, Bendt KM, Stahl RC. The cytoplasmic domain of syndecan-1 is required for cytoskeleton association but not detergent insolubility. Identification of essential cytoplasmic domain residues. J Biol Chem 1996; 271:15253–15260.

89. Lebakken CS, Rapraeger AC. Syndecan-1 mediates cell spreading in transfected human lymphoblastoid (Raji) cells. J Cell Biol 1996; 132:1209–1221.

90. McFall AJ, Rapraeger AC. Identification of an adhesion site within the syndecan-4 extracellular protein domain. J Biol Chem 1997; 272:12901–12904.

91. Woods A, Couchman JR, Johansson S, Höök M. Adhesion and cytoskeletal organization of fibroblasts in response to fibronectin fragments. EMBO J 1986; 5:665–670.

92. Baciu PC, Goetinck PF. Protein kinase C regulates the recruitment of syndecan-4 into focal contacts. Mol Biol Cell 1995; 6:1503–1513.

93. Elenius K, Maatta A, Salmivirta M, Jalkanen M. Growth factors induce 3T3 cells to express bFGF-binding syndecan. J Biol Chem 1992; 267:6345–6441.

94. Salmivirta M, Heino J, Jalkanen M. Basic fibroblast growth factor-syndecan complex at acell surface or immobilized to matrix promotes cell growth. J Biol Chem 1992; 267:17606–17610.

95. Chernousov MA, Carey DJ. N-syndecan (syndecan 3) from neonatal rat brain binds basic fibroblast growth factor. J Biol Chem 1993; 268:16810–16814.

96. Kojima T, Katsumi A, Yamazaki T, Muramatsu T, Nagasaka T, Ohsumi K, Saito H. Human ryudocan from endothelium-like cells binds basic fibroblast growth factor, midkine, and tissue factor pathway inhibitor. J Biol Chem 1996; 271:5914–5920.

97. Kinnunen T, Raulo E, Nolo R, Maccarana M, Lindahl U, Rauvala H. Neurite outgrowth in brain neurons induced by heparin-binding growth-associated molecule (HB-GAM) depends on the specific interaction of HB-GAM with heparan sulfate at the cell surface. J Biol Chem 1996; 271:2243–2248.

98. Rapraeger AC, Krufka A, Olwin BB. Requirement of heparan sulfate for bFGF-mediated fibroblast growth and myoblast differentiation. Science 1991; 252:1705–1708.

99. Yayon A, Klagsburn M, Esko JD, Leder P, Ornitz DM. Cell surface, heparin-like molecules are required for binding of basic fibroblast growth factor to its high affinity. Cell 1991; 64:841–848.

100. Olwin BB, Rapraeger A. Repression of myogenic differentiation by aFGF, bFGF, and K-FGF is dependent on cellular heparan sulfate. J Cell Biol 1992; 118:631–639.

101. Ornitz DM, Leder P. Ligand specificity and heparin dependence of fibroblast growth factor receptors 1 and 3. J Biol Chem 1992; 267:16305–16311.

102. Bernfield M, Hooper KC. Possible regulation of FGF activity by syndecan, an integral membrane heparan sulfate proteoglycan. Ann NY Acad Sci 1991; 638:182–194.

103. Klagsbrun M, Baird A. A dual receptor system is required for basic fibroblast growth factor activity. Cell 1991; 67:229–231.

104. Mali M, Elenius K, Miettinen HM, Jalkanen M. Inhibition of basic fibroblast growth factor-induced growth promotion by overexpression of syndecan-1. J Biol Chem 1993; 268:24215–24222.

105. Aviezer D, Levy E, Safran M, Svahn C, Buddecke E, Schmidt A, David G, Vlodavsky I, Yayon A. Differential structural requirements of heparin and heparan sulfate proteogycans that promote binding of basic fibroblast growth factor to its receptor. J Biol Chem 1994; 269:114–121.

106. Steinfeld R, Van Den Berghe H, David G. Stimulation of fribroblast growth factor receptor-1 occupancy and signalling by cell surface-associated syndecans and glypican. J Cell Biol 1996; 133:405–416.

107. Aviezer D, Hecht D, Safran M, Eisinger M, David G, Yayon A. Perlecan, basal lamina proteoglycan, promotes basic fibroblast growth factor-receptor binding, mitogenesis, and angiogenesis. Cell 1994; 79:1005–1013.

108. Penc SF, Pomahac B, Winkler T, Dorschner RA, Eriksson E, Gallo RL. Dermatan sulfate released after injury is a potent promoter of FGF-2 activity. J Biol Chem 1998; 273:28116–28121.

109. Kan M, Wang F, To B, Gabriel JL, McKeehan WL. Divalent cations and heparin/heparan sufate cooperate to control assembly and activity of the fibroblast growth factor receptor complex. J Biol Chem 1996; 271:26143–26148.

110. Schwall RH, Chang LY, Godowski PJ, Kahn DW, Hillan KJ, Bauer KD, Zioncheck TF. Heparin induces dimerization and confers proliferative activity onto the hepatocyte growth factor antagonists NK1 and NK2. J Cell Biol 1996; 133:709–718.

111. DiGabriele AD, Lax I, Chen DI, Svahn CM, Jaye M, Schlessinger J, Handrickson WA. Structure of a heparin-linked biologically active dimer of fibroblast growth factor. Nature 1998; 393:812–817.

112. Nurcombe V, Ford MD, Wildschut JA, Bartlett PF. Development regulation of neural response to FGF-1 and FGF-2 by heparan sulfate proteoglycan. Science 1993; 260:103–106.

113. Friedl A, Chang Z, Tierney A, Rapraeger AC. Differential binding of fibroblast growth factor-2 and -7 to basement membrane heparan sulfate: comparison of normal and abnormal human tissues. Am J Pathol 1997; 150:1443–1455.

114. Saxena U, Klein MG, Goldberg IJ. Identification and characterization of the endothelial cell surface lipoprotein lipase receptor. J Biol Chem 1991; 266:17516–17521.

115. Fuki IV, Kuhn KM, Lomazov IR, Rothman VL, Tuszynski GP, Iozzo RV, Swenson TL, Fisher EA. The syndecan family of proteoglycans. Novel receptors mediating

internalization of atherogenic lipoproteins in vitro. J Clin Invest 1997; 100:1611–1622.

116. Rosenberg RD, Schworak NW, Liu J, Schwartz JJ, Schwartz LZ. Heparan sulfate proteoglycans of the cardiovascular system. Specific structures emerge but how is synthesis regulated? J Clin Invest 1997; 99:2062–2070.

117. Kojima T, Leone CW, Marchildon GA, Marcum JA, Rosenberg RD. Isolation and characterization of heparan sulfate proteoglycans produced by cloned rat microvascular endothelial cells. J Biol Chem 1992; 267:4859–4869.

118. Stevens RL. Recent advances in the cellular and molecular biology of mast cells. Immunol Today 1989; 10:381–386.

119. Nishiyama A, Stallcup WB. Expression of NG2 proteoglycan causes retention of type VI collagen on the cell surface. Mol Biol Cell 1993; 4:1097–1108.

120. David G, Lories V, Decock B, Marynen P, Cassiman J-J, Van den Berghe H. Molecular cloning of a phosphatidylinositol-anchored membrane heparan sulfate proteoglycan from human lung fibroblasts. J Cell Biol 1990; 111:3165–3176.

121. Stipp CS, Litwack ED, Lander AD. Cerebroglycan: an integral membrane heparan sulfate proteoglycan that is unique to the developing nervous system and expressed specifically during neuronal differentiation. J Cell Biol 1994; 124:149–160.

122. Filmus J, Church JG, Buick RN. Isolation of a cDNA corresponding to a developmentally regulated transcript in rat intestine. Mol Cell Biol 1988; 8:4243–4249.

123. Watanabe K, Yamada H, Yamaguchi Y. K-glypican: a novel GPI-anchored heparan sulfate proteoglycan that is highly expressed in developing brain and kidney. J Cell Biol 1995; 130:1207–1218.

124. Veugelers M, Vermeesch J, Reekmans G, Steinfeld R, Marynen P, David G. Characterization of glypican-5 and chromosomal localization fo human GPC5, a new member of the glypican gene family. Genomics 1997; 40:24–30.

125. Haggerty JG, Bretton RH, Milstone LM. Identification and characterization of a cell surface proteoglycan on keratinocytes. J Invest Dermatol 1992; 99:374–380.

126. Wang X, Lin HY, Ng-Eaton E, Downward J, Lodish HF, Weinberg RA. Expression cloning and characterization of the TGF-B type III receptor. Cell 1991; 67:797–805.

127. Doege K, Sasaki M, Horigan E, Hassall JR, Yamada Y. Complete primary structure of the rat cartilage proteoglycan core protein deduced from cDNA clones. J Biol Chem 1987; 262:17757–17767.

128. Doege KJ, Sasaki M, Kimura T, Yamada Y. Complete coding sequence and deduced primary structure of the human cartilage large aggregating proteoglycan, aggrecan. Human-specific repeats, and additional alternatively spliced forms. J Biol Chem 1991; 266:894–902.

129. Zimmermann DR, Dours-Zimmermann MT, Schubert M, Bruckner-Tuderman L. Versican is expressed in the proliferating zone in the epidermis and in association with the elastic network of the dermis. J Cell Biol 1994; 124:817–825.

130. LeBaron RG, Zimmermann DR, Ruoslahti E. Hyaluronate binding properties of versican. J Biol Chem 1992; 267:10003–10010.

131. Kahari VM, Larjava H, Uitto J. Differential regulation of extracellular matrix proteoglycan (PG) gene expression. Transforming growth factor-beta 1 up-regulates biglycan (PG1), and versican (large fibroblast PG) but down-regulates decorin

(PGII) mRNA levels in human fibroblasts in culture. J Biol Chem 1991; 266: 10608–10615.

132. Yamada H, Watanabe K, Shimonaka M, Yamaguchi Y. Molecular cloning of brevican, a novel brain proteoglycan of the aggrecan/versican family. J Biol Chem 1994; 269:10119–10126.

133. Perides G, Rahemtulla F, Lane WS, Asher RA, Bignami A. Isolation of a large aggregating proteoglycan from human brain. J Biol Chem 1992; 267:23883–23887.

134. Rauch U, Karthikeyan L, Maurel P, Margolis RU, Margolis RK. Cloning and primary structure of neurocan, a developmentally regulated, aggregating chondroitin sulfate proteoglycan of brain. J Biol Chem 1992; 267:19536–19547.

135. Brennan MJ, Oldberg A, Pierschbacher MD, Ruoslahti E. Chondroitin/dermatan sulfate proteoglycan in human fetal membranes. Demonstration of an antigenically similar proteoglycan in fibroblasts. J Biol Chem 1984; 259:13742–13750.

136. Fisher LW, Termine JD, Young MF. Deduced protein sequence of bone small proteoglycan I (biglycan) shows homolgy with proteoglycan II (decorin) and several nonconnective tissue proteins in a variety of species. J Biol Chem 1989; 264:4571–4576.

137. Johnson HJ, Rosenberg L, Choi JU, Garza S, Hook M, Neame PJ. Characterization of epiphycan, a small proteoglycan with a leucine-rich repeat core protein. J Biol Chem 1997; 272:18709–18717.

138. Oldberg A, Antonsson P, Lindblom K, Henegard D. A collagen-binding 59-kd protein (fibromodulin) is structurally related to the small interstitial proteoglycans PG-S1 and PG-S2 (decorin). EMBO J 1989; 8:2601–2604.

139. Blochberger TC, Vergnes JP, Hempel J, Hassell JR. cDNA to chick lumican (corneal keratan sulfate proteoglycan) reveals homology to the small interstitial proteoglycan gene family and expression in muscle and intestine. J Biol Chem 1992; 267: 347–352.

140. Shinomura T, Kimata K. Proteoglycan-Lb, a small dermatan sulfate proteoglycan expressed in embryonic chick epiphyseal cartilage, is structurally related to osteoinductive factor. J Biol Chem 1992; 267:1265–1270.

141. Tsen G, Halfter W, Kroger S, Cole GJ. Agrin is a heparan sulfate proteoglycan. J Biol Chem 1995; 270:3392–3399.

142. Noonan DM, Fulle A, Valente P, Cai S, Horigan E, Sasaki M, Yamada Y, Hassall JR. The complete sequence of perlecan, a basement membrane heparan sulfate proteoglycan, reveals extensive similarity with laminin A chain, low density lipoprotein-receptor, and the neural cell adhesion molecule. J Biol Chem 1991; 266: 22939–22947.

143. Murdoch AD, Dodge GR, Cohen I, Tuan RS, Iozzo RV. Primary structure of the human heparan sulfate proteoglycan from basement membrane (HSPG2/perlecan). A chimeric molecule with multiple domains homologous to the low density lipoprotein receptor, laminin, neural cell adhesion molecules, and epidermal growth factor. J Biol Chem 1992; 267:8544–8557.

144. Couchman JR, Kapoor R, Sthanam M, Wu RR. Perlecan and basement membrane-chondroitin sulfate proteoglycan (bamacan) are two basement membrane chondroitin/dermatan sulfate proteoglycans in the Engelbreth-Holm-Swarm tumor matrix. J Biol Chem 1996; 271:9595–95602.

4
Integrin Regulation in Wound Repair

Jiahua Xu and Richard A. F. Clark
*School of Medicine, State University of New York at Stony Brook,
Stony Brook, New York*

I. INTRODUCTION

Normal wound healing processes follow specific time sequences and can be temporally categorized into three major groups: inflammation, tissue formation, and tissue remodeling. The three phases of wound repair, however, are not mutually exclusive but rather overlapping in time. Immediately after skin injury, a temporary repair is achieved in the form of a clot that plugs the defect, and over subsequent days steps to regenerate the missing parts are initiated. Inflammatory cells and then fibroblasts and capillaries invade the clot to form a contractile granulation tissue that draws the wound margins together; meanwhile, the cut epidermal edges migrate forward to cover the denuded wound surface. At the end of adult wound healing, the skin lesions are healed imperfectly, since epidermal appendages that have been lost at the site of damage do not regenerate. A connective tissue scar forms since the collagen matrix has been poorly reconstructed, in dense parallel bundles, unlike the mechanically efficient basketweave meshwork of collagen in nonwounded dermis (1). On the contrary, early gestational fetal skin wound healing occurs more efficiently and often perfectly. Therefore, one goal in wound healing research is to understand the difference between adult and fetal healing processes.

Molecular and cellular activities after injury that have been studied extensively include cell proliferation, cell adhesion, cell migration, extracellular matrix (ECM) production and reorganization, and cell apoptosis. Much effort has been devoted to searching for signals that trigger relatively sedentary cell lineages at

63

the wound margin to proliferate, to become invasive, and then to deposit new matrix in the wound gap. Molecules that belong to this list of signals include integrins, cytokines, growth factors, and matrix components. The integrin family in particular has emerged as a critical player since it is involved in all phases of wound healing by acting as a structural molecule for cells to adhere, a signal molecule for cells to function, and a signal processor for cells to respond correctly to other signals. The understanding of integrin regulation will undoubtedly lead to the comprehension of fundamental wound healing knowledge and the development of therapeutic approaches. A much improved, ultimately scarless, wound repair can be achieved. This chapter mechanistically examines the expression and function of integrins in the wound healing process by focusing on the regulation of integrin gene expression, integrin regulation of new tissue formation, and integrin regulation of tissue remodeling.

II. INTEGRIN GENE EXPRESSION AND WOUND HEALING

A. Temporal and Spatial Integrin Expression During Wound Healing

The profile of integrin expression during wound healing is finely tuned to fit the functional role of each cell type under temporal and spatial restraints. Migrating epidermis and capillary sprouts are two revealing examples of the temporal and spatial expression of wound integrins. Keratinocytes, a major cell type in epidermis, express collagen receptor integrin $\alpha_2\beta_1$ and laminin receptor integrins $\alpha_3\beta_1$ and $\alpha_6\beta_4$. In nonwounded skin, keratinocytes rest on the basal lamina through $\alpha_6\beta_4$ integrins linked to laminin. The $\alpha_2\beta_1$ is expressed in the stratum basal layer of the epidermis, whereas the $\alpha_3\beta_1$ is expressed in all epidermal layers. The $\alpha_6\beta_4$ is expressed exclusively at the basal pole of the basal keratinocytes and along the epidermal–dermal junction (2). Wounding is associated with alterations in extracellular matrix proteins, namely, loss of laminin and type IV collagen in the region of the wound and expression of tenascin, vitronectin, and fibronectin. As a result, a new set of integrins, provisional matrix integrins, are synthesized during reepithelialization. In response to the appearance of new ECM proteins, wound keratinocytes newly synthesize the $\alpha_5\beta_1$ and $\alpha_v\beta_6$ fibronectin/tenascin receptors and the $\alpha_v\beta_5$ vitronectin receptor to crawl over and grasp hold of the provisional wound matrix. In the meantime, they relocate $\alpha_2\beta_1$ collagen receptor integrin to get hold of the underlying wound dermis. These integrins were found in filopodia of migrating keratinocytes in several cell layers of the migrating sheet. The leading edge of keratinocytes travels between granulation tissue and the fibrin clot that is eventually dissolved. To avoid the fibrin clot while migrating granulation tissue, wound keratinocytes do not express surface $\alpha_v\beta_3$ fibrinogen/vitronectin receptor. Once the denuded wound surface has been covered by a monolayer of keratinocytes, epidermal migration ceases and a new stratified epidermis with basal lamina is reestablished from the margins of the wound inward. Suprabasal cells cease to express integrins and basal keratins, and instead undergo differentiation in the outlayers of nonwounded epidermis (3–6).

The endothelial cell–lined wall of blood vessels in normal tissue interacts with basal lamina while facing circulating blood. Severe tissue injury causes blood vessel disruption with concomitant extravasation of blood constituents. As a result of this trauma, endothelial cells express intercellular adhesion molecules that recognize the β_2 integrins, which are up-regulated on circulating leukocytes by chemoattractant factors. The cell–cell interaction mediated by these receptors is responsible for circulating leukocyte adherence at the site of injury (7). Endothelial cells themselves undergo active proliferation and migration after stimulation by injury-induced angiogenic signals, causing new blood vessel formation. In this process, the proteolytic fragmentation of the basement membrane allows endothelial cells to migrate to the injured site in response to angiogenic signals. Neovascularization occurs when wound endothelial cells invade fibrin clot from basement membrane to form granulation tissues. Three types of integrins, $\alpha_v\beta_3$, $\alpha_v\beta_5$, and $\alpha_v\beta_6$, are up-regulated briefly during wound angiogenesis with different patterns of expression (8). At the tips of the sprouting capillaries in the granulation tissue is $\alpha_v\beta_3$, an integrin receptor for fibrin, fibronectin, and vitronectin. The surface expression and activation of endothelial $\alpha_v\beta_3$ are crucial for neovascularization, since its functional inhibition by antibody or peptide blocked new vessel formation (8–10). In fact, the capillary regression after the withdrawal of angiogenic stimuli is promoted by the diminishing surface presence of integrin $\alpha_v\beta_3$ (11,12).

B. Regulation of Integrin Expression by Growth Factors and Extracellular Matrix Ligands

The correct expression of integrins in response to growth factors and their ECM ligands is an exquisite cell strategy in the progression of wound repair: inflammation, reepithelialization, angiogenesis, fibroplasia, and wound contraction. In the process three components, growth factors, ECM proteins, and their receptor integrins, are interdependent. Growth factors released during wound repair promote cell growth and migration that require cell adhesion to ECM components. The cell–ECM adhesive interaction, in turn, enables ECM proteins and their ligand integrins to impact on growth factor action and cell function. Furthermore, the environmental level of ECM proteins and surface presence of integrin receptors are partly controlled by growth factors. Therefore, the regulation of integrin expression is at the center of this highly organized wound control network.

The release of numerous soluble inflammatory factors is a characteristic of wound repair. Immediately following tissue injury, platelet aggregation is accompanied by the release of chemotactic factors for blood leukocytes and growth factors, such as platelet-derived growth factor (PDGF), transforming growth factor-α (TGF-α), and -β (TGF-β) (13–15). The emigration of neutrophils and monocytes into the injured tissue occurs in an environment densely populated with such inflammatory factors as interleukin-1 (IL-1) and -8 (IL-8), colony stimulating factor-1 (CSF-1), tumor necrosis factor-α (TNF-α), and γ-interferon (γ-IFN), other inflammatory cells, as well as activated neutrophils and monocytes themselves. Additional factors secreted during the inflammation or later phases include insulin-like growth factor-1 (IGF-1), fibroblast growth factor (FGF), epidermal growth factor (EGF), heparin-binding epidermal growth factor (HB-EGF), keratinocyte growth factor (KGF), Neu differentiation factor (NDF), and vascular endothelial growth factor (VEGF). While most of these factors function as mitogens and motogens, they have been shown to alter the expression patterns of cellular integrins. For example, PDGF can increase fibroblast proliferation (13), migration (16), and integrin expression (17–19). Considerable studies have been conducted to assess the role of soluble wound factors in integrin gene expression, predominantly by measuring surface integrin levels after treatment of cultured cells with soluble factors or transfection with growth factors. Some of these studies are summarized in Table 1.

However, in the wound environment, soluble factors function in the world of ECM, integrin ligands. Severe injury changes not only the local concentration of growth factors and cytokines, but also the constituents of ECM. For example, wound fibroblasts are surrounded by provisional matrix in granulation tissue rather than collagen matrix as in normal dermis. Correspondingly, the level of provisional matrix integrin receptors is elevated in wound fibroblasts (28). Therefore, the impact of ECM proteins on gene expression, particularly integrin expression, can not be ignored. Participation of ECM in regulating integrin expression can be summarized by two approaches. The first approach is direct regulation by themselves to provide a feedback loop, and the second is crosstalk with growth factors to provide another layer of control as a signal processor. The direct feedback regulation of integrin expression by ECM employs two types of mechanisms in current knowledge, posttranslational and pretranslational regulation. Posttranslational regulation is a mechanism by which the concentration of laminin determines the amount of receptor $\alpha_6\beta_1$ integrin expressed on the surface of sensory neurons. When ligand availability is low, surface amounts of receptor increase, whereas integrin ribonucleic acid (RNA) and total integrin protein decrease. Ligand concentration determines cell surface levels of integrin by altering the rate at which receptor is removed from the cell surface. The increased level of integrin at the cell surface is associated with increased neuronal cell adhesion and neurite outgrowth. This model suggests that the presence of available surface integrin maintains neuronal growth-cone motility over a broad range of ligand concentrations, allowing axons to invade different tissues during development and regeneration (29). Pretranslational regulation is proposed as a positive feedback mecha-

Table 1 Regulation of Integrin Expression by Growth Factors

Soluble factors	Cell types	Integrins	References
Lipopolysaccharide (LPS) and interferon -γ (IFN-γ)	Monocytes	$\alpha_1\beta_1$	Rubio et al. (20)
The combination of substance P and insulin-like growth factor-1 (IGF-1)	Rabbit corneal epithelial cells	α_5	Nakamura et al. (21)
TGF-β1	Keratinocytes	Up-regulation of $\alpha_5\beta_1$, $\alpha_v\beta_5$, $\alpha_2\beta_1$; down-regulation of $\alpha_3\beta_1$; induction of the de nova synthesis of $\alpha_v\beta_6$	Zambruno et al. (22)
Neu differentiation factor (NDF), a member of EGF family	Keratinocytes	α_5 and α_6	Danilenko et al. (23)
EGF or TGF-α	Keratinocytes	α_2	Chen et al. (24)
VEGF	Endothelial cells	$\alpha_1\beta_1$, $\alpha_2\beta_1$, and $\alpha_v\beta_3$	Senger et al. (11) and Klein et al. (25)
bFGF, TGF-β, and IFN-γ	Endothelial cells	$\alpha_v\beta_3$	Sepp et al. (26)
FGF-2	Fibroblasts	α_5	Sun et al. (27)
PDGF	Fibroblasts	α_1, α_2, α_3, α_5	Gailit et al. (19) and Rubio et al. (20)
IFN-γ, TNF-α, and IL-1β	Fibroblasts	α_1 and α_5	Gailit et al. (19)

nism for collagen to control its receptor integrin $\alpha_2\beta_1$. As the injury site progresses from blood clot to scar, the wound environment becomes increasingly collagenous. This transition from provisional matrix-predominant to collagen-rich environment is accompanied by increased surface collagen receptor $\alpha_2\beta_1$ levels on fibroblasts (28). The underlying molecular mechanisms have been further studied using a three-dimensional (3D) collagen lattice populated by fibroblasts, an in vitro system considered the simulation of wound contraction (30). The expression of fibroblast collagen receptor integrin α_2 subunit was increased by 3D collagen (31) at pretranslational level since α_2 promoter is transcriptionally activated by a transcription factor NF-κB (32).

A second approach for ECM proteins to impact on the integrin expression is to modulate growth factor regulation. The coinhabitation of ECM molecules with inflammatory factors in the wound environment allows the crosstalk to occur between the two groups of cell regulators. This ECM–growth factor coordination can be demonstrated by the temporal expression of fibroblasts integrins $\alpha_2\beta_1$, $\alpha_3\beta_1$, and $\alpha_5\beta_1$. Periwound fibroblasts on the day prior to granulation tissue formation, and infiltrating fibroblasts on early granulation tissue increased their provisional receptor integrins $\alpha_3\beta_1$ and $\alpha_5\beta_1$, whereas collagen receptor $\alpha_2\beta_1$ did not express appreciably (28). In vitro models of provisional matrix bed and collagen-rich dermis showed that the stimulation of PDGF on specific integrin receptor expression can be modified by their ECM ligands in a positive feedback manner. Platelet-derived growth factor together with the 3D fibrin-fibronectin bed, a model of provisional matrix wound bed in the early phase of the granulation tissue, up-regulates provisional matrix integrins $\alpha_3\beta_1$ and $\alpha_5\beta_1$ (28). When the ECM partner of PDGF is switched from provisional matrix proteins to collagen, the PDGF up-regulation of $\alpha_3\beta_1$ and $\alpha_5\beta_1$ is attenuated, whereas that of $\alpha_2\beta_1$, the collagen receptor integrin, is further enhanced (28). Therefore, ECM proteins appear to influence the growth factor regulation of their receptor integrins in order to insure the correct balance between ligands and integrin receptors by acting as a signal processor. Similar types of signal processing by ECM proteins can also be observed in the attenuation of TGF-β–stimulated type I collagen production by a 3D collagen gel (33) and PDGF-induced cell proliferation by a relaxed 3D collagen gel (34).

How ECM and growth factors conduct their crosstalk is an intensively pursued research area. Since growth factor and integrin signal transduction pathways overlap with one another, there are many potential converging points for the interaction to occur. Although final functional outcomes of such studies are mostly cell growth and migratory activity instead of integrin gene expression, the delineation of the ECM–growth factor crosstalk will provide the fundamental knowledge of injury-altered patterns of tissue integrins. Several mechanisms have been proposed to explain such interactions potentially related to the wound cellular activities. Two inducible integrin ligands, Cyr61 and osteopontin, have suggested that growth factors newly synthesize ligands for integrins as an intermediary to initiate the signaling process. Cyr61, a growth factor–induced immediate–early gene identified in fibroblasts, promotes cell adhesion, migration, and proliferation. A ligand for $\alpha_1\beta_3$, it encodes a secreted cysteine-rich, heparin-binding protein associated with the ECM or with cell surface through integrins (35). Similar fashion might also be employed by angiotensin II (AII), a factor that modulates cardiac hypertrophy, fibroblast proliferation, and ECM production. AII induces the expression of osteopontin, a phosphoprotein that binds $\alpha_v\beta_1$, $\alpha_v\beta_3$, $\alpha_v\beta_5$ (36), $\alpha_4\beta_1$ (37), and $\alpha_9\beta_1$ (38) integrins and is involved in the vascular cell remodeling process (36,39,40). The ligation of osteopontin to β_3 integrin rapidly increased

NF-κB activity, which is crucial for osteopontin-mediated cell survival (41). Insulin-like growth factor-1, on the other hand, might use preexisting protein factors as liaison between influx growth factors and membrane integrins. Insulin-like growth factor-1 is dependent on the presence of IGF binding protein-1 (IGFBP-1) to act as a wound healing agent. IGFBP-1 binds to $\alpha_5\beta_1$ as well as IGFBP-1. The activation of both IGF-1 receptor and $\alpha_5\beta_1$ is required for IGF-1 to stimulate wound healing (42).

Another potential mechanism for the crosstalk to occur is that integrin activation might potentiate the growth factor action by enhancing autophosphorylation of receptors for growth factors such as PDGF and EGF (43,44). Integrins might achieve this synergism with growth factors after activation by aggregation and occupancy, triggering tyrosine phosphorylation of EGF, PDGF, and FGF receptors (45). The association between integrins and tyrosine protein kinases has been observed between $\alpha_6\beta_4$ and ErbB-2 (46). In fact, tyrosine phosphorylation has been linked to wound healing by several studies. In normal epidermis, β_1 and β_4 localized primarily to basal cells, where both integrin subunits were generally distributed over all parts of the cell periphery. Except for a modest presence in suprabasal cells and a minimal presence adjacent to the epidermal basement membrane, phosphotyrosine had a similar distribution. In migrating keratinocytes, β_1, β_4, and phosphotyrosine localized most heavily at the interface between the forming wound epithelium and the wound bed (47). Fibroblast growth factor-2 (FGF-2)–induced capillary-like tube formation inside collagen lattice is regulated by tyrosine phosphorylation, but not mediated through protein kinase C pathway (48).

Furthermore, other signal molecules downstream of growth factor receptors could provide converging points where growth factor- and integrin-initiated signals meet. An adapter protein, Shc, known in growth factor signal transduction, has proven an essential component in the integrin $\alpha_1\beta_1$ signaling pathway by gene knockout studies. The integrin α_1-null mouse fibroblasts fail to recruit and activate Shc. The failure to activate Shc is accompanied by a downstream deficiency in recruitment of Grb2 and subsequent mitogen-activated protein kinase activation. Taken together with the growth deficiency observed on collagens, this finding indicates that $\alpha_1\beta_1$ is the sole collagen receptor that can activate the Shc-mediated growth pathway (49). The crosstalk regulation will be further discussed in the next section.

III. INTEGRIN REGULATION OF TISSUE FORMATION IN WOUND REPAIR

Cell proliferation and migration are inseparable partners that shape the tissue formation phase of wound repair process. Numerous reports in the literature have stated the requirement of integrins for cell growth activities. A recent report showed the critical role of $\alpha_1\beta_1$ in cell proliferation (49). The integrins $\alpha_5\beta_1$ and $\alpha_v\beta_3$ in particular have been implicated in growth factor–stimulated cell proliferation (50,51). Collagen matrix has been shown to affect PDGF-stimulated cell proliferation by mechanical force (34), fibrillar structure (52), and ligand property for PDGF (53). For a detailed discussion of the underlying mechanism the reader is referred to other exhaustive reviews on the role of integrins in cell growth (54–57).

This section focuses on the role of integrins in cell migration. The early response to the injury is marked by the deposition of platelets and the migration of macrophages and neutrophils to the site of wounding. A distinctive feature of granulation tissue formation is migration of fibroblasts, macrophages, and endothelial cells to a bed of provisional matrix. The migration of keratinocytes is an essential feature of reepithelialization. Increasing evidence has shown the involvement of integrins in these migratory processes. For example, the function of $\alpha_3\beta_1$ integrin and the α_6-containing integrins is identified in epithelial wound closure after blocking antibodies specific for the integrin subunits β_1, α_3, and α_6 potently inhibited epithelial cell migration into wounds (58). Current studies of integrin-mediated migratory processes have mostly focused on the identification of integrin signal transduction pathways in cell migration, the integrin-mediated expression and activity of proteases, and the feedback regulation of ECM and integrins by proteolytic activities.

A.   Integrin Signal Transduction Pathway in Wound Migratory Cellular Activities

Platelets are activated by contact with ECM proteins, apparently by the triggering of signal events via integrins. Contact of platelets with collagen in the subendothelial matrix, as occurs during wound healing, is a potent stimulus triggering protein tyrosine phosphorylation, secretion, and hemostatis (59). Once activated by initial stimuli, the platelet integrin $\alpha_{IIb}\beta_3$ binds fibrinogen, induces platelet aggregation (60,61), triggers protein phosphorylation (62,63), generates phosphatidylinositol 3,4-bisphosphate (64), activates factors that are involved in overlapping signal transduction pathways (65), and causes further platelet activation. The activation (ligand-binding affinity) of $\alpha_{IIb}\beta_3$ is controlled by intracellular biochemical events including the activity of small GTPases of the Rho and Ras families. The active H-Ras and Raf-1 kinase are the suppressors of the $\alpha_{IIb}\beta_3$ activation (66,67). An extensive body of research has resulted in the identification of two regions of the β plasmic domains that are important in the regulation of $\alpha_{IIb}\beta_3$-affinity states (68).

The recruitment of neutrophils and monocytes to the site of the wound is stimulated by a variety of chemoattractants, including the degradation products of fibrinogen, fibrin, collagen, elastin, and fibronectin; growth factors, such as PDGF and TGF-β; cytokines, such as IL-1 and IL-8; and peptides cleaved from bacterial proteins. Integrin-mediated signal transduction pathways are involved in migratory processes of both neutrophils and monocytes (69). For example, stimulation of the respiratory burst in neutrophils by cytokines such as TNF-α and f-met-leu-phe is enhanced by adhesion to the ECM and blocked by integrin antibodies (70). Further study has shown that integrin-mediated adhesion via $\alpha_L\beta_2$ and $\alpha_X\beta_2$, but not $\alpha_M\beta_2$, triggers the respiratory burst in neutrophils (71). More recently, bacterial LPA and TNF have been found to activate p38 mitogen-activated protein (MAP) kinase and induce β_2 integrin–dependent neutrophil adhesion (72), probably by modifying β_2 cytoplasmic domain where cytoskeletal and signal transducing proteins are located (73). In another example, β_2 integrin–mediated adhesion in lymphoid cells seems to be regulated by RhoGTPase, although it is unclear if changes in affinity or in avidity are involved (74). The activated β_2 may in turn initiate the signal transduction pathway (75), since β_2 integrin, receptor for urokinase plasminogen activator (uPAR), and protein tyrosine kinases Fyn, Lyn, Hck and Fgr are assembled into one complex after the activation of monocytes (76). The activation of β_2 may involve multi-integrins since the β_2 integrin–dependent transendothelial migration of monocytes is mediated by $\alpha_v\beta_3$ as well as integrin-associated protein (IAP), a protein functionally associated with $\alpha_v\beta_3$ (77). Once neutrophils arrive at the wound site, fibrin clot could affect the effectiveness of cytokines that initiate the migration of neutrophils. In vitro culture has shown that fibrin clot modulates the cytokine-stimulated migration of neutrophils through the clot (78,79). The task to eliminate wound neutrophils, once their mission is accomplished, may be performed by integrin-mediated cell apoptosis (80).

The migration of endothelial cells occurs in response to angiogenic signals and is dependent on the activation of $\alpha_v\beta_3$, $\alpha_2\beta_1$ and $\alpha_1\beta_1$ (11,81). Angiogenic factors identified include vascular endothelial growth factor (11), basic fibroblast growth factor (bFGF) (82,83), angiopoietin-1 (84), transferrin (85), and tetraspan molecules CD81/TAPA-1 and CD151/PETA-3 (86). Other soluble factors, such as TNF-α, cooperate with angiogenic factors in inducing human microvascular endothelial cells in vitro to invade a three-dimensional fibrin matrix and to form capillary-like tubular structures (87). The $\alpha_v\beta_3$ is thus far the most extensively studied integrin involved in endothelial cell migration. The activation of $\alpha_v\beta_3$ requires the presence of both subunits since the α_v integrin cytoplasmic tail is the premise for the inducible tyrosine phosphorylation of the cytoplasmic domain of β_3 subunit (88). The phosphorylation of β_3 cytoplasmic domain is followed by the activation of focal adhesion kinase and mediates cytoskeletal assembly (89–91). The ligation of $\alpha_v\beta_3$ to its ligand is crucial for angiogenic factor bFGF to induce sustained activity of MAP kinase kinase (MEK) and MAP kinase (ERK) (92), which further phosphorylate myosin light chain kinase (MLCK) and MLC

(93). The ligation between osteopontin and $\alpha_v\beta_3$ activates pp60c-src in association with $\alpha_v\beta_3$ (94) followed by a rapid increase of NF-κB activity via the Ras pathway (41). Increased protein tyrosine phosphorylation was also observed in FGF-2–induced vascular formation (48).

Fibroblast migration constitutes granulation tissue formation. Integrin-mediated adhesion and proteolysis are two elements that control fibroblast migration. Ligand properties govern the occurrence of cell migration as well as the migration speed (95). Fibronectin, a predominant type of provisional matrix protein, directs wound fibroblast migration into the fibrin clot (96,97). Fibroblasts express several fibronectin receptor integrins that interact with fibronectin at primarily two binding sites. While $\alpha_3\beta_1$, $\alpha_5\beta_1$, $\alpha_v\beta_1$, $\alpha_v\beta_3$ and $\alpha_v\beta_5$ recognize the Arg-Gly-Asp-Ser (RGDS) tetrapeptide within the cell binding domain, $\alpha_4\beta_1$ rests on the IIICs domain (1). The adhesion of fibroblasts to fibronectin induces a cascade of signaling events, including the activation of focal adhesion kinase (98), recruitment of significant amounts of p190-B and Rho to the plasma membrane (99), the increase of membrane lipid biosynthesis (100), and the association and phosphorylation of paxillin by c-Abl (101). An in vitro wound healing model has established the direct role of a tumor suppressor gene, PTEN, in the wound fibroblast migration. The PTEN encodes the catalytic signature motif of protein tyrosine phosphatase, which has sequence similarity to tensin, a cytoskeletal protein that binds to actin filaments at focal adhesions and is tyrosine-phosphorylated upon integrin-mediated adhesion. Transfection of NIH 3T3 cell lines demonstrated that PTEN inhibited cell migration in the in vitro wound healing model, cell spreading on fibronectin, and focal adhesion formation of transfected human foreskin fibroblasts plated on fibronectin (102).

B. Integrin-Mediated Wound Protease Expression and Function

The migratory activities of wound cells can be viewed as a tissue remodeling process that involves a proteolytic degradation of ECM in the surrounding normal tissue. In particular, the serine protease plasmin and a variety of matrix metalloproteinases (MMPs) have been implicated in the degradation. These enzymes, usually undetectable under normal circumstances, are prominently expressed during wound healing. The same proteinases are also involved in matrix degradation in a number of tissue remodeling processes, such as cancer invasion, involution, and implantation. The activity of proteases is controlled by a family of inhibitors called tissue inhibitors of metalloproteinases (TIMPs). The expression pattern of TIMPs is also altered along with MMPs during wound healing in comparison with normal skin. Efforts have been made to identify the protease genes that are affected by injury. Six MMP genes, stromelysin 1 (MMP-3), stromelysin 3 (MMP-11), collagenase 3, gelatinase A (MMP-2), gelatinase B (MMP-9), and membrane type-1 matrix matalloproteinase (MT1-MMP), are highly expressed during rat skin wound healing after cDNA libraries were screened (103). MMP-2 can be detected at high levels in its mature form in the granulation tissue, but not in the regenerating epidermis following MT1-MMP activation. The role of these protease-related proteins in wound healing is being actively identified by gene-targeting experiments. Deficiency in MMP-2 and MMP-9 reduces angiogenesis (104,105), whereas disruption in plasminogen gene impairs keratinocyte migration from incisional wound edges due to the diminished ability to proteolytically dissect their way through ECM beneath the wound crust (106). The MT1-MMP directly mediates angiogenesis through a plasminogen activator–independent pathway (107). The expression of wound proteases is not only temporally but also spatially controlled. This is best demonstrated by the expression of MMP-1 in basal keratinocytes at the leading edge of migration bordering the sites of active reepithelialization in both normally healing wounds and chronic ulcers (108–110). Expression of MMP-1 is rapidly induced in wound edge keratinocytes after injury, persists during the healing phase, and ceases following wound closure (111), indicating that collagenolytic activity is a characteristic response of the epidermis to wounding. Similarly, in new blood vessels, tips of the vessel sprouts are rich in integrin $\alpha_v\beta_3$ (10), which colocalizes with MMP-2 (112).

The expression and function of wound proteases is under control by a number of molecules, including ECM proteins and integrins. The ligation of integrins to their antibodies has been reported to induce protease expression and/or activity. Antibodies against β_1 and α_3 integrin subunits were found to stimulate the expression of the 92-kDa type IV collagenase in human mucosal keratinocytes severalfold in a dose-dependent manner (113), whereas anti-α_3 integrin antibody induces the activated form of MMP-2 in human rhabdomyosarcoma cells (114,115). Furthermore, ECM proteins as integrin ligands induce protease expression. Laminin, a major component of basement membrane, stimulates both uPA and MMP-9 expression in macrophages in a time-dependent manner, suggesting that macrophage binding to laminin plays an important role in the regulation of their degradative phenotype via the up-regulation of uPA and MMP-9 (116). Vitronectin increases the secretion of both MMP-2 and TIMP-2 in melanoma cells (117). Type I collagen in a three-dimensional structure stimulates the expression of MMP-1 in fibroblasts (118), expression of MT1-MMP and MMP2 in microvascular endothelial cells (119), and activation of MMP-2 in fibroblasts (120). The requirement of specific integrins for the induction of proteases by ECM proteins is established by eliminating either integrin function using blocking antibodies or integrin surface proteins using antisense inhibition. Several integrins have been identified. Integrins $\alpha_5\beta_1$ and $\alpha_4\beta_1$ cooperatively regulate metalloproteinase gene expression in fibroblasts adhering to fibronectin (121). The interaction between $\alpha_6\beta_1$ and two peptides derived from laminin-1 α chain, laminin G peptides, induces the surface expression of the 170-kDa membrane-bound gelatinase, separase, as well as cell invasiveness of LOX human melanoma cells (122). The co-clustering of antigen receptor and integrin β_1 or β_2 in normal T-lymphocytes during inflammation (123) or in monocytoid cell lines THP and U937 (124) induces the expression of receptors for urokinase plasminogen activator, which is undetectable in rest normal T-cells (123). Antisense removal of integrin α_2 subunit in osteoblasts inhibits MMP-1 expression induced by a 3D collagen lattice (125).

How do integrins modulate the expression and activation of proteases? Several mechanisms have been proposed to address the question. The integrin-induced cytoskeletal changes present a strong candidate to modulate cellular proteolytic activities. At the margin of the embryonic wound there was a cable of actin running in the front row of basal epidermal cells (126). The reepithelialization of the wound was completely inhibited by the disruption of actin cable assembly at the embryonic wound margin by cytochalasin D (127) and C3 transferase, a bacterial exoenzyme that inactivates endogenous Rho (128). Myosin II is localized to the actin pursestring, providing contractile motors necessary for the epithelial movement (129). The cytoplasmic domain of an integrin molecule directly or spatially associates with cytoskeletal proteins, including plectin, talin, filamin, tensin, vinculin, paxillin, actin, F-actin, and α-actinin (73). The integrin-mediated change in cytoskeletal structure can alter the activity of small GTPases including Rho, Ras, Rac, and Cdc42 (130) that could signal a cascade of events leading to protease expression and cell migration. Specifically, MMP-1 expression induced by ligation of the $\alpha_5\beta_1$ integrin was found to be dependent on the small GTPase Rac1 when cells adopted a rounded morphology in response to soluble $\alpha_5\beta_1$ antibodies, but not when cells were allowed to spread fibronectin-bound $\alpha_5\beta_1$ antibodies (131). Phosphatidylinositide 3-kinase (PI3K) is required in the cell migration process as a downstream component of Rac1 and Cdc42 (132). The direct link of $\alpha_6\beta_4$ to cytoskeletal protein plectin (133) induces cell migration via PI3K (134). The focal adhesion complexes caused by the integrin ligation can also induce movement of messenger RNA (mRNA) and ribosomes to focal adhesions and thus locally increase the concentration of messenger for translation (135).

Another mechanism that addresses the need of the coordination between integrins and growth factor signal transduction pathways in controlling cell proteolytic activity is based on the requirement of both growth factors and integrin receptors in angiogenesis (136). For example, uPA interacts with its cell surface receptor uPAR to provide cells an inducible, localized surface proteolytic activity. The induction of cell surface expression of uPA–uPAR by growth factors or phorbol esters was necessary for vitronectin-dependent cell migration, an event mediated by $\alpha_v\beta_5$ (137). It is hypothesized that the growth factors or phorbol esters activate protein kinase C to increase phosphorylation of focal adhesion kinase and recruitment of cytoskeletal proteins by $\alpha_v\beta_5$ (138). Integrin $\alpha_v\beta_3$, on the other hand, has been found to associate with activated insulin and PDGF-β receptors to induce PDGF-β–dependent protease activation and chemotaxis (51). The similar migration-inducing mechanism has also been observed by TNF-α and $\alpha_5\beta_1$ (139), bFGF with $\alpha_v\beta_3$ (92), and IL-1 with chondrocyte integrins (140).

Protease activity is often found in association with cell membrane. Some proteases are membrane-bound proteins, such as MT1-MMP, that contain a putative membrane domain (141–143), while others apparently rely on the membrane anchors as seen in the uPA–uPAR complex (144). Integrins have been reported to function as cell membrane anchors for proteases to be localized in a proteolytically active form on the surface of invasive cells. Integrin $\alpha_v\beta_3$ is found in the invasive cells at the tips of newly formed blood vessels in wound healing or cancer formation (10). MMP-2 and $\alpha_v\beta_3$ were specifically co-localized on angiogenic blood vessels and melanoma cells in vivo (112). Cell migration and angiogenesis are inhibited when MMP-2 fails to form a complex with $\alpha_v\beta_3$ in the membrane. In vitro MMP-2 and $\alpha_v\beta_3$ form an SDS-stable complex that depends on the noncatalytic C-terminal hemopexin-like domain of MMP-2 (145). This fragment is able to prevent MMP-2 from binding to $\alpha_v\beta_3$ and to block cell surface collagenolytic activity. A naturally occurring form of this fragment can be detected in vivo in conjunction with $\alpha_v\beta_3$ expression in tumors and during developmental retinal neovascularization, suggesting its physiological role in regulating the invasive behavior of new blood vessels. Therefore, the anchorage localization of protease activity is an important mechanism for angiogenesis.

The competitive binding to ECM ligands between protease inhibitors and integrins or protease receptors is a novel mechanism to assess cell migration. During wound healing, migrating cells increase expression of both the vitronectin receptor integrins and plasminogen activators. Vitronectin significantly enhances the migration of smooth muscle cells, a process mediated by $\alpha_v\beta_3$. The uPA increases vitronectin binding to endothelial cells due to an increase in the affinity of vitronectin for the uPA receptor mediated by the amino terminal fragment of the uPA. Active plasminogen activator inhibitor-1 (PAI-1), but not inactivated PAI-1, inhibited vitronectin binding to cells (146,147). The $\alpha_v\beta_3$ attachment site on vitronectin overlaps with the binding site for PAI-1. It is hypothesized that the serpin PAI-1 inhibits cell migration by blocking integrin $\alpha_v\beta_3$ binding to vitronectin (97).

C. Feedback Regulation of Extracellular Matrix, Integrins, and Plasminogen by Proteases

Increased protease activity will result in not only wound cell migration, but also accumulation of proteolytic products in the environment. ECM and integrins are regulators as well as substrates of proteases. The feedback regulation presents itself yet another level of control mechanisms for a delicate proteolytic system that requires precision.

The proteolysis of ECM is not only a way for cells to open up a route to migrate, but also to produce a variety of fragments to mediate physiological activities distinct from one another and from their intact parental molecules. Fibronectin degradation products, but not intact fibronectin, have been found to induce MMP-1, MMP-3 and MMP-9 gene expression (148–151). Different domains of fibronectin, cell adhesion RGD site and amino terminal matrix assembly site, are recognized by $\alpha_5\beta_1$ but crosscompete against each other for the $\alpha_5\beta_1$ binding. As a result, these two domains induce distinct $\alpha_5\beta_1$-mediated signaling pathways (152). The proteolytic fragments of laminin produced by different enzymes can differentially impact on epithelial cell migration. Plasmin proteolysis of laminin results in apoptosis of hippocampal neurons (153) and impaired epithelial cell motility as compared with the intact laminin, possibly by promoting assembly of hemidesmosomes (154). On the other hand, MMP-2 digestion of laminin-5 exposes a putative migratory signal and, as a result, promotes migration of breast epithelial cells (155). In other instances, proteolytic processing and exposure of cryptic sites in ECM result in changes in the binding specificity of integrins. MMP matrilysin (MMP-7) cleaves entactin, a basement membrane protein. The E-domain released by digestion can ligate β_3-like integrins of neutrophils and signal chemotaxis (156). The MMP-2–dependent processing of type I collagen exposes a site that allows cells to utilize $\alpha_v\beta_3$ rather than $\alpha_2\beta_1$. In melanoma cells, this change allows cells to receive survival signals via $\alpha_v\beta_3$, whereas in vascular smooth muscle cells the result is increased cell proliferation (157).

The cleavage of native collagen is proposed to have marked effects on integrin $\alpha_2\beta_1$-mediated cell migration on type I collagen. Interaction of keratinocyte $\alpha_2\beta_1$ integrin with native type I collagen in a provisional wound matrix induces MMP-1 expression (158). It is hypothesized that by cleaving collagen, the initial high-affinity contact is loosened, releasing the cell that then migrates to ''grab'' high-affinity $\alpha_2\beta_1$ integrin bonds with undigested collagen ahead in the open wound. Indeed keratinocytes can migrate on native collagen, but not on a collagenase-resistant collagen matrix (159). In vitro cleavage of type I collagen by collagenase-3 has also demonstrated a drastically altered $\alpha_2\beta_1$ integrin-mediated cell adhesion as compared with native collagen (160). Cryptic sites within ECM molecules can also be exposed by applying mechanical tension to cells. The increased contractility by Rho overexpression or stretching fibronectin covalently linked to rubber culture dishes exposes a cryptic site in fibronectin molecules in fibroblasts. Fibronectin matrix assembly is consequentially enhanced (161). Different domains of fibronectin can affect the matrix assembly. While the RGD cell-binding site is essential for the matrix assembly, the first type III repeats plays a regulatory role since the intact and the repeats-deleted fibronectin differ in their rate of fibrillar matrix formation (162).

Integrins are subjected to proteolytic degradation which, as a result, will impair integrin-mediated signaling transduction. Both β_1 and β_4 subunits have been found to be cleaved by MMPs, jararhagin and matrilysin, respectively (163,164). The cleavage of $\alpha_2\beta_1$ by jararhagin results in the generation of a 115-kDa β_1 fragment and inhibits collagen-induced platelet aggregation (165). A protein consisting of disintegrin and MMP domain, jararhagin might bind to platelet α_2 subunit via the disintegrin domain followed by proteolysis of the β_1 subunit with loss of the integrin structure (conformation) necessary for the binding of collagen ligands. The cleavage also interferes with collagen-stimulated phosphorylation of pp72 (syk), a protein tyrosine kinase (163).

Proteases themselves can also be the target of proteolysis. As a result, the degradation products of proteases can modulate the parental protease activity and have significant consequences in wound repair as well as other pathological processes, such as cancer formation. The importance of this mode of regulation has been a recurrent theme in the angiogenesis. For instance, the conversion of plasminogen to angiostatin (166), collagen XVIII to endostatin (167), and MMP-2 to PEX (145) by proteolysis produces angiogenic inhibitors that impair neovascularization. Enzymes, including MMP-7 (168), MMP-9 (168), macrophage elastase (169), and plasmin reductase (170), have been shown to cleave plasminogen for the release of angiostatin. The MMP-2–and MMP-9–null mice demonstrated the decreased angiogenesis (104,105).

IV. INTEGRIN REGULATION OF TISSUE REMODELING IN WOUND REPAIR

A. Integrin-Mediated Wound Contraction

Fibroblasts undergo a series of phenotypic changes during granulation tissue formation and assume some characteristics of smooth muscle cells to become actin-rich myofibroblasts. The appearance of myofibroblasts corresponds to the commencement of collagen-rich granulation tissue contraction. Wound contraction involves the reorganization of extracellular matrix and intracellular actin cytoskeleton. Integrins have been increasingly recognized as critical components in the regulation of wound contraction. Conversely, wound contraction affects integrin function by altering cell geometry through cytoskeletal structure. Thus, wound contraction represents a complex and masterfully orchestrated process of reciprocal control between integrins and ECM compaction. How integrins affect wound contraction has been studied from these angles: the identification of integrin receptors required in wound contraction, the role of integrins in extracellular factor-induced collagen contraction, and mechanisms underlying integrin-mediated wound contraction. While some work may be performed in vivo, most studies in wound contraction are conducted in vitro with various three-dimensional ECM, most notably type I collagen, culture systems.

Integrin $\alpha_2\beta_1$, a collagen receptor in fibroblasts, is probably the first integrin recognized as a wound contraction regulatory integrin. Using a well-characterized in vitro model, collagen lattice contraction mediated by fibroblasts, Schiro et al. (171) demonstrated that the transfection of an $\alpha_2\beta_1$-negative cell line, rhabdomyosarcoma (RD), with α_2 cDNA restored its ability to contract collagen matrices. Similar findings in the role of $\alpha_2\beta_1$ in collagen contraction have also been made in other cell types: human dermal fibroblasts (172), human vascular smooth muscle cells (173), and human colonic carcinoma (174). In addition to $\alpha_2\beta_1$, the $\alpha_1\beta_1$ collagen receptor and $\alpha_6\beta_1$ laminin receptor have also been suggested to modulate matrix contraction (175–178). The laminin receptor $\alpha_6\beta_4$, on the other hand, has been shown to reduce $\alpha_2\beta_1$-mediated collagen gel contraction in a breast carcinoma cell line (179).

Several wound growth factors and exogenous factors have been found to mediate the contraction of collagen matrices. Among these factors that induce the collagen gel contraction are PDGF (180), TGF-β (125,181), MUC1 mucin (182), and angiotensin II and osteopontin (36,183). On the other hand, prostaglandins, cigarette smoke extract (184) and hydroxy radicals (185,186) inhibit collagen gel contraction. Integrins appear to participate in the collagen gel contraction mediated by these factors. For example, TGF-β induces collagen gel contraction by increasing cellular $\alpha_2\beta_1$ level (125). Several laboratories have also found that PDGF-BB induced $\alpha_2\beta_1$ in human dermal fibroblasts (17,29). A ligand for $\alpha_v\beta_3$, $\alpha_v\beta_1$, $\alpha_v\beta_5$ (39,40), $\alpha_4\beta_1$ (37), and $\alpha_9\beta_1$ (38), osteopontin mediates gel contraction directly or as an intermediary for angiotensin II (183). The ligation of osteopontin to $\alpha_v\beta_3$ integrin stimulated pp60c-src kinase activity (94) and NF-κB (41). Our laboratory also found that NF-κB activity is required for collagen gel contraction (32). Cigarette smoke extract inhibits collagen gel contraction as well as fibronectin production (184).

Several mechanisms have been proposed in the understanding of integrin-mediated wound contraction. Induced protein tyrosine phosphorylation has been observed following cell–collagen interaction and is obviously required for collagen gel contraction. The integrin β_1 induces PDGF-independent tyrosine phosphorylation of PDGF-β receptors in human fibroblasts by type I collagen (187). The use of tyrosine inhibitors abrogated the collagen gel contraction (188). Further downstream, signaling events that might occur include tyrosine phosphorylation of focal adhesion (189), ERK1, ERK2, and PLC-gamma-1 (190), and activation of protein kinase C and NF-κB (32,172).

The cytoplasmic domain, but not the extracellular domain, of integrin α_2 subunit may contain information to regulate wound contraction (171). In light of this finding, the fact that the α_2 plasmic domain directly binds to F-actin (191) is of considerable interest since collagen gel contraction has been found to be accompanied by changes in actin cytoskeletal architecture (192). Therefore, integrin $\alpha_2\beta_1$-mediated wound contraction could result from the $\alpha_2$chain–initiated actin cytoskeleton reorganization. Another example from muscle integrin β_1D-mediated contraction further supports this hypothesis (193). In muscle cells β_1D and β_1A are alternatively spliced variants in their cytoplasmic domains. The β_1D integrin significantly enhanced contractility compared with β_1A. The enhanced contractility by β_1D is accompanied by forming extremely stable association with the detergent-insoluble cytoskeleton, elevated stability of focal adhesion, binding to talin instead of α-actinin, increased ligand binding, and fibronectin assembly. Thus, it appears that the cytoskeletal organization plays a key role in integrin-mediated wound contraction. Extensive studies have been conducted to identify cytoskeleton-associated components involved in cell contraction. Integrin-engagement in mouse results in the rapid recruitment to the cytoskeleton of RasGAP (p120RasGAP), its associated protein the GTPase activating protein for RhoA (p190RhoGAP), and the focal adhesion kinase (p125FAK) (194). Small GTPases Rho, Rac, and Cdc42 are required either for the formation of actin filament-based structures or for the assembly of adhesion sites to ECM (195,196), which in turn could affect integrin-mediated wound contraction (192). Furthermore, microtubule cytoskeleton appears to have a significant role in wound contraction, since its disruption activates the integrin-dependent signaling cascade, which leads to the assembly of matrix adhesions and the induction of DNA synthesis. The increase in cell contractility is an indispensable intermediary step in this signaling process (197).

The inseparable partnership between integrins and proteases is a characteristic of not only cell migratory process, but also wound contraction. The collagen gel contraction process has been observed with accompanying changes in the expression or activation of MMP-1, MMP-2, and MMP-9 (118,120). In this model, the activity of cell surface–associated MMP-2, but not soluble active MMP-2, plays a critical role in mediating collagen gel contraction (198). Therefore, the contraction process itself seems to be the recipient of protease-associated signals. It is unclear, however, whether there is a link between collagen gel contraction and the contraction-associated changes in the expression of collagen alpha(I) and MMP-1. Most tyrosine phosphorylation inhibitors, including genistein, have been reported to prevent the contraction of collagen gels. Genistein, however, failed to abrogate the induction of MMP-1 by collagen. Furthermore, none of these inhibitors prevented the down-regulation of collagen expression (188). Obviously, the collagen gel contraction and gene expression do not have a simple relationship of cause and consequence.

B. Integrin-Mediated Scar Formation and Scarless Wound Healing

Wound contraction is followed by scar formation in the adult, but not in the embryo. Thus, the organ is patched rather than restored in adult wound repair, whereas early gestation fetal tissue heals perfectly. In scar, the collagen matrix is poorly reconstituted in dense parallel bundles unlike the mechanically efficient basketweave meshwork of collage in normal dermis. Several cellular activities, including integrin expression, protease activity, collagen matrix deposition, and cell apoptosis, have been proposed to mediate scar formation. In the search for a scarless wound repair approach, many studies discovered that integrins once again emerge as a prominent player in the scar formation process.

The rapid reepithelialization as a result of early up-regulation of integrin expression in fetal wounds is hypothesized to limit the induction of inflammatory factors and scar (199). In an in vitro fetal wound model, fetal skin from six human abortuses was transplanted subcutaneously into severe combined immunodeficient mice. Wounded human fetal skin grafts reepithelialized rapidly within 24 to 36 hr and healed scarlessly with increased suprabasal expression within 4 hr of α_2, α_3, α_6, and β_4 or new synthesis of α_5, α_v, and β_6 integrins at the epidermal wound edge. This increased integrin expression persisted until reepithelialization was complete.

TGF-β1 is expressed transiently and at low levels in the embryo after injury (200,201) but persistently high in the adult wounds (202). In fact, TGF-β1 has been implicated in the induction of scarring of skin wounds (203–205). Integrins may contribute to scar formation as a mediator of TGF-β–induced phenotypes linked to scarring: the conversion from fibroblasts to myofibroblasts (206), ECM deposition (205), and cell apoptosis (207). Although TGF-β is a known regulator of integrin expression, it is unclear whether TGF-β increases scarring by regulating integrin expression, since TGF-β can both stimulate and inhibit integrin expression depending on cell types (208,209) or specific integrins (22). For example, TGF-β stimulates the integrin expression in monocytes, but inhibits it in microvascular endothelial cells (208,209). In keratinocytes, TGF-β up-regulates the expression of $\alpha_5\beta_1$, $\alpha_v\beta_5$, $\alpha_2\beta_1$, induces the de nova synthesis of $\alpha_v\beta_6$, but down-regulates $\alpha_3\beta_1$ (22). In fibroblasts, TGF-β can induce the expression of $\alpha_2\beta_1$ (125), a collagen receptor integrin that increases its expression during wound contraction (28), modulates TGF-β–induced wound contraction (125), and mediates MMP-1 expression induced by 3D collagen gel (210). Therefore, it is possible that integrins might act as both a functional modulator and an intermediary of TGF-β.

The conversion from fibroblasts to myofibroblasts is a phenotype that is apparently absent in embryos but characterizes the evolution of granulation tissue to scar in adult wounds (126,127,211). Myofibroblasts are characterized by large bundles of actin-containing microfilaments disposed along the cytoplasmic face of the plasma membrane and the establishment of cell–cell and cell–matrix lineages (212). TGF-β is a major promoter of myofibroblast differentiation by inducing α-smooth muscle actin (213–215). The accumulation of α-smooth muscle actin requires the TGF-β1–induced deposition and polymerization of ED-A fibronectin, an isoform de novo expressed during wound healing and fibrotic changes (206). It appears that both ED-A fibronectin and TGF-β1 are necessary for myofibroblast conversion. In vitro, TGF-β1 increases total fibronectin levels by preferentially promoting accumulation of ED-A fibronectin (216,217) on which cells adhere and migrate more actively than other splicing variants of fibronectin (218), probably because of the altered accessibility of the RGD motif of ED-A fibronectin to integrin $\alpha_5\beta_1$. It is hypothesized that ED-A fibronectin could transduce signals by TGF-β1 and/or synergize with them. The integrins are involved in this process at two levels: receptors for fibronectin and essential components in the fibronectin matrix. The interaction between fibronectin and $\alpha_5\beta_1$ initiates signal transduction pathways that overlap with growth factor signal transduction pathways and lead to many physiological process (152,219). The fibronectin matrix assembly, the only fibronectin structure in which ED-A domain can exert its permissive function on TGF-β activity (206), requires the activation of integrins $\alpha_3\beta_1$ and $\alpha_4\beta_1$, and the interaction between integrins and cytoskeletal proteins (220–222).

The cellular proteolytic level directly influences the extracellular matrix deposition. The exogenous application of TGF-β to fetal wounds in an in vitro model resulted in scarring associated with reduced MMP-1 level (205). The TGF-β also reduced uPA level in fetal cell culture (223). The TGF-β1–null fibroblasts from knockout mice accumulated and synthesized lower constitutive levels of pro–alpha1(I) collagen, fibronectin, and PAI-1 mRNA, indicating that TGF-β1 acts as a positive autocrine regulator of ECM biosynthesis (224). Although integrin activation and protease down-regulation by TGF-β have not been directly connected, interaction between dermal fibroblasts and type I collagen has been reported to attenuate TGF-β–induced type I collagen synthesis (33). Additionally, the elevated levels of ECM proteins could prevent cells from undergoing apoptosis since type VI collagen, fibronectin, vitronectin, and type I collagen can modulate apoptotic cell death mediated by integrins β_1, $\alpha_5\beta_1$, $\alpha_v\beta_3$, $\alpha_2\beta_1$, and $\alpha_6\beta_4$ (225–229). In fact, apoptosis has been hypothesized as a mechanism by which granulation tissue is evolved into a scar since the transition between granulation tissue and scar is accompanied by the increased number of myofibroblasts and vascular cells that undergo apoptosis (230). On the other hand, excessive scarring (hypertrophic scar or fibrosis) may indicate that the process of apoptosis could not take place (231). Therefore, the regulation of apoptotic phenomena during wound healing may be important in the establishment and development of pathological scarring.

REFERENCES

1. Clark RAF. The Molecular and Cellular Biology of Wound Repair. 2d ed. New York: Plenum. 1996.
2. Zhang Z, Monteiro-Riviere NA. Comparison of integrins in human skin, pig skin,

and perfused skin: an in vitro skin toxicology model. J Appl Toxicol 1997; 17: 247–253.

3. Juhasz I, Murphy GF, Yan HC, Herlyn M, Albelda SM. Regulation of extracellular matrix proteins and integrin cell substratum adhesion receptors on epithelium during cutaneous human wound healing in vivo. Am J Pathol 1993; 143:1458–1469.

4. Cavani A, Zambruno G, Marconi A, Manca V, Marchetti M, Giannetti A. Distinctive integrin expression in the newly forming epidermis during wound healing in humans. J Invest Dermatol 1993; 101:600–604.

5. Larjava H, Salo T, Haapasalmi K, Kramer RH, Heino J. Expression of integrins and basement membrane components by wound keratinocytes. J Clin Invest 1993; 92:1425–1435.

6. Hertle MD, Kubler MD, Leigh IM, Watt FM. Aberrant integrin expression during epidermal wound healing and in psoriatic epidermis. J Clin Invest 1992; 89:1892–1901.

7. Tonnesen MG. Neutrophil-endothelial cell interactions: mechanisms of neutrophil adherence to vascular endothelium. J Invest Dermatol 1989; 93:53S–58S.

8. Christofidou-Solomidou M, Bridges M, Murphy GF, Albelda SM, DeLisser HM. Expression and function of endothelial cell α_v integrin receptors in wound-induced human angiogenesis in human skin/SCID mice chimeras. Am J Pathol 1997; 151: 975–983.

9. Swerlick RA, Brown EJ, Xu Y, Lee KH, Manos S, Lawley TJ. Expression and modulation of the vitronectin receptor on human dermal microvascular endothelial cells. J Invest Dermatol 1992; 99:715–722.

10. Clark RA, Tonnesen MG, Gailit J, Cheresh DA. Transient functional expression of $\alpha_v\beta_3$ on vascular cells during wound repair. Am J Pathol 1996; 148:1407–1421.

11. Senger DR, Claffey KP, Benes JE, Perruzzi CA, Sergiou AP, Detmar M. Angiogenesis promoted by vascular endothelial growth factor: regulation through $\alpha_1\beta_1$ and $\alpha_2\beta_1$ integrins. Proc Natl Acad Sci USA 1997; 94:13612–13617.

12. Brooks PC, Clark RA, Cheresh DA. Requirement of vascular integrin $\alpha_v\beta_3$ for angiogenesis. Science 1994; 64:569–571.

13. Heldin CH, Westermark B. Platelet-derived growth factor: mechanism of action and possible in vivo function. Cell Regul 1990; 1:555–566.

14. Assoian RK, Fleurdelys BE, Stevenson HC, Miller PJ, Madtes DK, Raines EW, Ross R, Sporn MB. Expression and secretion of type β transforming growth factor by activated human macrophages. Proc Natl Acad Sci USA 1987; 84:6020–6024.

15. Rappolee DA, Mark D, Banda MJ, Werb Z. Wound macrophages express TGF-α and other growth factors in vivo: analysis by mRNA phenotyping. Science 1988; 241:708–712.

16. Seppa H, Grotendorst G, Seppa S, Schiffmann E, Martin GR. Platelet-derived growth factor in chemotactic for fibroblasts. J Cell Biol 1982; 92:584–588.

17. Ahlen K, Rubin K. Platelet-derived growth factor-BB stimulates synthesis of the integrin α_2-subunit in human diploid fibroblasts. Exp Cell Res 1994; 215:347–353.

18. Xu J, Zutter MM, Santoro SA, Clark RA. PDGF induction of α_2 integrin gene expression is mediated by protein kinase C-ζ. J Cell Biol 1996; 134:1301–1311.

19. Gailit J, Xu J, Bueller H, Clark RA. Platelet-derived growth factor and inflammatory cytokines have differential effects on the expression of integrins $\alpha_1\beta_1$ and $\alpha_5\beta_1$ by human dermal fibroblasts in vitro. J Cell Physiol 1996; 169:281–289.

20. Rubio MA, Sotillos M, Jochems G, Alvarez V, Corbi AL. Monocyte activation: rapid induction of $\alpha_1\beta_1$ (VLA-1) integrin expression by lipopolysaccharide and interferon-γ. Eur J Immunol 1995; 25:2701–2705.

21. Nakamura M, Chikama T, Nishida T. Up-regulation of integrin α_5 expression by combination of substance P and insulin-like growth factor-1 in rabbit corneal epithelial cells. Biochem Biophys Res Commun 1998; 246:777–782.

22. Zambruno G, Marchisio PC, Marconi A, Vaschieri C, Melchiori A, Giannetti A, De Luca M. Transforming growth factor-β_1 modulates β_1 and β_5 integrin receptors and induces the de novo expression of the $\alpha_v\beta_6$ heterodimer in normal human keratinocytes: implications for wound healing. J Cell Biol 1995; 129: 853–865.

23. Danilenko DM, Ring BD, Lu JZ, Tarpley JE, Chang D, Liu N, Wen D, Pierce GF. Neu differentiation factor upregulates epidermal migration and integrin expression in excisional wounds. J Clin Invest 1995; 95:842–851.

24. Chen JD, Kim JP, Zhang K, Sarret Y, Wynn KC, Kramer RH, Woodley DT. Epidermal growth factor (EGF) promotes human keratinocyte locomotion on collagen by increasing the α_2 integrin subunit. Exp Cell Res 1993; 209:216–223.

25. Klein S, Bikfalvi A, Birkenmeier TM, Giancotti FG, Rifkin DB. Integrin regulation by endogenous expression of 18-kDa fibroblast growth factor-2. J Biol Chem 1996; 271:22583–22590.

26. Sepp NT, Li LJ, Lee KH, Brown EJ, Caughman SW, Lawley TJ, Swerlick RA. Basic fibroblast growth factor increases expression of the $\alpha_v\beta_3$ integrin complex on human microvascular endothelial cells. J Invest Dermatol 1994; 103:295–299.

27. Sun L, Xu L, Chang H, Henry FA, Miller RM, Harmon JM, Nielsen TB. Transfection with aFGF cDNA improves wound healing. J Invest Dermatol 1997; 108:313–318.

28. Xu J, Clark RA. Extracellular matrix alters PDGF regulation of fibroblast integrins. J Cell Biol 1996; 132:239–249.

29. Condic ML, Letourneau PC. Ligand-induced changes in integrin expression regulate neuronal adhesion and neurite outgrowth. Nature 1997; 389:852–856.

30. Grinnell F. Fibroblasts, myofibroblasts, and wound contraction. J Cell Biol 1994; 124:401–404.

31. Klein CE, Dressel D, Steinmayer T, Mauch C, Eckes B, Krieg T, Bankert RB, Weber L. Integrin $\alpha_2\beta_1$ is upregulated in fibroblasts and highly aggressive melanoma cells in three-dimensional collagen lattices and mediates the reorganization of collagen I fibrils. J Cell Biol 1991; 115:1427–1436.

32. Xu J, Zutter MM, Santoro SA, Clark RA. A three-dimensional collagen lattice activates NF-κB in human fibroblasts: role in integrin α_2 gene expression and tissue remodeling. J Cell Biol 1998; 140:709–719.

33. Clark RA, Nielsen LD, Welch MP, McPherson JM. Collagen matrices attenuate the collagen-synthetic response of cultured fibroblasts to TGF-β. J Cell Sci 1995; 108:1251–1261.

34. Lin YC, Grinnell F. Decreased level of PDGF-stimulated receptor autophosphorylation by fibroblasts in mechanically relaxed collagen matrices. J Cell Biol 1993; 122:663–672.

35. Kireeva ML, Lam SC, Lau LF. Adhesion of human umbilical vein endothelial cells to the immediate-early gene product Cyr61 is mediated through integrin $\alpha_v\beta_3$. J Biol Chem 1998; 273:3090–3096.

36. Ashizawa N, Graf K, Do YS, Nunohiro T, Giachelli CM, Meehan WP, Tuan TL, Hsueh WA. Osteopontin is produced by rat cardiac fibroblasts and mediates A(II)-induced DNA synthesis and collagen gel contraction. J Clin Invest 1996; 98:2218–2227.

37. Bayless KJ, Meininger GA, Scholtz JM, Davis GE. Osteopontin is a ligand for the $\alpha_4\beta_1$ integrin. J Cell Sci 1998; 111:1165–1174.

38. Smith LL, Cheung HK, Ling LE, Chen J, Sheppard D, Pytela R, Giachelli CM. Osteopontin N-terminal domain contains a cryptic adhesive sequence recognized by $\alpha_9\beta_1$ integrin. J Biol Chem 1996; 271:28485–28491.

39. Liaw L, Skinner MP, Raines EW, Ross R, Cheresh DA, Schwartz SM, Giachelli CM. The adhesive and migratory effects of osteopontin are mediated via distinct cell surface integrins. Role of $\alpha_v\beta_3$ in smooth muscle cell migration to osteopontin in vitro. J Clin Invest 1995; 95:713–724.

40. Giachelli CM, Liaw L, Murry CE, Schwartz SM, Almeida M. Osteopontin expression in cardiovascular diseases. Ann NY Acad Sci 1995; 760:109–126.

41. Scatena M, Almeida M, Chaisson ML, Fausto N, Nicosia RF, Giachelli CM. NF-κB mediates $\alpha_v\beta_3$ integrin-induced endothelial cell survival. J Cell Biol 1998; 141:1083–1093.

42. Galiano RD, Zhao LL, Clemmons DR, Roth SI, Lin X, Mustoe TA. Interaction between the insulin-like growth factor family and the integrin receptor family in tissue repair processes. Evidence in a rabbit ear dermal ulcer model. J Clin Invest 1996; 98:2462–2468.

43. Burridge K, Turner CE, Romer LH. Tyrosine phosphorylation of paxillin and pp125FAK accompanies cell adhesion to extracellular matrix: a role in cytoskeletal assembly. J Cell Biol 1992; 119:893–903.

44. Cybulsky AV, McTavish AJ, Cyr MD. Extracellular matrix modulates epidermal growth factor receptor activation in rat glomerular epithelial cells. J Clin Invest 1994; 94:68–78.

45. Miyamoto S, Teramoto H, Gutkind JS, Yamada KM. Integrins can collaborate with growth factors for phosphorylation of receptor tyrosine kinases and MAP kinase activation: roles of integrin aggregation and occupancy of receptors. J Cell Biol 1996; 135:1633–1642.

46. Falcioni R, Antonini A, Nistico P, Di Stefano S, Crescenzi M, Natali PG, Sacchi A. $\alpha_6\beta_4$ and $\alpha_6\beta_1$ integrins associate with ErbB-2 in human carcinoma cell lines. Exp Cell Res 1997; 236:76–85.

47. Donaldson DJ, Mahan JT, Yang H, Yamada KM. Integrin and phosphotyrosine expression in normal and migrating newt keratinocytes. Anatom Rec 1995; 241:49–58.

48. Satake S, Kuzuya M, Ramos MA, Kanda S, Iguchi A. Angiogenic stimuli are essen-

tial for survival of vascular endothelial cells in three-dimensional collagen lattice. Biochem Biophys Res Commun 1998; 244:642–646.

49. Pozzi A, Wary KK, Giancotti FG, Gardner HA. Integrin $\alpha_1\beta_1$ mediates a unique collagen-dependent proliferation pathway in vivo. J Cell Biol 1998; 142:587–594.

50. Guilherme A, Torres K, Czech MP. Cross-talk between insulin receptor and integrin $\alpha_5\beta_1$ signaling pathways. J Biol Chem 1998; 273:22899–22903.

51. Schneller M, Vuori K, Ruoslahti E. $\alpha_v\beta_3$ Integrin associates with activated insulin and PDGFβ receptors and potentiates the biological activity of PDGF. EMBO J 1997; 16:5600–5607.

52. Koyama H, Raines EW, Bornfeldt KE, Roberts JM, Ross R. Fibrillar collagen inhibits arterial smooth muscle proliferation through regulation of Cdk2 inhibitors. Cell 1996; 87:1069–1078.

53. Somasundaram R, Schuppan D. Type I, II, III, IV, V, and VI collagens serve as extracellular ligands for the isoforms of platelet-derived growth factor (AA, BB, and AB). J Biol Chem 1996; 271:26884–26891.

54. Howe A, Aplin AE, Alahari SK, Juliano RL. Integrin signaling and cell growth control. Curr Opin Cell Biol 1998; 10:220–231.

55. Schwartz MA. Integrins, oncogenes, and anchorage independence. J Cell Biol 1997; 139:575–578.

56. Assoian RK, Marcantonio EE. The extracellular matrix as a cell cycle control element in atherosclerosis and restenosis. J Clin Invest 1996; 98:2436–2439.

57. Faux MC, Scott JD. Molecular glue: kinase anchoring and scaffold proteins. Cell 1996; 85:9–12.

58. Lotz MM, Nusrat A, Madara JL, Ezzell R, Wewer UM, Mercurio AM. Intestinal epithelial restitution. Involvement of specific laminin isoforms and integrin laminin receptors in wound closure of a transformed model epithelium. Am J Pathol 1997; 150:747–760.

59. Nakamura SI, Yamamura H. Thrombin and collagen induce rapid phosphorylation of a common set of cellular proteins on tyrosine in human platelets. J Biol Chem 1989; 264:7089–7091.

60. Torti M, Festetics ET, Bertoni A, Sinigaglia F, Balduini C. Thrombin induces the association of cyclic ADP-ribose-synthesizing CD38 with the platelet cytoskeleton. FEBS Lett 1998; 428:200–204.

61. Derrick JM, Loudon RG, Gardner JK. Peptide LSARLAF activates $\alpha_{IIb}\beta_3$ on resting platelets and causes resting platelet aggregate formation without platelet shape change. Thromb Res 1998; 89:31–40.

62. Ferrell JE, Martin GS. Tyrosine-specific phosphorylation is regulated by glycoprotein IIb/IIIa in platelets. Proc Natl Acad Sci USA 1989; 86:2234–2238.

63. Golden A, Brugge JS, Shattil SJ. Role of platelet membrane glycoprotein IIb-IIIa in agonist-induced tyrosine phosphorylation of platelet proteins. J Cell Biol 1990; 120:1509–1517.

64. Banfic H, Tang X, Batty IH, Downes CP, Chen C, Rittenhouse SE. A novel integrin-activated pathway forms PKB/Akt-stimulatory phosphatidylinositol 3, 4-bisphosphate via phosphatidylinositol 3-phosphate in platelets. J Biol Chem 1998; 273:13–16.

65. Hamazaki Y, Kojima H, Mano H, Nagata Y, Todokoro K, Abe T, Nagasawa T. Tec is involved in G protein-coupled receptor- and integrin-mediated signaling in human blood platelets. Oncogene 1998; 16:2773–2779.

66. Hughes PE, Renshaw MW, Pfaff M, Forsyth J, Keivens VM, Schwartz MA, Ginsberg MH. Suppression of integrin activation: a novel function of a Ras/Raf-initiated MAP kinase pathway. Cell 1997; 88:521–530.

67. O'Toole TE, Mandelman D, Forsyth J, Shattil SJ, Plow EF, Ginsberg MH. Modulation of the affinity of integrin $\alpha_{IIb}\beta_3$ (GPIIb-IIIa) by the cytoplasmic domain of α_{IIb}. Science 1991; 254:845–847.

68. O'Toole TE, Ylanne J, Culley BM. Regulation of integrin affinity states through an NPXY motif in the β subunit cytoplasmic domain. J Biol Chem 1995; 270: 8553–8558.

69. Romanic AM, Graesser D, Baron JL, Visintin I, Janeway CAJ, Madri JA, Marra F, Pastacaldi S, Romanelli RG, Pinzani M, Ticali P, Carloni V, Laffi G, Gentilini P. T cell adhesion to endothelial cells and extracellular matrix is modulated upon transendothelial cell migration: integrin-mediated stimulation of monocyte chemotactic protein-1 expression. Lab Invest 1997; 76:11–23.

70. Nathan C, Srimal S, Farber C, Sanchez E, Kabbash L, Asch A, Gailit J, Wright SD. Cytokine-induced respiratory burst of human neutrophils: dependence on extracellular matrix proteins and CD11/CD18 integrins. J Cell Biol 1989; 109:1341–1349.

71. Berton G, Laudanna C, Sorio C, Rossi F. Generation of signals activating neutrophil functions by leukocyte integrins: LFA-1 and gp150/95, but not CR3, are able to stimulate the respiratory burst of human neutrophils. J Cell Biol 1992; 116:1007–1017.

72. Detmers PA, Zhou D, Polizzi E, Thieringer R, Hanlon WA, Vaidya S, Bansal V. Role of stress-activated mitogen-activated protein kinase (p38) in β_2-integrin-dependent neutrophil adhesion and the adhesion-dependent oxidative burst. J Immunol 1998; 161:1921–1929.

73. Dedhar S, Hannigan GE. Integrin cytoplasmic interactions and bidirectional transmembrane signalling. Curr Opin Cell Biol 1996; 8:657–669.

74. Laudanna C, Campbell JJ, Butcher EC. Role of Rho in chemoattractant-activated leukocyte adhesion through integrins. Science 1996; 271:981–983.

75. Berton G, Fumagalli L, Laudanna C, Sorio C. β_2 Integrin-dependent protein tyrosine phosphorylation and activation of the FGR protein tyrosine kinase in human neutrophils. J Cell Biol 1994; 126:1111–1121.

76. Bohuslav J, Horejsi V, Hansmann C, Stockl J, Weidle UH, Majdic O, Bartke I, Knapp W, Stockinger H. Urokinase plasminogen activator receptor, β_2-integrins, and Src-kinases within a single receptor complex of human monocytes. J Exp Med 1995; 181:1381–1390.

77. Weerasinghe D, McHugh KP, Ross FP, Brown EJ, Gisler RH, Imhof BA. A role for the $\alpha_v\beta_3$ integrin in the transmigration of monocytes. J Cell Biol 1998; 142: 595–607.

78. Loike JD, el Khoury J, Cao L, Richards CP, Rascoff H, Mandeville JT, Maxfield FR, Silverstein SC. Fibrin regulates neutrophil migration in response to interleukin

8, leukotriene B4, tumor necrosis factor, and formyl-methionyl-leucyl-phenylalanine. J Exp Med 1995; 181:1763–1772.

79. Moghe PV, Nelson RD, Tranquillo RT. Cytokine-stimulated chemotaxis of human neutrophils in a 3-D conjoined fibrin gel assay. J Immunol Methods 1995; 180: 193–211.

80. Dransfield I, Stocks SC, Haslett C. Regulation of cell adhesion molecule expression and function associated with neutrophil apoptosis. Blood 1995; 85:3264–3273.

81. Davis GE, Camarillo CW. An $\alpha_2\beta_1$ integrin-dependent pinocytic mechanism involving intracellular vacuole formation and coalescence regulates capillary lumen and tube formation in three-dimensional collagen matrix. Exp Cell Res 1996; 224: 39–51.

82. Gualandris A, Rusnati M, Belleri M, Nelli EE, Bastaki M, Molinari-Tosatti MP, Bonardi F, Parolini S, Albini A, Morbidelli L, Ziche M, Corallini A, Possati L, Vacca A, Ribatti D, Presta M. Basic fibroblast growth factor overexpression in endothelial cells: an autocrine mechanism for angiogenesis and angioproliferative diseases. Cell Growth Diff 1996; 7:147–160.

83. Bastaki M, Nelli EE, Dell'Era P, Rusnati M, Molinari-Tosatti MP, Parolini S. Auerbach R, Ruco LP, Possati L, Presta M. Basic fibroblast growth factor-induced angiogenic phenotype in mouse endothelium. A study of aortic and microvascular endothelial cell lines. Arterioscler Thromb Vasc Biol 1997; 17:454–464.

84. Koblizek TI, Weiss C, Yancopoulos GD, Deutsch U, Risau W. Angiopoietin-1 induces sprouting angiogenesis in vitro. Curr Biol 1998; 8:529–532.

85. Carlevaro MF, Albini A, Ribatti D, Gentili C, Benelli R, Cermelli S, Cancedda R, Cancedda FD. Transferrin promotes endothelial cell migration and invasion: implication in cartilage neovascularization. J Cell Biol 1997; 136:1375–1384.

86. Yanez-Mo M, Alfranca A, Cabanas C, Marazuela M, Tejedor R, Ursa MA, Ashman LK, de Landazuri MO, Sanchez-Madrid F. Regulation of endothelial cell motility by complexes of tetraspan molecules CD81/TAPA-1 and CD151/PETA-3 with $\alpha_3\beta_1$ integrin localized at endothelial lateral junctions. J Cell Biol 1998; 141:791–804.

87. Koolwijk P, van Erck MG, de Vree WJ, Vermeer MA, Weich HA, Hanemaaijer R, van Hinsbergh VW. Cooperative effect of TNFα, bFGF, and VEGF on the formation of tubular structures of human microvascular endothelial cells in a fibrin matrix. Role of urokinase activity. J Cell Biol 1996; 132:1177–1188.

88. Blystone SD, Lindberg FP, Williams MP, McHugh KP, Brown EJ. Inducible tyrosine phosphorylation of the α_3 integrin requires the α_v integrin cytoplasmic tail. J Biol Chem 1996; 271:31458–31462.

89. Schaffner-Reckinger E, Gouon V, Melchior C, Plancon S, Kieffer N. Distinct involvement of β_3 integrin cytoplasmic domain tyrosine residues 747 and 759 in integrin-mediated cytoskeletal assembly and phosphotyrosine signaling. J Biol Chem 1998; 273:12623–12632.

90. Jenkins AL, Nannizzi-Alaimo L, Silver D, Sellers JR, Ginsberg MH, Law DA, Phillips DR. Tyrosine phosphorylation of the β_3 cytoplasmic domain mediates integrin-cytoskeletal interactions. J Biol Chem 1998; 273:13878–13885.

91. Tahiliani PD, Singh L, Auer KL, LaFlamme SE. The role of conserved amino acid

motifs within the integrin β_3 cytoplasmic domain in triggering focal adhesion kinase phosphorylation. J Biol Chem 1997; 272:7892–7898.

92. Eliceiri BP, Klemke R, Stromblad S, Cheresh DA. Integrin $\alpha_v\beta_3$ requirement for sustained mitogen-activated protein kinase activity during angiogenesis. J Cell Biol 1998; 140:1255–1263.

93. Klemke RL, Cai S, Giannini AL, Gallagher PJ, de Lanerolle P, Cheresh DA. Regulation of cell motility by mitogen-activated protein kinase. J Cell Biol 1997; 137:481–492.

94. Chellaiah M, Fitzgerald C, Filardo EJ, Cheresh DA, Hruska KA. Osteopontin activation of c-src in human melanoma cells requires the cytoplasmic domain of the integrin α_v-subunit. Endocrinology 1996; 137:2432–2440.

95. Palecek SP, Loftus JC, Ginsberg MH, Lauffenburger DA, Horwitz AF. Integrin-ligand binding properties govern cell migration speed through cell-substratum adhesiveness. Nature 1997; 385:537–540.

96. Greiling D, Clark RA. Fibronectin provides a conduit for fibroblast transmigration from collagenous stroma into fibrin clot provisional matrix. J Cell Sci 1997; 110:861–870.

97. Stefansson S, Lawrence DA. The serpin PAI-1 inhibits cell migration by blocking integrin $\alpha_v\beta_3$ binding to vitronectin. Nature 1996; 383:441–443.

98. Guan JL, Trevithick JE, Hynes RO. Fibronectin/integrin interaction induces tyrosine phosphorylation of a 120-kDa protein. Cell Regul 1991; 2:951–964.

99. Burbelo PD, Miyamoto S, Utani A, Brill S, Yamada KM, Hall A, Yamada Y. p190-B, a new member of the Rho GAP family, and Rho are induced to cluster after integrin cross-linking. J Biol Chem 1995; 270:30919–30926.

100. Page K, Lange Y. Cell adhesion to fibronectin regulates membrane lipid biosynthesis through 5′-AMP-activated protein kinase. J Biol Chem 1997; 272:19339–19342.

101. Lewis JM, Schwartz MA. Integrins regulate the association and phosphorylation of paxillin by c-Abl. J Biol Chem 1998; 273:14225–14230.

102. Tamura M, Gu J, Matsumoto K, Aota S, Parsons R, Yamada KM. Inhibition of cell migration, spreading, and focal adhesions by tumor suppressor PTEN. Science 1998; 280:1614–1617.

103. Okada A, Tomasetto C, Lutz Y, Bellocq JP, Rio MC, Basset P. Expression of matrix metalloproteinases during rat skin wound healing: evidence that membrane type-1 matrix metalloproteinase is a stromal activator of pro-gelatinase A. J Cell Biol 1997; 137:67–77.

104. Itoh T, Tanioka M, Yoshida H, Yoshioka T, Nishimoto H, Itohara S. Reduced angiogenesis and tumor progression in gelatinase A-deficient mice. Cancer Res 1998; 58:1048–1051.

105. Vu TH, Shipley JM, Bergers G, Berger JE, Helms JA, Hanahan D, Shapiro SD, Senior RM, Werb Z. MMP-9/gelatinase B is a key regulator of growth plate angiogenesis and apoptosis of hypertrophic chondrocytes. Cell 1998; 93:411–422.

106. Romer J, Bugge TH, Pyke C, Lund LR, Flick MJ, Degen JL, Dano K. Impaired wound healing in mice with a disrupted plasminogen gene. Nature Med 1996; 2:287–292.

107. Hiraoka N, Allen E, Apel I, Gyetko M, Weiss S. Matrix metalloproteinases regulate neovascularization by acting as pericellular fibrinolysins. Cell 1998; 95:365–377.

108. Saarialho-Kere UK, Kovacs SO, Pentland AP, Olerud JE, Welgus HG, Parks WC. Cell-matrix interactions modulate interstitial collagenase expression by human keratinocytes actively involved in wound healing. J Clin Invest 1993; 92:2858–2866.
109. Stricklin GP, Li L, Jancic V, Wenczak BA, Nanney LB. Localization of mRNAs representing collagenase and TIMP in sections of healing human burn wounds. Am J Pathol 1993; 143:1657–1666.
110. Saarialho-Kere UK, Crouch EC, Parks WC. Matrix metalloproteinase matrilysin is constitutively expressed in adult human exocrine epithelium. J Invest Dermatol 1995; 105:190–196.
111. Inoue M, Kratz G, Haegerstrand A, Stahle-Backdahl M. Collagenase expression is rapidly induced in wound-edge keratinocytes after acute injury in human skin, persists during healing, and stops at re-epithelialization. J Invest Dermatol 1995; 104:479–483.
112. Brooks PC, Stromblad S, Sanders LC, von Schalscha TL, Aimes RT, Stetler-Stevenson WG, Quigley JP, Cheresh DA. Localization of matrix metalloproteinase MMP-2 to the surface of invasive cells by interaction with integrin $\alpha_v\beta_3$. Cell 1996; 85:683–693.
113. Larjava H, Lyons JG, Salo T, Makela M, Koivisto L, Birkedal-Hansen H, Akiyama SK, Yamada KM, Heino J. Anti-integrin antibodies induce type IV collagenase expression in keratinocytes. J Cellul Physiol 1993; 157:190–200.
114. Kubota S, Ito H, Ishibashi Y, Seyama Y. Anti-α_3 integrin antibody induces the activated form of matrix metalloprotease-2 (MMP-2) with concomitant stimulation of invasion through matrigel by human rhabdomyosarcoma cells. Int J Cancer 1997; 70:106–111.
115. Chintala SK, Sawaya R, Gokaslan ZL, Rao JS. Modulation of matrix metalloprotease-2 and invasion in human glioma cells by $\alpha_3\beta_1$ integrin. Cancer Lett 1996; 103:201–208.
116. Khan KF, Falcone DJ. Role of laminin in matrix induction of macrophage urokinase-type plasminogen activator and 92-kDa metalloproteinase expression. J Biol Chem 1997; 272:8270–8275.
117. Bafetti LM, Young TN, Itoh Y, Stack MS. Intact vitronectin induces matrix metalloproteinase-2 and tissue inhibitor of metalloproteinases-2 expression and enhanced cellular invasion by melanoma cells. J Biol Chem 1998; 273:143–149.
118. Unemori EN, Werb Z. Reorganization of polymerized actin: a possible trigger for induction of procollagenase in fibroblasts cultured in and on collagen gels. J Cell Biol 1986; 103:1021–1031.
119. Haas TL, Davis SJ, Madri JA. Three-dimensional type I collagen lattices induce coordinate expression of matrix metalloproteinases MT1-MMP and MMP-2 in microvascular endothelial cells. J Biol Chem 1998; 273:3604–3610.
120. Tomasek JJ, Halliday NL, Updike DL, Ahern-Moore JS, Vu TK, Liu RW, Howard EW. Gelatinase A activation is regulated by the organization of the polymerized actin cytoskeleton. J Biol Chem 1997; 272:7482–7487.
121. Huhtala P, Humphries MJ, McCarthy JB, Tremble PM, Werb Z, Damsky CH. Cooperative signaling by $\alpha_5\beta_1$ and $\alpha_4\beta_1$ integrins regulates metalloproteinase gene expression in fibroblasts adhering to fibronectin. J Cell Biol 1995; 129:867–879.

122. Nakahara H, Nomizu M, Akiyama SK, Yamada Y, Yeh Y, Chen WT. A mechanism for regulation of melanoma invasion. Ligation of $\alpha_6\beta_1$ integrin by laminin G peptides. J Biol Chem 1996; 271:27221–27224.

123. Bianchi E, Ferrero E, Fazioli F, Mangili F, Wang J, Bender JR, Blasi F, Pardi R. Integrin-dependent induction of functional urokinase receptors in primary T lymphocytes. J Clin Invest 1996; 98:1133–1141.

124. Kim SO, Plow EF, Miles LA. Regulation of plasminogen receptor expression on monocytoid cells by β_1-integrin-dependent cellular adherence to extracellular matrix proteins. J Biol Chem 1996; 271:23761–23767.

125. Riikonen T, Koivisto L, Vihinen P, Heino J. Transforming growth factor-β regulates collagen gel contraction by increasing $\alpha_2\beta_1$ integrin expression in osteogenic cells. J Biol Chem 1995; 270:376–382.

126. Martin P, Lewis J. Actin cables and epidermal movement in embryonic wound healing. Nature 1992; 360:179–183.

127. McCluskey J, Martin P. Analysis of the tissue movements of embryonic wound healing—DiI studies in the limb bud stage mouse embryo. Dev Biol 1995; 170: 102–114.

128. Brock J, Midwinter K, Lewis J, Martin P. Healing of incisional wounds in the embryonic chick wing bud: characterization of the actin purse-string and demonstration of a requirement for Rho activation. J Cell Biol 1996; 135:1097–1107.

129. Bement WM, Forscher P, Mooseker MS. A novel cytoskeletal structure involved in purse string wound closure and cell polarity maintenance. J Cell Biol 1993; 121: 565–578.

130. Hall A. Rho GTPases and the actin cytoskeleton. Science 1998; 279:509–514.

131. Kheradmand F, Werner E, Tremble P, Symons M, Werb Z. Role of Rac1 and oxygen radicals in collagenase-1 expression induced by cell shape change. Science 1998; 280:898–902.

132. Keely PJ, Westwick JK, Whitehead IP, Der CJ, Parise LV. Cdc42 and Rac1 induce integrin-mediated cell motility and invasiveness through PI(3)K. Nature 1997; 390: 632–636.

133. Rezniczek GA, de Pereda JM, Reipert S, Wiche G. Linking integrin $\alpha_6\beta_4$-based cell adhesion to the intermediate filament cytoskeleton: direct interaction between the β_4 subunit and plectin at multiple molecular sites. J Cell Biol 1998; 141:209–225.

134. Shaw LM, Rabinovitz I, Wang HH, Toker A, Mercurio AM. Activation of phosphoinositide 3-OH kinase by the $\alpha_6\beta_4$ integrin promotes carcinoma invasion. Cell 1997; 91:949–960.

135. Chicurel ME, Singer RH, Meyer CJ, Ingber DE. Integrin binding and mechanical tension induce movement of mRNA and ribosomes to focal adhesions. Nature 1998; 392:730–733.

136. Friedlander M, Brooks PC, Shaffer RW, Kincaid CM, Varner JA, Cheresh DA. Definition of two angiogenic pathways by distinct α_v integrins. Science 1995; 270: 1500–1502.

137. Yebra M, Parry GN, Stromblad S, Mackman N, Rosenberg S, Mueller BM, Cheresh DA. Requirement of receptor-bound urokinase-type plasminogen activator for integrin $\alpha_v\beta_5$-directed cell migration. J Biol Chem 1996; 271:29393–29399.

138. Lewis JM, Cheresh DA, Schwartz MA. Protein kinase C regulates $\alpha_v\beta_5$-dependent cytoskeletal associations and focal adhesion kinase phosphorylation. J Cell Biol 1996; 134:1323–1332.

139. Xie B, Laouar A, Huberman E. Autocrine regulation of macrophage differentiation and 92-kDa gelatinase production by tumor necrosis factor-α via $\alpha_5\beta_1$ integrin in HL-60 cells. J Biol Chem 1998; 273:11583–11588.

140. Arner EC, Tortorella MD. Signal transduction through chondrocyte integrin receptors induces matrix metalloproteinase synthesis and synergizes with interleukin-1. Arthrit Rheumat 1995; 38:1304–1314.

141. Sato H, Takino T, Okada Y, Cao J, Shinagawa A, Yamamoto E, Seiki M. A matrix metalloproteinase expressed on the surface of invasive tumour cells. Nature 1994; 370:61–65.

142. Will H, Hinzmann B. cDNA sequence and mRNA tissue distribution of a novel human matrix metalloproteinase with a potential transmembrane segment. Eur J Biochem 1995; 231:602–608.

143. Takino T, Sato H, Shinagawa A, Seiki M. Identification of the second membrane-type matrix metalloproteinase (MT-MMP-2) gene from a human placenta cDNA library. MT-MMPs form a unique membrane-type subclass in the MMP family. J Biol Chem 1995; 270:23013–23020.

144. Werb Z. ECM and cell surface proteolysis: regulating cellular ecology. Cell 1997; 91:439–442.

145. Brooks PC, Silletti S, von Schalscha TL, Friedlander M, Cheresh DA. Disruption of angiogenesis by PEX, a noncatalytic metalloproteinase fragment with integrin binding activity. Cell 1998; 92:391–400.

146. Kanse SM, Kost C, Wilhelm OG, Andreasen PA, Preissner KT. The urokinase receptor is a major vitronectin-binding protein on endothelial cells. Exp Cell Res 1996; 224:344–353.

147. Lawrence DA, Palaniappan S, Stefansson S, Olson ST, Francis-Chmura AM, Shore JD, Ginsburg D. Characterization of the binding of different conformational forms of plasminogen activator inhibitor-1 to vitronectin. Implications for the regulation of pericellular proteolysis. J Biol Chem 1997; 272:7676–7680.

148. Werb Z, Tremble PM, Behrendtsen O, Crowley E, Damsky CH. Signal transduction through the fibronectin receptor induces collagenase and stromelysin gene expression. J Cell Biol 1989; 109:877–889.

149. Tremble PM, Lane TF, Sage EH, Werb Z. SPARC, a secreted protein associated with morphogenesis and tissue remodeling, induces expression of metalloproteinases in fibroblasts through a novel extracellular matrix-dependent pathway. J Cell Biol 1993; 121:1433–1444.

150. Tremble P, Chiquet-Ehrismann R, Werb Z. The extracellular matrix ligands fibronectin and tenascin collaborate in regulating collagenase gene expression in fibroblasts. Mol Biol Cell 1994; 5:439–453.

151. Xie B, Laouar A, Huberman E. Fibronectin-mediated cell adhesion is required for induction of 92-kDa type IV collagenase/gelatinase (MMP-9) gene expression during macrophage differentiation. The signaling role of protein kinase C-β. J Biol Chem 1998; 273:11576–11582.

152. Hocking DC, Sottile J, McKeown-Longo PJ. Activation of distinct $\alpha_5\beta_1$-mediated

signaling pathways by fibronectin's cell adhesion and matrix assembly domains. J Cell Biol 1998; 141:241–253.

153. Chen ZL, Strickland S. Neuronal death in the hippocampus is promoted by plasmin-catalyzed degradation of laminin. Cell 1997; 91:917–925.

154. Goldfinger LE, Stack MS, Jones JC. Processing of laminin-5 and its functional consequences: role of plasmin and tissue-type plasminogen activator. J Cell Biol 1998; 141:255–265.

155. Giannelli G, Falk-Marzillier J, Schiraldi O, Stetler-Stevenson WG, Quaranta V. Induction of cell migration by matrix metalloprotease-2 cleavage of laminin-5. Science 1997; 277:225–228.

156. Gresham HD, Graham IL, Griffin GL, Hsieh JC, Dong LJ, Chung AE, Senior RM. Domain-specific interactions between entactin and neutrophil integrins. G2 domain ligation of integrin $\alpha_3\beta_1$ and E domain ligation of the leukocyte response integrin signal for different responses. J Biol Chem 1996; 271:30587–30594.

157. Montgomery AM, Reisfeld RA, Cheresh DA. Integrin $\alpha_v\beta_3$ rescues melanoma cells from apoptosis in three-dimensional dermal collagen. Proc Natl Acad Sci USA 1994; 91:8856–8860.

158. Sudbeck BD, Pilcher BK, Welgus HG, Parks WC. Induction and repression of collagenase-1 by keratinocytes is controlled by distinct components of different extracellular matrix compartments. J Biol Chem 1997; 272:22103–22110.

159. Pilcher BK, Dumin JA, Sudbeck BD, Krane SM, Welgus HG, Parks WC. The activity of collagenase-1 is required for keratinocyte migration on a type I collagen matrix. J Cell Biol 1997; 137:1445–1457.

160. Messent AJ, Tuckwell DS, Knauper V, Humphries MJ, Murphy G, Gavrilovic J. Effects of collagenase-cleavage of type I collagen on $\alpha_2\beta_1$ integrin-mediated cell adhesion. J Cell Sci 1998; 111:1127–1135.

161. Zhong C, Chrzanowska-Wodnicka M, Brown J, Shaub A, Belkin AM, Burridge K. Rho-mediated contractility exposes a cryptic site in fibronectin and induces fibronectin matrix assembly. J Cell Biol 1998; 141:539–551.

162. Sechler JL, Takada Y, Schwarzbauer JE. Altered rate of fibronectin matrix assembly by deletion of the first type III repeats. J Cell Biol 1996; 134:573–583.

163. Kamiguti AS, Markland FS, Zhou Q, Laing GD, Theakston RD, Zuzel M. Proteolytic cleavage of the β_1 subunit of platelet $\alpha_2\beta_1$ integrin by the metalloproteinase jararhagin compromises collagen-stimulated phosphorylation of pp72. J Biol Chem 1997; 272:32599–32605.

164. von Bredow DC, Nagle RB, Bowden GT, Cress AE. Cleavage of β_4 integrin by matrilysin. Exp Cell Res 1997; 236:341–345.

165. Kamiguti AS, Hay CR, Zuzel M. Inhibition of collagen-induced platelet aggregation as the result of cleavage of $\alpha_2\beta_1$-integrin by the snake venom metalloproteinase jararhagin. Biochem J 1996; 320:635–641.

166. O'Reilly MS, Holmgren L, Shing Y, Chen C, Rosenthal RA, Moses M, Lane WS, Cao Y, Sage EH, Folkman J. Angiostatin: a novel angiogenesis inhibitor that mediates the suppression of metastases by a Lewis lung carcinoma. Cell 1994; 79:315–328.

167. O'Reilly MS, Boehm T, Shing Y, Fukai N, Vasios G, Lane WS, Flynn E, Birkhead

JR, Olsen BR, Folkman J. Endostatin: an endogenous inhibitor of angiogenesis and tumor growth. Cell 1997; 88:277–285.

168. Patterson BC, Sang QA. Angiostatin-converting enzyme activities of human matrilysin (MMP-7) and gelatinase B/type IV collagenase (MMP-9). J Biol Chem 1997; 272:28823–28825.

169. Dong Z, Kumar R, Yang X, Fidler IJ. Macrophage-derived metalloelastase is responsible for the generation of angiostatin in Lewis lung carcinoma. Cell 1997; 88:801–810.

170. Stathakis P, Fitzgerald M, Matthias LJ, Chesterman CN, Hogg PJ. Generation of angiostatin by reduction and proteolysis of plasmin. Catalysis by a plasmin reductase secreted by cultured cells. J Biol Chem 1997; 272:20641–20645.

171. Schiro JA, Chan BM, Roswit WT, Kassner PD, Pentland AP, Hemler ME, Eisen AZ, Kupper TS. Integrin $\alpha_2\beta_1$ (VLA-2) mediates reorganization and contraction of collagen matrices by human cells. Cell 1991; 67:403–410.

172. Xu J, Clark RA. A three-dimensional collagen lattice induces protein kinase C-zeta activity: role in α_2 integrin and collagenase mRNA expression. J Cell Biol 1997; 136:473–483.

173. Lee RT, Berditchevski F, Cheng GC, Hemler ME. Integrin-mediated collagen matrix reorganization by cultured human vascular smooth muscle cells. Circul Res 1995; 76:209–214.

174. Kirkland SC, Henderson K, Liu D, Pignatelli M. Organisation and gel contraction by human colonic carcinoma (HCA-7) sublines grown in 3-dimensional collagen gel. Int J Cancer 1995; 60:877–882.

175. Racine-Samson L, Rockey DC, Bissell DM. The role of $\alpha_1\beta_1$ integrin in wound contraction. A quantitative analysis of liver myofibroblasts in vivo and in primary culture. J Biol Chem 1997; 272:30911–30917.

176. Gotwals PJ, Chi-Rosso G, Lindner V, Yang J, Ling L, Fawell SE, Koteliansky VE. The $\alpha_1\beta_1$ integrin is expressed during neointima formation in rat arteries and mediates collagen matrix reorganization. J Clin Invest 1996; 97:2469–2477.

177. Carver W, Molano I, Reaves TA, Borg TK, Terracio L. Role of the $\alpha_1\beta_1$ integrin complex in collagen gel contraction in vitro by fibroblasts. J Cell Physiol 1995; 165:425–437.

178. Hierck BP, Poelmann RE, van Iperen L, Brouwer A, Gittenberger-de Groot AC. Differential expression of α-6 and other subunits of laminin binding integrins during development of the murine heart. Dev Dynam 1996; 206:100–111.

179. Sun H, Santoro SA, Zutter MM. Downstream events in mammary gland morphogenesis mediated by reexpression of the $\alpha_2\beta_1$ integrin: the role of the α_6 and β_4 integrin subunits. Cancer Res 1998; 58:2224–2233.

180. Clark RA, Folkvord JM, Hart CE, Murray MJ, McPherson JM. Platelet isoforms of platelet-derived growth factor stimulate fibroblasts to contract collagen matrices. J Clin Invest 1989; 84:1036–1040.

181. Thieszen SL, Dalton M, Gadson PF, Patterson E, Rosenquist TH. Embryonic lineage of vascular smooth muscle cells determines responses to collagen matrices and integrin receptor expression. Exp Cell Res 1996; 227:135–145.

182. Hudson MJ, Stamp GW, Hollingsworth MA, Pignatelli M, Lalani EN. MUC1 ex-

pressed in PanC1 cells decreases adhesion to type 1 collagen but increases contraction in collagen lattices. Am J Pathol 1996; 148:951–960.

183. Nunohiro T, Ashizawa N, Graf K, Do YS, Hsueh WA, Yano K. Angiotensin II promotes remodelling-related events in cardiac fibroblasts. Heart Vessels 1997; Suppl 12:201–204.

184. Carnevali S, Nakamura Y, Mio T, Liu X, Takigawa K, Romberger DJ, Spurzem JR, Rennard SI. Cigarette smoke extract inhibits fibroblast-mediated collagen gel contraction. Am J Physiol 1998; 274:L591–L598.

185. Arisawa S, Arisawa T, Ohashi M, Nitta Y, Ikeya T, Asai J. Effect of the hydroxyl radical on fibroblast-mediated collagen remodelling in vitro. Clin Exp Pharmacol Physiol 1996; 23:222–228.

186. Buffoni F, Pino R, Dal Pozzo A. Effect of tripeptide-copper complexes on the process of skin wound healing and on cultured fibroblasts. Arch Intl Pharmacodynam Therap 1995; 330:345–360.

187. Sundberg C, Rubin K. Stimulation of β_1 integrins on fibroblasts induces PDGF independent tyrosine phosphorylation of PDGF β-receptors. J Cell Biol 1996; 132: 741–752.

188. Broberg A, Heino J. Integrin $\alpha_2\beta_1$-dependent contraction of floating collagen gels and induction of collagenase are inhibited by tyrosine kinase inhibitors. Exp Cell Res 1996; 228:29–35.

189. Roeckel D, Krieg T. Three-dimensional contact with type I collagen mediates tyrosine phosphorylation in primary human fibroblasts. Exp Cell Res 1994; 211:42–48.

190. Langholz O, Roeckel D, Petersohn D, Broermann E, Eckes B, Krieg T. Cell-matrix interactions induce tyrosine phosphorylation of MAP kinases ERK1 and ERK2 and PLCgamma-1 in two-dimensional and three-dimensional cultures of human fibroblasts. Exp Cell Res 1997; 235:22–27.

191. Kieffer JD, Plopper G, Ingber DE, Hartwig JH, Kupper TS. Direct binding of F actin to the cytoplasmic domain of the α_2 integrin chain in vitro. Biochem Biophys Res Commun 1995; 217:466–474.

192. Stephens P, Genever PG, Wood EJ, Raxworthy MJ. Integrin receptor involvement in actin cable formation in an in vitro model of events associated with wound contraction. Int J Biochem Cell Biol 1997; 29:121–128.

193. Belkin AM, Retta SF, Pletjushkina OY, Balzac F, Silengo L, Fassler R, Koteliansky VE, Burridge K, Tarone G. Muscle β_1D integrin reinforces the cytoskeleton-matrix link: modulation of integrin adhesive function by alternative splicing. J Cell Biol 1997; 139:1583–1595.

194. Sharma SV. Rapid recruitment of p120RasGAP and its associated protein, p190RhoGAP, to the cytoskeleton during integrin mediated cell-substrate interaction. Oncogene 1998; 17:271–281.

195. Allen WE, Jones GE, Pollard JW, Ridley AJ. Rho, Rac and Cdc42 regulate actin organization and cell adhesion in macrophages. J Cell Sci 1997; 110:707–720.

196. Machesky LM, Hall A. Role of actin polymerization and adhesion to extracellular matrix in Rac- and Rho-induced cytoskeletal reorganization. J Cell Biol 1997; 138: 913–926.

197. Bershadsky A, Chausovsky A, Becker E, Lyubimova A, Geiger B. Involvement

of microtubules in the control of adhesion-dependent signal transduction. Curr Biol 1996; 6:1279–1289.

198. Deryugina EI, Bourdon MA, Reisfeld RA, Strongin A. Remodeling of collagen matrix by human tumor cells requires activation and cell surface association of matrix metalloproteinase-2. Cancer Res 1998; 58:3743–3750.

199. Cass DL, Bullard KM, Sylvester KG, Yang EY, Sheppard D, Herlyn M, Adzick NS. Epidermal integrin expression is upregulated rapidly in human fetal wound repair. J Pediat Surg 1998; 33:312–316.

200. Whitby DJ, Ferguson MW. Immunohistochemical localization of growth factors in fetal wound healing. Dev Biol 1991; 147:207–215.

201. Martin P, Dickson MC, Millan FA, Akhurst RJ. Rapid induction and clearance of TGFβ1 is an early response to wounding in the mouse embryo. Dev Genet 1993; 14:225–238.

202. Frank S, Madlener M, Werner S. Transforming growth factors β1, β2, and β3 and their receptors are differentially regulated during normal and impaired wound healing. J Biol Chem 1996; 271:10188–10193.

203. Shah M, Foreman DM, Ferguson MW. Neutralising antibody to TGF-β1,2 reduces cutaneous scarring in adult rodents. J Cell Sci 1994; 107:1137–1157.

204. Shah M, Foreman DM, Ferguson MW. Neutralisation of TGF-β1 and TGF-β2 or exogenous addition of TGF-β3 to cutaneous rat wounds reduces scarring. J Cell Sci 1995; 108:985–1002.

205. Bullard KM, Cass DL, Banda MJ, Adzick NS. Transforming growth factor β1 decreases interstitial collagenase in healing human fetal skin. J Pediat Surg 1997; 32: 1023–1027.

206. Serini G, Bochaton-Piallat ML, Ropraz P, Geinoz A, Borsi L, Zardi L, Gabbiani G. The fibronectin domain ED-A is crucial for myofibroblastic phenotype induction by transforming growth factor-β1. J Cell Biol 1998; 142:873–881.

207. Rich S, Van Nood N, Lee HM. Role of $\alpha_5\beta_1$ integrin in TGF-β1-costimulated CD8+ T cell growth and apoptosis. J Immunol 1996; 157:2916–2923.

208. Frank R, Adelmann-Grill BC, Herrmann K, Haustein UF, Petri JB, Heckmann M. Transforming growth factor-β controls cell-matrix interaction of microvascular dermal endothelial cells by downregulation of integrin expression. J Invest Dermatol 1996; 106:36–41.

209. Bauvois B, Van Weyenbergh J, Rouillard D, Wietzerbin J. TGF-β1-stimulated adhesion of human mononuclear phagocytes to fibronectin and laminin is abolished by IFN-γ: dependence on $\alpha_5\beta_1$ and β_2 integrins. Exp Cell Res 1996; 222:209–217.

210. Langholz O, Rockel D, Mauch C, Kozlowska E, Bank I, Krieg T, Eckes B. Collagen and collagenase gene expression in three-dimensional collagen lattices are differentially regulated by $\alpha_1\beta_1$ and $\alpha_2\beta_1$ integrins. J Cell Biol 1995; 131:1903–1915.

211. Estes JM, Vande BJ, Adzick NS, MacGillivray TE, Desmouliere A, Gabbiani G. Phenotypic and functional features of myofibroblasts in sheep fetal wounds. Differentiation 1994; 56:173–181.

212. Welch MP, Odland GF, Clark RA. Temporal relationships of F-actin bundle formation, collagen and fibronectin matrix assembly, and fibronectin receptor expression to wound contraction. J Cell Biol 1990; 110:133–145.

213. Desmouliere A, Geinoz A, Gabbiani F, Gabbiani G. Transforming growth factor-

β1 induces α-smooth muscle actin expression in granulation tissue myofibroblasts and in quiescent and growing cultured fibroblasts. J Cell Biol 1993; 122:103–111.

214. Ronnov-Jessen L, Petersen OW. Induction of α-smooth muscle actin by transforming growth factor-β1 in quiescent human breast gland fibroblasts. Implications for myofibroblast generation in breast neoplasia. Lab Invest 1993; 68:696–707.

215. Yokozeki M, Moriyama K, Shimokawa H, Kuroda T. Transforming growth factor-β1 modulates myofibroblastic phenotype of rat palatal fibroblasts in vitro. Exp Cell Res 1997; 231:328–336.

216. Borsi L, Castellani P, Risso AM, Leprini A, Zardi L. Transforming growth factor-β regulates the splicing pattern of fibronectin messenger RNA precursor. FEBS Lett 1990; 261:175–178.

217. Kocher O, Kennedy SP, Madri JA. Alternative splicing of endothelial cell fibronectin mRNA in the IIICS region. Functional significance. Am J Pathol 1990; 137: 1509–1524.

218. Manabe R, Ohe N, Maeda T, Fukuda T, Sekiguchi K. Modulation of cell-adhesive activity of fibronectin by the alternatively spliced EDA segment. J Cell Biol 1997; 139:295–307.

219. Burridge K, Chrzanowska-Wodnicka M. Focal adhesions, contractility, and signaling. Annu Rev Cell Dev Biol 1996; 12:463–518.

220. Wu C, Chung AE, McDonald JA. A novel role for $\alpha_3\beta_1$ integrins in extracellular matrix assembly. J Cell Sci 1995; 108:2511–2523.

221. Wu C, Fields AJ, Kapteijn BA, McDonald JA. The role of $\alpha_4\beta_1$ integrin in cell motility and fibronectin matrix assembly. J Cell Sci 1995; 108:821–829.

222. Wu C, Keivens VM, O'Toole TE, McDonald JA, Ginsberg MH. Integrin activation and cytoskeletal interaction are essential for the assembly of a fibronectin matrix. Cell 1995; 83:715–724.

223. Cullen B, Silcock D, Brown LJ, Gosiewska A, Geesin JC. The differential regulation and secretion of proteinases from fetal and neonatal fibroblasts by growth factors. Int J Biochem Cell Biol 1997; 29:241–250.

224. Sudarshan C, Yaswen L, Kulkarni A, Raghow R. Phenotypic consequences of transforming growth factor β 1 gene ablation in murine embryonic fibroblasts: autocrine control of cell proliferation and extracellular matrix biosynthesis. J Cell Physiol 1998; 176:67–75.

225. Howell SJ, Doane KJ. Type VI collagen increases cell survival and prevents anti-β1 integrin-mediated apoptosis. Exp Cell Res 1998; 241:230–241.

226. Fukai F, Mashimo M, Akiyama K, Goto T, Tanuma S, Katayama T. Modulation of apoptotic cell death by extracellular matrix proteins and a fibronectin-derived antiadhesive peptide. Exp Cell Res 1998; 242:92–99.

227. Isik FF, Gibran NS, Jang YC, Sandell L, Schwartz SM. Vitronectin decreases microvascular endothelial cell apoptosis. J Cellul Physiol 1998; 175:149–155.

228. Bozzo C, Bellomo G, Silengo L, Tarone G, Altruda F. Soluble integrin ligands and growth factors independently rescue neuroblastoma cells from apoptosis under nonadherent conditions. Exp Cell Res 1997; 237:326–337.

229. Clarke AS, Lotz MM, Chao C, Mercurio AM. Activation of the p21 pathway of growth arrest and apoptosis by the β_4 integrin cytoplasmic domain. J Biol Chem 1995; 270:22673–22676.

230. Desmouliere A, Redard M, Darby I, Gabbiani G. Apoptosis mediates the decrease in cellularity during the transition between granulation tissue and scar. Am J Pathol 1995; 146:56–66.
231. Desmouliere A, Badid C, Bochaton-Piallat ML, Gabbiani G. Apoptosis during wound healing, fibrocontractive diseases and vascular wall injury. Int J Biochem Cell Biol 1997; 29:19–30.

5
Collagen Considerations in Scarring and Regenerative Repair

H. Paul Ehrlich
Milton S. Hershey Medical Center, Hershey, Pennsylvania

I. INTRODUCTION

Skin loss by burns, abrasions, surgical incisions, infection, or the termination of the local blood supply initiates the wound healing response. Irreversible cell death coupled with dermal disruption in burns usually requires replacement with a skin graft containing viable cells and a new connective tissue matrix. In the absence of skin grafting, the host's response is to replace or repair lost tissues by either tissue regeneration or scar deposition. Skin repair by regeneration in mammals is limited to the epidermal layer. The restoration of lost dermis is by scarring, with the exception of fetal repair at specific gestational ages of specific species (1). Regenerative repair is the ideal modality for the restoration of lost skin, but cellular necrosis coupled with the disruption of the connective tissue matrix of dermis initiates the deposition of granulation tissue and its maturation of that transitional tissue into scar (2). Histological differences define scar from skin. Scar lacks both subepidermal appendages as well as rété pegs at the epidermal–dermal interface. The normal basketweave pattern of collagen fiber bundles from lost dermis is replaced with collagen fiber bundles arranged in arrays parallel to the skin surface. The basketweave pattern allow the flexibility of skin dermis associated with tissue strength. In scar, the parallel arrangement of the collagen fiber bundles accounts for the lack of tissue malleability and suppleness. Functionally, normal scar is less elastic.

The gross appearance of scar leads to cosmetic consequences, such as a lack of a color match with surrounding skin and an unevenness of the skin's surface with either a dimple or a ridge. The location of scar may contribute to a scar's cosmetic morbidity; a scar on the face or hands is more serious than a scar on parts of the body that can be covered with clothing.

Excessive scarring conditions are either hypertrophic scar or keloid scar, which have different types of pathologies. Hypertrophic scars are more common and result from deep injuries involving delayed wound closure often associated with wound infection. They stay within the boundaries of the original injury and contain characteristic nodules that can be identified by light microscopy (3). Hypertrophic scars resulting from burns that develop over joints disrupt joint function and movement as a consequence of scar contractures. These scars can be improved functionally and cosmetically by reconstructive surgery. Keloid scars differ from hypertrophic scars. They often occur as a result of superficial injuries, they exceed the boundaries of the initial injury, and do not contain nodules. By light microscopy, their collagen fiber bundles are arranged in a ribbon pattern in which these ribbons run in parallel arrays. They respond poorly to reconstructive surgery and in response to surgery they often become larger. A keloid can be considered to be like a benign tumor.

The depth of tissue loss dictates the repair response. A first-degree burn injury (a sunburn) results in the loss of the epidermal cell surface, but little or no damage to the underlying dermis. Through the migration of epidermal cells and their proliferation, such a shallow skin defect is resurfaced and healing proceeds by regeneration. The synthesis and deposition of collagen and reorganization of a new connective tissue is not a component of this type of trauma. Healing only requires the regeneration of the epidermal surface. With deeper tissue damage in which disruption and tissue loss includes the dermis, the repair process will require both the regenerative repair of the epidermal surface as well as the replacement of the lost dermal matrix. The dermal replacement, a scar whose chemical components are similar to that of dermis, differs from dermis by its reduced vascular supply and organization of the newly deposited collagen fiber bundles in parallel arrays. The size of a scar will depend upon the volume of tissue loss, its location, and what role wound contraction plays in closure.

Incisional, suture-closed wounds, healing by the first intention, that do not follow skin tension lines are prominent compared with those that follow the skin tension lines. Surgical incisions made to follow Langer's skin lines of tension will show minimal scarring because the collagen fiber bundles' deposition in parallel arrays is an acceptable orientation of collagen fiber bundles in such areas of the skin (4). Normally, the closure of deep incision wounds is by the approximation of the wound edges, which reduces the volume of scar tissue needed to replace lost dermis. The important component for the development of increasing wound breaking strength with incisional wounds is the welding of the new granulation tissue deposited within the wound site with the collagen fiber bundles of the dermis at the cut edge of the wound. The welding of the old collagen fibers with the new collagen fibers of granulation tissue is the weakest point in a suture-closed incisional wound.

A deep, full-thickness wound in which the wound edges are too far apart to be approximated and sutured closed, is healing by second intention. The closure of such a defect requires both a new epidermal surface as well as a new connective tissue matrix. In patients, the size of a second-intention wound in terms of volume loss will increase the chances for complications of excess scarring. A wound whose depth does not eliminate subepidermal appendages (such as hair follicles and sweat glands) will undergo rapid epithelialization by the migration of epidermal cells residing in the surviving subepidermal structures within the defect. From these many loci, epidermal cells migrate out and rapidly grow over the denuded area. Since the amount of dermal loss is minimal, the volume of new connective tissue needed to replace that loss is modest. Defects such as uncomplicated second-degree burns or abrasions are typically closed within two weeks, and produce minimal cosmetic or functional scar problems. However, with full-thickness dermal loss and the annihilation of subepidermal appendages, the regeneration of the epidermis is restricted to epidermal cell migration from the wound edges. Because of the size of the area needed to be covered with viable epidermal cells, the time requirement for wound closure by the regeneration of the epidermis will be greater than two weeks. Such retarded closure of open wounds in healthy individuals leads to excess scar formation and its functional as well as cosmetic consequences. It appears that the absence of an epidermal roof over granulation tissue retards maturation of this tissue and leads to the overabundance of connective tissue deposition, often in a disorganized state.

II. CONNECTIVE TISSUE

Adult wound healing involves the maturation of granulation tissue into scar tissue. The connective tissue matrix of granulation tissue shares characteristics of fetal dermis. Both are quite plastic, collagen fiber bundles are finer than adult dermal fiber bundles, and both lack tensile strength, having low resistance to tearing. Wound remodeling involves some reductions in cell number and decrease in vascular density as well as reorganization and reorientation of the newly deposited connective tissue matrix. The maturation of the granulation tissue matrix requires further organization of collagen fiber bundles into a pattern that characterizes scar matrix. Contrasted to scar, the granulation tissue connective tissue matrix has a high density of blood vessels, capillaries, fibroblasts, myofibroblasts, macrophages, and fine loosely organized collagen fibrils. The metabolic activity of granulation tissue is elevated with increased cell density, more abundant protein synthesis, and a high generation of adenosine triphosphate (ATP). Initially, the volume of granulation tissue expands until the defect is filled. When granulation tissue becomes covered with a viable epidermal surface, the remodeling phase of the repair process is underway. During the remodeling phase of repair, populations of inflammatory cells and mesenchymal cells both decline. Blood flow to the area moderates, the metabolic activity of the tissue decreases, and the density of capillaries as well as blood vessels declines. The collagen fibers of maturing granulation tissue undergo a condensation, becoming thicker and more insoluble.

The major protein component of granulation tissue and dermis is collagen. The chemical structure of native collagen is responsible for its biological activity. It is the glue that holds tissues together. At least 19 unique gene products or types of collagen have been described (5). Collagen is a rod-shaped molecule composed of three polypeptide chains that form a rigid triple helical structure that is 15 Å in diameter and 300 Å in length. The process of denaturing of collagen usually involves heat energy separating the three polypeptide chains. Denatured collagen is gelatin, having biological and physical chemical characteristics opposite to those of native collagen. At body temperature, native collagen is in the form of a gel resulting from the polymerization of collagen fibrils. Gelatin at body temperature is unpolymerized in a liquid state. At neutral pH under cold conditions (4°C) native collagen is a viscous liquid. Gelatin at neutral pH at 4°C polymerizes and forms a gel. Gelatin is an excellent substrate for numerous proteinases, while the triple helical configuration of native collagen is resistant to attack by most proteinases. Native collagen requires a specialized metaloproteinase called interstitial collagenase or metaloproteinase-1 to cleave its polypeptide chains. Collagen is cleaved at a single site, where all three chains are severed, creating one-quarter and three-quarter pieces that undergo rapid unraveling and the loss of its triple helical structure. The nonhelical peptide products are susceptible to further breakdown by other proteinases.

The amino acid makeup of collagen peptides is highly conserved; 33% of the amino acid residues are glycine and 20% are derived from incorporated proline. The abundance of glycine and proline residues is essential for the triple helical folding of the three polypeptide chains that form the ridgid rodlike structure of interstitial collagens. The amino acid sequence of collagen polypeptide chains is also highly conserved, having the repeating units of the tripeptide sequence glycine-x-y. The y residue is often proline or hydroxyproline, which is a posttranslational oxidation of select proline residues by the enzyme peptidyl proline hydroxylase, which requires specific cofactors. The presence of hydroxyproline in the y position is critical for the hydrogen bonding required for maintaining the triple helical structure of native collagen. The secretion of collagen requires the posttranslational hydroxylation of proline and selected lysine residues. Molecular oxygen, ferrous iron, α-ketoglutarate, and ascorbate are the cofactors required for selected proline and lysine hydroxylation. Deficiencies of any of these cofactors, e.g., hypoxia or no ascorbate (scurvy), results in reduced collagen synthesis and impaired wound healing.

Besides synthesizing collagen, the fibroblast has been reported to pack collagen molecules into collagen fibers within specialized cellular clefts (6). These clefts are part of the extracellular compartment. Within this compartment collagen molecules undergo self-assembly, polymerize into fibrils, and these fibrils are organized into packets of fiber bundles. The packets of collagen fiber bundles are released from the cellular compartment and are integrated into thicker collagen fibers. It is possible that the self-assembly of collagen fibrils and the release of collagen packets from embryonic fibroblasts and wound fibroblasts are different and that difference is responsible for the distinction between the orientation of the connective tissues of fetal dermis and granulation tissue. A better understanding of those differences may reveal a process whereby the organization of scar collagen fiber bundles can be controlled and collagen fiber bundles can be laid down in a basketweave pattern.

The strength of a scar relies upon the increasing packing of the newly deposited collagen fibrils and their stabilization by chemical covalent crosslinks. The further processing of lysine amino acid residues in collagen makes collagen more insoluble by forming intramolecular and intermolecular covalent crosslinks. The action of an interstitial enzyme, lysyl oxidase, catalyzes these covalent crosslinks between collagen peptides at the nonhelical ends of the molecules. The inhibition of the formation of collagen covalent crosslinks leads to reduced incision wound tensile strength. At one time, an attempt to control scarring involved the elimination of collagen crosslink formation by inhibiting the enzyme lysyl oxidase by the compound β-amino propionitrile (7). The compound is found in chickpeas and blocks lysyl oxidase by chelating its cofactor copper ions. That drug and another collagen cross-link inhibitor, D-penicillamine have been shown to be ineffective in the clinic. A possible reason for this failure is that formation of collagen fibers precedes the formation of these covalent crosslinks. The organization of collagen within fiber bundles is the basis of fibrosis and comes before the formation of collagen covalent cross-links. Modulating the organization of collagen fibers will impact fibrosis more than altering the formation of collagen crosslinks.

An immediate function of the newly deposited connective tissue matrix is to support the sprouting blood vessels that permeate out from beneath the wound site. The new vessels are essential for supplying nutrients to the newly developing tissue. The establishment of new blood vessels occurs by a process of budding or sprouting beneath the wound site. This arborization process allows for the ingrowth of new vessels with minimal hemorrhage as new vessel growth progresses as blood flows in a closed system (8). Numerous growth factors modulate the process, and manipulation of angiogenesis growth factors may prove to have clinical value in the future (9).

A scar is a ''patch'' that covers, seals, and fills a wound defect. The volume of tissue needed to fill a defect should equal the volume that was lost. Initially, granulation tissue usually occupies a greater volume than the tissue it replaces. During the maturation process, there is a reduction in granulation tissue volume in which the tissue volume loss occurs by the breakdown of a portion of newly synthesized connective tissue and the condensation of collagen fibers. In dermis, the collagen fiber bundles are arranged in a basketweave pattern; in granulation tissue, the collagen fiber bundles are randomly organized; and in normal scar, they are arranged in parallel arrays. The remodeling of granulation tissue into scar involves the establishment of an intact epidermal surface, a reduced cell density, termination of the outgrowth of capillaries, moderation of blood flow to the area, and decline in the level of metabolic activity.

III. COLLAGEN FEATURES

Suture-closed wounds in experimental animals show that wound breaking strength reaches about 3% of its final strength at one week, a time when sutures are commonly removed. The final breaking strength acquired by a healed wound one year after injury is about 80% of that of intact skin. The inability of a scar to obtain the equivalent strength of intact skin is mostly due to the flaw in the reestablishment of the collagen fiber bundles between the residual dermis and the newly deposited scar. The junction formed between the scar tissue collagen fibers and dermal collagen fibers is suboptimal. The reweaving of the collagen fibers at the interface between the two tissues is incomplete. Testing wounds for wound breaking strength shows the point of cleavage occurs at that junction.

Testing the breaking strength of a rabbit intestinal anastomosis, in which cut ends of the intestine are rejoined by suturing the two edges together, showed rupture at intestinal wall distant from the suture line. The expected weakest area of an anastomosis is the suture line. However, the weakest region was distant from the cut edge of the intestinal wall and developed as a consequence of reutilizing collagen at the healing anastomosis site. The loss of collagen is due to local increased collagenolytic activity (10). The speculation is that formed collagen fibers are released from fiber bundles and soluble collagen molecules are recruited to the suture line and utilized to seal and secure the defect. The concept of intact collagen reutilization has been proposed (11). Using radioisotope incorporation studies, intact collagen molecules were recruited to the wound site and reincorporated into granulation tissue collagen fibers. The reutilization of intact collagen molecules in vivo within granulation tissue was demonstrated by injecting fluorescent-tagged soluble collagen into 5-day-old polyvinyl alcohol (PVA) sponge implants in rats. The PVA sponges were harvested two days later, frozen, cryosections cut, fixed, mounted, and viewed with a fluorescent microscope. Figure 1 shows the presence of autofluorescent collagen fibers within the

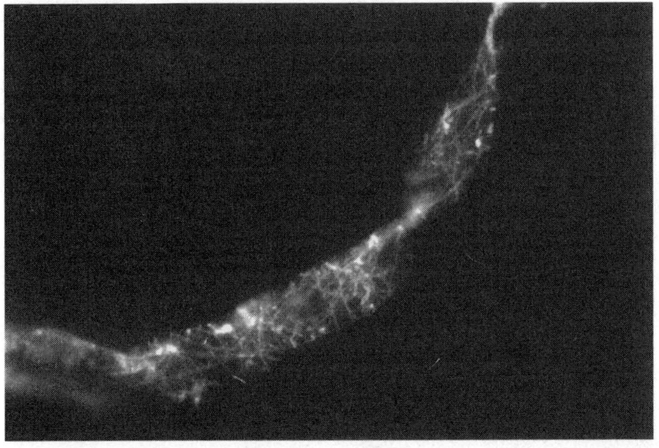

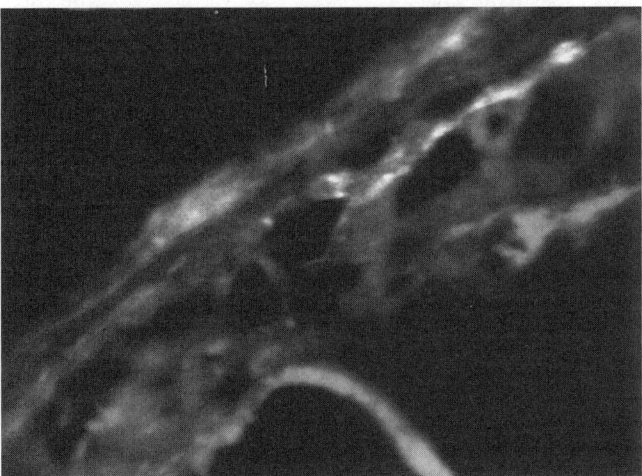

Figure 1 Autofluorescent collagen fibers derived from fluorescent-tagged soluble collagen injected into implanted PVA sponge implants. Fluorescein isothiocyanate (FITC)-tagged soluble collagen was made from isolated and purified from rat rail tendons incubated with FITC isothiocyanate. The tagged collagen was injected into PVA sponge implants that had been implanted within subcutaneous pockets of 350-g rats for 5 days. The rats were returned to their cages and sponges harvested 2 days later (day 7 after implantation). Sponges were frozen, cryosections cut, fixed, and viewed with a fluorescent microscope. (Top) autofluorescent collagen fibers within the interstices of the sponge implant. (Bottom) a similar cut section that has been counterstained with Evans blue and viewed with a fluorescent microscope with FITC filters. (Courtesy of GEM Willow©.)

granulation tissue. Counterstaining sections showed that the autofluorescent collagen fibers are associated with fibroblasts within the granulation tissue. If the collagen was heat denatured before being injected into the implants, no fluorescent fibers appear. Only native collagen could be incorporated into collagen fibers. Since the fluorescent tag is covalently linked to collagen lysine residues, the breakdown of collagen into its amino acid components would produce fluorescein-tagged lysine amino acid residues, which cannot be taken up by transfer ribonucleic acid (tRNA) and reincorporated into newly synthesized proteins. It is proposed that intact collagen is recruited at the wound site and reincorporated into collagen fibers, hence, the concept that scar tissue is composed of both newly synthesized collagen as well as recruited residual collagen within the wound site. It should be considered in scarless fetal repair that the collagen deposited at the repair site is due to reutilization as well as synthesis.

The major collagen types of interstitial tissues are types I and III collagens. Type I collagen is the most prevalent form of collagen, found in virtually all major connective tissues and in the stroma of most organs. It is composed of three chains, $[\alpha1(I)]_2\,\alpha2(I)$, which make it a hybrid molecule with two identical chains and one homologous chain. It is almost the exclusive collagen type of bone, tendon, and dentin collagen fiber bundles. Type I collagen forms thick collagen fiber bundles. The major support elements of connective tissues are composed of type I collagen, showing minimal distensibility under mechanical load. Type III collagen is made up of three identical chains, $[\alpha1(III)]_3$. Its amino acid composition is unusual, having two cysteinyl residues per chain and the greatest hydroxyproline to proline ratio of any collagen type. Type III collagen–enriched tissues include blood vessels, visceral organs, and dermis, having fine reticular fibers. In general, soft tissues, which include visceral organs, contain type III collagen. Experimentally, type III collagen is relatively insoluble and difficult to solubilize from adult tissues. Limited proteinase digestion is necessary to extract it from adult tissues. In contrast, fetal tissues exhibit a portion of their type III collagen extractable in neutral salt solutions. In addition to this increased solubility of fetal type III collagen, appreciable quantities of it are in the form of type III procollagen. In fetal dermis, type III procollagen is released from cells in its precursor form. A pool of type III procollagen as well as the adult forms of type III collagen accumulate in fetal dermis. Since procollagen can not polymerize, it is incapable of forming collagen fibrils and is absent from collagen fiber bundles. It is proposed that the pool of type III procollagen reluctant to form collagen fibers may contribute to enhanced fetal dermal pliability and plasticity.

In normal dermis, 20% of the collagen fibers are composed of type III collagen. The collagen fiber bundles of granulation tissue contain 30% type III collagen, an increase of 50% (12). A mature, normal scar has only 10% type III collagen, a reduction of 50% compared with dermis. The differences in type III collagen concentrations between dermis, scar, and granulation tissue may be related to the organization of the collagen fiber bundles in those tissues. These differences in type III collagen content may contribute to the character of the tissues. With dermis, the collagen fibers are arranged in a basketweave pattern as demonstrated by the birefringence pattern by polarized light and have 20% type III collagen. In granulation tissue, having 30% type III collagen, the collagen is in the form of fine, disorganized fibers demonstrating minimal birefringence. In mature scar, the type III collagen content is 10% and the collagen fibers are packed into thick bundles that are arranged in parallel arrays as demonstrated by birefringence. It is important to differentiate among collagen polymerization, the collagen fibrils, and collagen fiber bundles. In vitro, under physiological conditions, native collagen solution polymerizes and forms fine collagen fibrils. In vivo, the organization of collagen fibrils into collagen fiber bundles requires cellular intervention. The cellular organization of collagen fibrils into fiber bundles is important for the integrity of skin and scar in terms of volume, stability, and strength.

IV. WOUND CONTRACTION

In loose-skinned laboratory animals and in certain parts of the human body, open wounds will close spontaneously by the process of wound contraction. The healing of second intention wounds occurs with minimal scarring because intact normal skin is pulled into the defect, thus the volume of newly synthesized tissue filling the defect is minimal. The process of wound contraction entails the inward movement of intact whole skin. The movement of skin occurs through cellularly generated forces residing within granulation tissue. The granulation tissue becomes a contractile unit that generates the pulling force. The surrounding skin is stretched. The proposed mechanism for generating the force of wound contraction is through the reorientation of collagen fibers and their compaction (13). The compaction of granulation tissue produces the force that pulls in the surrounding tissues. The contraction of cells is not involved in wound contraction. The organization of collagen fibers is the force that pulls on the surrounding tissues (14).

The proposed mechanism for generating the force of wound contraction is fibroblast reorganizing collagen fiber bundles by the physical translocation of the collagen fibers (15). Collagen organization results in fine collagen fibrils condensed into thicker and longer collagen fibers. The degree of organization of collagen fibers can be followed by the intensity and pattern of polarized light–induced birefringence. The granulation tissue within an open contracting rat wound shows minimal birefringence at 7 days. By 14 days, rat granulation tissue contains collagen fibrils that demonstrate fine green birefringence. At 7 days, wound contraction has progressed to 50% of its initial size. At 14 days, the wound area is reduced to 30% of its initial area. Between days 7 and 14 the rate of wound contraction has slowed. It appears that a rapid rate of wound contraction occurs when collagen fibrils are in their most disorganized state. As the collagen becomes more organized, the rate of wound contraction slows.

V. FETAL REPAIR

The repair of fetal wounds shows a variety of responses in regard to wound healing and scarless repair. Open wounds made in the fetal sheep of midgestation close and show scarless repair (16). A late-term fetal rabbit open wound does not close. It increases in size as the fetus grows (17). In the late-term fetal sheep, an open wound closes by contraction (16). Suture-closed wounds (first-intention wounds) heal in a scarless manner depending upon the species of the animal as well as its gestational age when the fetus was wounded (18,19). A mouse (gestation about 20 to 22 days) shows scarless repair of first-intention wounds at midtrimester, which is 14 to 15 days. In the third trimester, at 18 days, the fetal mouse suture-closed wound heals by scarring. In contrast, a first-intention, suture-closed wound made in a fetal rabbit during the third trimester heals without scarring. An open fetal rabbit wound (a second-intention wound) that is covered with a piece of silastic, which prevents contact between the wound and the surrounding amniotic fluid, closes by wound contraction (20). In vivo, an open wound in contact with fetal rabbit amniotic fluid demonstrated inhibition of wound contraction. There is limited information on the collagen composition or the organization of collagen fiber bundles in either the closed or healing open wound of the fetal rabbit.

An organ culture system was introduced in which the healing of incisional wounds made in 14- and 18-day-gestation fetal mice was followed, while maintained in serum-free culture medium (21). Both the epidermis and dermis from a 14-day fetus healed in a scarless manner by regenerative repair. The repaired tissue from the disrupted dermis and epidermis was indistinguishable from the surrounding skin. In contrast, a similar wound made in an older fetal mouse limb (18-day gestation) maintained in culture for 7 days healed by scarring (Fig. 2). The healed, 18-day cultured fetal limb explant revealed collagen fiber bundles arranged in parallel arrays. Collagen fibers arranged in parallel arrays are characteristic of scar, which develops from the maturation of granulation tissue. In organ culture, fetal repair occurs in the absence of granulation tissue, but the pattern of deposited collagen fibers appears as a consequence of granulation tissue maturation. The fetal mouse limb organ culture model facilitates the investigation of the repair process in the absence of an inflammatory response or the influx of systemic factors from the blood. It shows that tissue repair can proceed without the participation of invading inflammatory cells or the diffusion of soluble factors from the circulation (21).

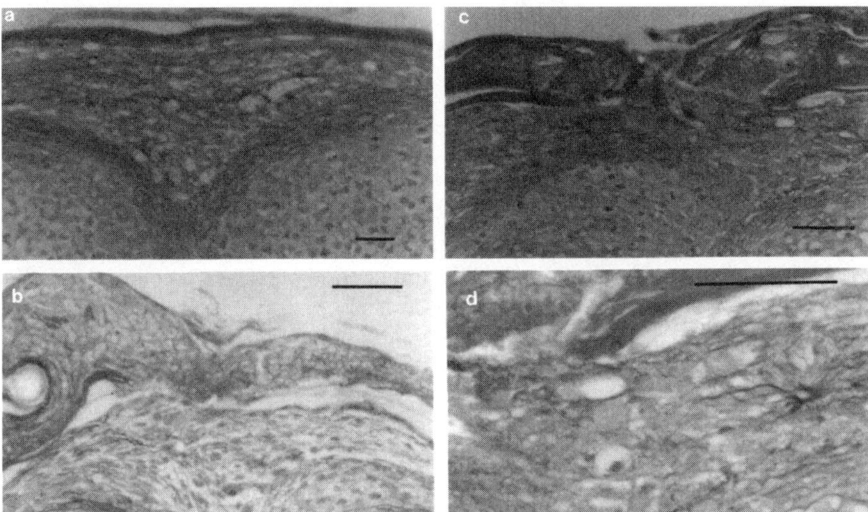

Figure 2 Repair of 14- and 18-day mouse fetal limb in organ culture for 4 days. Fetuses were harvested from either a 14- or 18-day pregnant mouse and the limbs removed, wounded, and sutured closed. After being maintained in organ culture for 4 days, the limbs were fixed, embedded, sectioned, and stained with Sirius red and viewed with a light microscope (bar is 50 μm). (a) A low-power view of a section taken from a healing 14-day fetal mouse limb with fine red collagen fiber arranged in a basketweave pattern. (b) The 14-day healed fetal mouse limb at higher power with the collagen fibers arranged in a basketweave pattern. (c) A Sirius red–stained section from a healed 18-day fetal mouse limb. The red-stained collagen fibers are denser and thicker within the healed wound site. (d) A higher-power view of panel c showing the thick collagen fiber bundles arranged in parallel arrays. (Courtesy of GEM Willow©.)

There is circumstantial evidence that collagen synthesis plays a role in scarless fetal repair. Glucocorticoids specifically inhibit the synthesis of dermal collagen (22). Rat skin collagen synthesis is inhibited by glucocorticoids, while fibronectin synthesis is increased (23). The transcription of procollagen messenger ribonucleic acids (mRNAs) is decreased by added corticosteroids, hence glucocorticoid retardation of repair involves the inhibition of collagen synthesis (24). Transforming growth factor-β (TGF-β), which is not a proinflammatory agent but has been demonstrated to increase collagen synthesis, reversed some of glucocorticoid's inhibiting effects of wound healing (25). It was shown with organ-cultured 14-day fetal limbs that added glucocorticoids inhibited repair. The implication is that collagen synthesis is needed for scarless repair. Adding TGF-β1 to glucocorticoid-treated limb explants reversed the inhibition of wound healing (26). Again, this implies a need for collagen synthesis in scarless fetal repair.

VI. FPCL MODEL

An in vitro model that investigates the organization of collagen fibers by fibroblast is the fibroblast-populated collagen lattice (FPCL) contraction model (Fig. 3). It was introduced by Bell et al. (27) and is composed of cultured fibroblasts suspended in a collagen lattice. The fibroblasts reorganize the surroundings collagen fibrils through their physical translocation to new locations (28). This model demonstrates that the forces for the translocation of collagen fibrils and their condensation is through tractional forces and not by forces of cell contraction (29). During FPCL contraction, the fine, unorganized nonbirefringent collagen fibrils become organized as thicker, more prominent birefringent collagen fiber bundles. The organization of collagen and the contraction of FPCL does not require cell division but involves functional microfilaments and microtubules as well as the continued synthesis of new protein (13).

The collagen makeup of a FPCL will influence the rate and degree of FPCL contraction. FPCL made with type III collagen contracted faster and to a greater

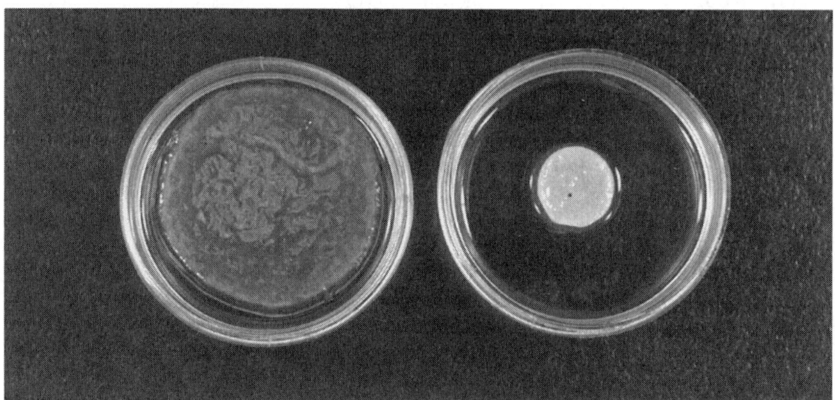

Figure 3 A contracting fibroblast-populated collagen lattice. Fibroblast-populated collagen lattices (FPCL) were made with 2.5 mg of acid-soluble rat tail tendon collagen, Dulbecco's modified Eagle's medium (DMEM) with 10% fetal bovine serum in a total volume of 2 ml contained within a 35-mm Petri dish. Human dermal fibroblasts at 10.0×10^4 cells per 2 ml of mixture were incorporated into the collagen matrix. (Left) The FPCL was made 6 hr prior to photographing. (Right) The smaller FPCL was made 30 hr prior to photographing. (Courtesy of GEM Willow©.)

degree than lattices made with type I collagen (30). This finding agrees with in vivo wound contraction studies in adult open wounds in which the granulation tissue of contraction open wounds is enriched with type III collagen (12). Stabilized, normal scar tissue does not exhibit contractile forces and has a reduced quantity of type III collagen. In the FPCL contraction model, the packing of collagen fibrils is enhanced with a high proportion of type III collagen. The removal of type III collagen or reducing its accumulation in granulation tissue will limit the contractile process. Fetal dermis has elevated levels of type III collagen, but wound contraction in some animals is not a feature of fetal scarless repair. It appears that collagen–fibroblast interactions are influenced by external environment, e.g., amniotic fluid (17,20).

Including rabbit amniotic fluid during the manufacture of FPCL inhibited FPCL contraction in a dose responsive manner (31). There is no direct evidence suggesting that the collagen makeup of fetal rabbit wounds influenced wound closure by wound contraction. The addition of TGF-β1 was shown to enhance wound contraction in open fetal rabbit wounds by instilling an inflammatory response and increasing the expression of collagen mRNA (32). In contrast to fetal rabbits, the contraction of FPCL containing sheep fetal fibroblasts was enhanced when sheep-derived amniotic fluid was included in its manufacture (33). Alterations in collagen synthesis between fetal rabbit and sheep fetal healing wounds may be influenced by the presence or absence of amniotic fluid. The identification or characterization of amniotic factors have not been done.

Fetal repair and adult repair involve the synthesis, deposition, and organization of collagen. A major difference between adult and fetal repair is the organization of the collagen within the wound site. In fetal repair, there is less new collagen synthesized and less deposited. However, wounds can heal with scar or in a scarless manner. The organization of the collagen within the wound site defines scarless repair from repair by scarring. There are three possibilities that may influence the organization of collagen fiber bundles in the fetal wound site: the amount of unprocessed type III procollagen, the proportion of type III collagen deposited, and fibroblast organization of collagen fiber bundles. Knowledge of how the collagen fiber bundles are organized within the wound site may point out a strategy for controlling scarring and the promotion of scarless repair in the injured adult.

REFERENCES

1. Dostal GH, Gamelli RL. Fetal wound healing. [Review] Surg Gynecol Obstet 1993; 176(3):299–306.
2. Edwards LC, Dunphy JE. Wound healing: injury and abnormal repair. N Engl J Med 1958; 259:275–280.

3. Ehrlich HP, et al. Morphological and immunochemical differences between keloids and hypertrophic scar. Am J Pathol 1994; 145:105–113.

4. Jackson JS, Flickeringer DB, Dunphy JE. Biochemical studies of connective tissue repair. Ann NY Acad Sci 1960; 86:943.

5. van der Rest M, Garrone R. Collagen family of proteins. FASEB J 1991; 5:2814–2823.

6. Birk DE, Zycband EI, Winkelmann DA, Trelstad RL. Collagen fibrillogenesis in situ: discontinuous segmental assembly in extracellular compartments. Ann NY Acad Sci 1990; 580:176–194.

7. Tanzer ML. Cross-linking of collagen. Science 1973; 180:561–566.

8. Clark ER, Clark EL. Microscopic observations on the growth of blood capillaries in the living mammal. Am J Anat 1939; 64:251–301.

9. Folkman J, Klagsbrun M. Vascular physiology. A family of angiogenic peptides. Nature 1987; 329:671–672.

10. Hawley PR. Collagenase activity and colonic anastomotic breakdown. Br J Surg 1970; 57:388–391.

11. Klein L, Rudolph R. H^3-collagen turnover in skin grafts. Surg Gynecol Obstet 1970; 35:49–57.

12. Bailey AJ, Sims TJ, LeLouis M, Bazin S. Collagen polymorphism in experimental granulation tissue. Biochem Biophys Res Commun 1975; 66(4):1160–1165.

13. Ehrlich HP, Rajaratnam, JRM. Cell locomotion forces versus cell contraction forces for collagen lattice contraction: An in vitro model of wound contraction. Tissue Cell 1990; 22(4):407–417.

14. Ehrlich HP. Wound closure: evidence of cooperation between fibroblasts and collagen matrix. Eye 1988; 2:149–157.

15. Berry DP, Harding KG, Stanton M, Jasani B, Ehrlich HP. Human wound contraction: collagen organization, fibroblast and myofibroblasts. Plast Reconstr Surg 1998; 102:124–131.

16. Burrington JD. Wound healing in the fetal lamb. J Pediatr Surg 1971; 6:523–528.

17. Krummel TM, Nelson J, Diegelmann RF, Lindblad WJ, Salzberg AM, Greenfield LJ, Cohen IK. Fetal response to injury in the rabbit. J Pediatr Surg 1987; 22:640–644.

18. Bleacher JC, Adolph VR, Dillon PW, Krummel TM. Isolated fetal mouse limbs: gestational effects on tissue repair in an unperfused system. J Pediatr Surg 1993; 28:1312–1315.

19. Lanning DA, Nwomeh BC, Nontante SJ, Maragh HA, Yager DR, Diegelmann RF, Cohen IK, Haynes JH. Differential effects of transforming growth factor β1 and β3 on excisional fetal rabbit wounds. Surg Forum 1998; 49:660–661.

20. Somasundaram K, Prathap K. 1970 Intra-uterine healing of skin wounds in rabbits foetuses. J Pathol 1970; 100:81–86.

21. Chopra V, Blewett CJ, Ehrlich HP, Krummel TM. The transition from fetal to adult repair occurring in forelimbs maintained in organ culture. Wound Repair Regen 1997; 5:47–51.

22. Newman RA, Cutroneo KR. Glucocorticoids selectively decrease the synthesis of hydroxylated collagen peptides. Mol Pharmacol 1978; 14:185–198.

23. Cockayne D, Sterling KM Jr, Shull S, Mintz KP, Illeyne S, Cutroneo KR. Glucocor-

ticoids decrease the synthesis of type I procollagen mRNAs. Biochemistry 1986; 25:3202–3209.

24. Sterling KM Jr, Harris MJ, Mitchell JJ, DePetrillo TA, Delaney G, Cutroneo, KR. Dexamethasone decreases the amounts of type I procollagen mRNAs in vivo and in fibroblast cell cultures. J Biol Chem 1983; 258:7644–7647.

25. Pierce GF, Mustoe TA, Lingelbach J, Masakowski VR, Gramates P, Deuel TF. GFβ reverses the glucocorticoid-induced wound-healing deficit in rats: possible regulation in macrophages by platelet-derived growth factor. Proc Natl Acad Sci USA 1989; 86:2229–2233.

26. Ehrlich HP, Blewett CJ, Krummel TM, Cutroneo KR. Inhibition of wound closure by transforming growth factor-β and dexamethasone in a fetal mouse limb organ culture model. Wound Repair Regen 1996; 4:482–488.

27. Bell E, Ivarson B, Merril C. Production of a tissue-like structure by contraction of collagen lattices by human fibroblasts of different proliferative potential in vitro. Proc Natl Acad Sci USA 1979; 76:1274–1278.

28. Yamato M, Adachi E, Yamamoto K, Hayashi T. Condensation of collagen fibrils to the direct vicinity of fibroblasts as a cause of gel contraction. J Biochem 1995; 117:940–946.

29. Harris AK, Wild P, Stopak D. Silicone rubber substrate: a new wrinkle in the study of cell locomotion. Science 1980; 280:177–179.

30. Ehrlich HP. The modulation of contraction of fibroblast populated collagen lattices by types I, II, and III collagen. Tissue Cell 1988; 20:47–50.

31. Krummel TM, Ehrlich HP, Nelson JM, Michna BA, Thomas BL, Haynes JH, Cohen K, Diegelmann RF. Fetal wounds do not contract in utero. Surg Form 1989; 11: 613–615.

32. Krummel TM, Michna BA, Thomas BL, Sporn MB, Nelson JM, Salzberg AM, Cohen IK, Diegelmann RF. Transforming growth factor beta (TGF beta) induces fibrosis in a fetal wound model. J Pediatr Surg 1988; 23(7):647–652.

33. Rittenberg T, Longaker MT, Adzick NS, Ehrlich HP. Sheep amniotic fluid has a protein factor which stimulates human fibroblast populated collagen lattice contraction. J Cell Physiol 1991; 149:444–450.

6
The Role of Hyaluronan–Receptor Interactions in Wound Repair

Rashmin C. Savani
University of Pennsylvania School of Medicine and Children's Hospital of Philadelphia, Philadelphia, Pennsylvania

Darius J. Bagli, Rene E. Harrison, and Eva A. Turley
University of Toronto and The Hospital for Sick Children, Toronto, Ontario, Canada

I. INTRODUCTION

Accumulating evidence suggests that interaction and signaling between the cell and the extracellular matrix (ECM) is critical to homeostasis following injury. Responses to injury appear to universally involve remodeling of ECM molecules. For example, arterial stretch injury stimulates expression of fibrillar proteins, type I collagen, and elastin, as well as proteoglycans, such as syndecan, versican, perlecan, and the glycosaminoglycan, hyaluronan (HA) (1). The restoration of tissue structure and function following injury invariably involves a balance between repair that is suitable for continued normal function and repair in which the fibrosis or the deposition of scar modifies tissue architecture sufficiently to compromise normal function. From a clinical point of view, the biological process of fibrosis is, therefore, a double-edged sword. The ability to modify this balance in repair in favor of more normal function and architecture would represent an important advance in tissue engineering and restoration of tissue integrity.

The remarkable observation that fetal wounds heal without scar formation has led to intense study of the differences between fetal and adult wound repair to uncover molecular mechanisms that regulate fibrosis (2–5). Fetal wounds demonstrate faster reepithelialization, occur in a sterile environment, and have a reduced inflammatory response and decreased angiogenesis. Such scarless healing is also notably associated with a prolonged increased HA content as compared with scar-forming wounds. Nevertheless, both adult and fetal wounds increase their HA content after injury. For example, in adult tissue, HA production is associated with fibrotic repair following acute injury to a number of organ systems, including the heart (6,7), lungs (8–10), and kidneys (11), as well as skin (12). However, fetal wounds maintain their elevated HA content throughout the repair process, while HA accumulation is transient in adult wounds, decreasing as the fibrotic response progresses. In further support of a role for HA in scarless fetal wound healing, treatment of fetal rabbit wounds with hyaluronidase results in increased granulation tissue and enhanced collagen deposition with fibrosis (13). Conversely, exogenous HA dampens the fibrotic healing response in injured fetal mouse limb organ cultures (14) and inhibits fetal fibroblast proliferation (15). Exogenous administration of high concentrations of high-molecular-weight HA to adult tissue injuries also promotes rapid healing and decreased fibrosis that normally occurs in skin burns (16), ruptured tympanic membranes (17), and abraded corneas (18). Although HA appears to be involved in scarless healing in these instances, it is obviously not the sole regulator of this process. Nevertheless, this glycosaminoglycan (GAG) appears to function as a dominant and multiforous regulator of tissue repair that occurs under normal cytokine exposure (19).

The molecular mechanisms by which HA alters repair responses are not yet completely understood, but HA exerts direct effects on cells and on the extracellular matrix that may be relevant to its role in wound repair. High-molecular-weight HA ($>10^3$–10^6 kDa) can trap large amounts of water, contributing to tissue viscosity and edema that follow tissue injury. The ability of HA to coil and self-associate may also contribute to tissue elasticity (20,21). In addition, an inverse relationship has been noted between collagen and HA localization during ECM remodeling (22), and HA may facilitate new collagen assembly by possibly loosening the early tissue matrix, indirectly allowing fibroblast influx following injury (23).

HA also directly affects cell behavior. Low amounts of HA fragments (10,000–600,000 Da) promote monocyte activation into macrophages (24), mediate adhesion of inflammatory cells to the endothelium (25,26), and also stimulate the migration and proliferation of smooth muscle cells, fibroblasts, immune cells, and endothelial cells responding to injury (27–30). Furthermore, HA increases cytokine gene expression by macrophages and fibroblasts (31,32). Some controversy exists in the literature about these effects of HA. Inconsistencies may be related to the differing molecular weights, purity, and concentrations of HA used in the various studies. For instance, high concentrations of high-molecular-weight HA inhibit white cell functions (33,34), while lower molecular weights of HA can enhance white cell functions (35). Clearly, the effect of HA on cells and matrix remodeling is complex and it will be important to document changes in molecular weight and concentration of HA during repair in order to assess more clearly the function of this interesting polysaccharide in wounding responses.

The finding that HA-mediated cell responses can be dose-dependent and context-specific predicts that HA bioactivity is regulated, at least in part, at a receptor level, and a growing list of cell-associated HA-binding proteins that interact with HA with high affinity, termed hyaladherins (36), has been characterized (Fig. 1) (37–50). Hyaladherins can be grouped as at least two classes of cellular HA-binding proteins. CD44 is a prototype of the type I transmembrane HA receptor, that can also be shed, but is predominately present at the cell surface. It binds to HA via a complex site known as the link module (51) (Fig. 2). RHAMM is a prototype of cell-associated hyaladherins that occur at multiple cellular loci, including the cell surface, cytoplasm, and nucleus, and are characterized by lack of transmembrane signal sequence or link module. Rather, HA binds to hyaladherins via simple motifs of basic amino acids (see Fig. 2) (51,52). The mechanism(s) by which these proteins are released and bound to the cell surface are unknown. Both classes of hyaladherins have been implicated in mediating some of the effects of HA in regulating wound repair.

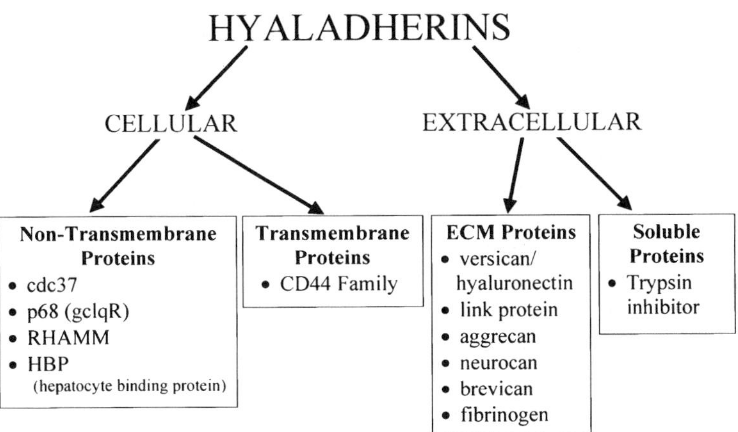

Figure 1 The family of hyaladherins. These proteins bind to HA with high affinity and although the function of ligand binding has not been determined for many of these proteins, HA interactions with CD44, RHAMM, cdc37 and p68 are important for cell attachment, motility, and control of cell cycle. Cellular hyaladherins include: cdc37, p68, RHAMM, HBP, and the transmembrane receptor CD44. Extracellular HA receptors include versican, link protein, aggrecan, neurocan, brevican, fibrinogen, and trypsin inhibitor.

HA BINDING

HYALADHERINS	LINK MODULE CONTRIBUTION	[B(X7)B] MOTIF CONTRIBUTION	COVALENT LINKAGE
cdc37	none	major	none apparent
P68	none	major	none apparent
RHAMM	none	major	none apparent
HBP (hepatocyte binding protein)	not determined	not determined	none apparent
CD44	major	present, minor	none apparent
Versican/Hyaluronectin	major	present, minor	none apparent
Aggrecan	major	present, minor	none apparent
Neurocan	major	present, minor	none apparent
Brevican	major	present, minor	none apparent
Link protein	major	present, minor	none apparent
Fibrinogen	not determined	not determined	none apparent
Trypsin inhibitor	none	present but importance not determined	major

Figure 2   The binding mechanism and affinities of the hyaladherins to hyaluronan via the link module, small basic amino acid motifs, or covalent linkages (see text).

II. CD44

Both RHAMM and CD44 are encoded as single genes (53–55), but occur as multiple protein forms due to extensive alternative ribonucleic acid (RNA) splicing and posttranslational modification (Fig. 3) (56–61).

CD44 was first described as a cell surface molecule of T lymphocytes, granulocytes, and cortical thymocytes (59), rediscovered as the phagocytic glycoprotein 1 (Pgp-1) (62) GP90Hermes (63), and later identified as a widely expressed protein that functions as a major receptor for HA (43,44). CD44 is a multifunctional receptor involved in cell–cell and cell–ECM adhesion, i.e., cell motility, trafficking, lymph node homing, lymphocyte activation, presentation of chemokines and growth factors to traveling cells, and transmission of these growth signals (reviewed in 64). In addition, CD44 participates in the endocytic uptake and intracellular degradation of HA (65,66) and transmission of signals mediating hematopoiesis and apoptosis (67–69) that are relevant to wound repair.

CD44 ligands other than HA include the ECM components collagen I and IV (70), fibronectin (71), laminin (72), and the chondroitin sulfate–modified invariant chain of class II major histocompatibility complex (MHC) (73), mucosal addressin (74), serglycin (75), and osteopontin (76). Constitutively, the molecule is predominantly expressed in regions of active cell growth (77), and is, notably,

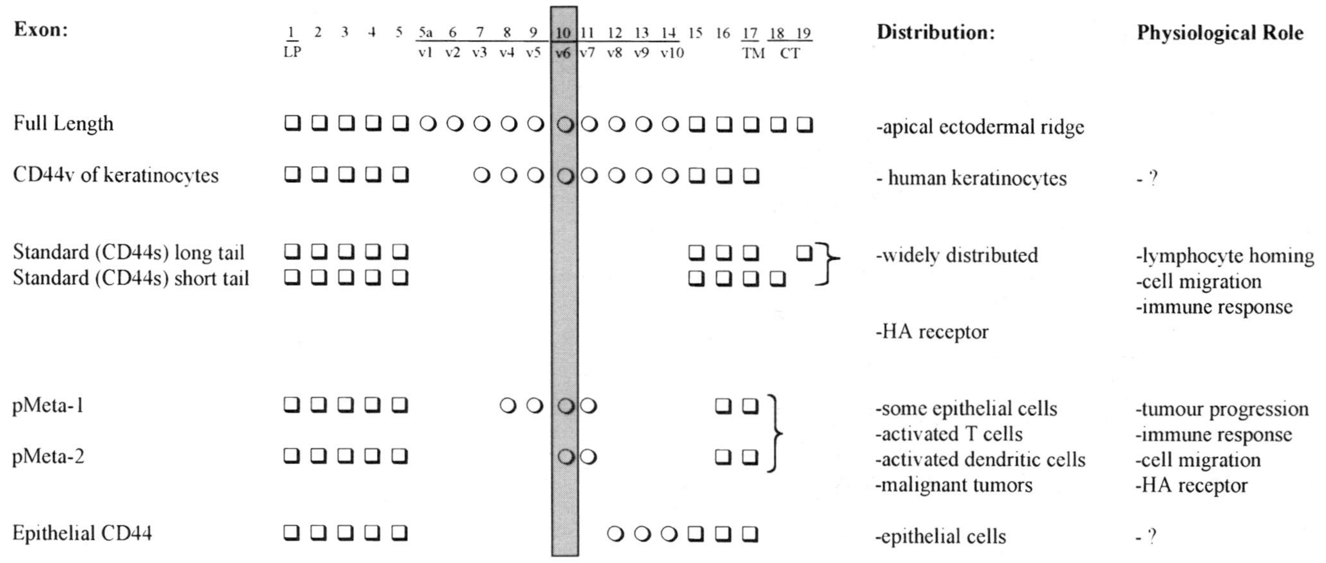

Figure 3 CD44 exon structure and RNA splicing in normal and diseased tissue showing known tissue distributions and potential physiological roles. The leader peptide (LP), transmembrane domain (TM), and cytoplasmic tail (CT) portions are indicated. The shaded exon 10 is believed to be important in conferring invasive abilities in transformed cells.

highly expressed in skin (78). CD44 is elevated in a variety of tissues following wounding, including skin (79).

A. Structure

Sequence conservation of CD44 among rat, mouse, horse, dog, cow, hamster, baboon, and human exceeds 70% (reviewed in 80). The human CD44 gene contains 50 to 60 kB of genomic DNA and consists of at least 20 known exons (see Fig. 3) (55,56). Exons 1 to 16 encode the extracellular domain of the protein, exon 18 encodes a short transmembrane domain, and exons 19 and 20 encode the cytoplasmic domain (see Fig. 3). Exons 5a to 14 are alternatively spliced, leading to a number of different potential isoforms with tremendous variability in the sequence of their extracellular domain (81). Exons 19 and 20 are also alternatively spliced, leading to two potential cytoplasmic tails (82). Posttranslational modification by N-glycosylation (63,83), O-glycosylation (84,85), and glycosaminoglycanation with heparin sulfate (86) and chondroitin sulfate (87) creates additional structural and functional diversity. In total, there are 20 known isoforms of different molecular sizes (85–230 kDa) (reviewed in 80).

The smallest CD44 isoform, known as CD44s, lacks all of the 10 variant exons and has a predicted core protein size of 37 to 38 kDa (see Fig. 3). This appears to be the major isoform that binds to HA. The larger variant (CD44v) transcripts encode proteins similar to the standard (CD44s) protein, but have sequences selected from the variant exons located in the membrane proximal region in the extracellular domain (see Fig. 3).

B. Domains of CD44 Related to Cell Motility and Cell Cycle Control

A key domain relevant to cell cycle/motility mediated by CD44 is the HA-binding domain. This domain of CD44 is homologous to the HA-binding structure recently characterized in link protein by NMR (see Fig. 2) (88). Interestingly, mutation of key basic amino acids within this structure that resemble RHAMM HA-binding sites (52) blocks the ability of CD44 to sustain proliferation (88) but has little effect on HA binding. This is in contrast to RHAMM, where mutation of these basic amino acids ablates HA binding (52,89). The solution structure of the link module from human TSG-6 consists of two alpha helices and two antiparallel beta sheets arranged around a large hydrophobic core (51). Interestingly, not all CD44-expressing cells are able to bind HA, but this property can be acquired or can occur transiently (90). The ability of HA to bind to CD44 is regulated by both protein conformation, rather like integrin activation, and glycosylation patterns. Thus, CD44 can be stimulated to bind HA by phorbol esters, anti-CD44 antibodies, or deglycosylation (reviewed in 91). Blocking anti-CD44 monoclonal antibodies (mAbs) studies suggest that topography of the CD44 epitopes and their orientation toward the HA-binding site determine the ability of antibodies to interfere with HA binding (64,92). Clustering of CD44 proteins, which is dependent upon cytoskeletal proteins, also seems important to its ability to bind HA (93). Certain cells (including some B and T cell lines) appear constitutively able to bind HA. However, further studies are required to define the molecular mechanisms that result in CD44–HA interactions as well as to assess the impact that these interactions have on cell behavior relevant to wound repair. Additionally, because CD44 has the capacity to bind various ECM molecules, it is possible that this diversifies its function in wound healing. Currently, little is known both of the structural requirements for binding and the biological consequence of these additional ligand interactions during wound repair.

C. CD44 Signaling

Signaling through CD44 involves protein tyrosine kinase (PTK), transcription factor, and cytoskeletal components (Fig. 4). This diversification of signaling is not surprising given the multiple effects CD44 has on cells. For instance, substrate-attached cells, such as fibroblasts and keratinocytes, use HA–CD44 interactions for cell adhesion and motility, as well as proliferation and HA metabolism. In white cells, HA–CD44 interactions are required for lymphocyte homing and activation by cytokines during infiltration into tissues, events necessary for wound repair. However, the individual signaling pathways that are responsible for these effects are only beginning to be understood.

In T and B cells, natural killer (NK) cells, polymorphonuclear leukocytes (PMLs), and macrophages, HA-bound CD44 stimulates protein tyrosine phosphorylation, calcium influx, and gene activation (35,94,95). Blocking monoclonal CD44 antibody studies indicate that HA–CD44 interactions are important for cytotoxic effector functions in these cells, as well as for cell proliferation and cytokine secretion, which are responses that are key to tissue repair (94–98). The cytoplasmic domain of CD44 binds to active Lck and Fyn kinases within protein-rich glycosyl phosphoinositide (GPI) islands in T cells and endothelial cells (99,100), and these islands appear to be necessary for CD44 to generate a protein tyrosine kinase signal. In both substrate-attached cells and in lymphocytes, CD44 also participates in the transmission of growth factor–mediated signals (reviewed in 80,91) (98,101–103). For instance, CD44 antibodies can inhibit interleukin-2 (IL-2) production normally induced by HA in T cells (104), probably by regulating NFK-β activation that causes expression of this cytokine, as well as IL-1β, tumor necrosis factor-α (TNF-α) and insulin-like growth factor-1 (IGF-1) in macrophages (24,35). CD44 is also required for signaling through growth factors such as her2/neu (105).

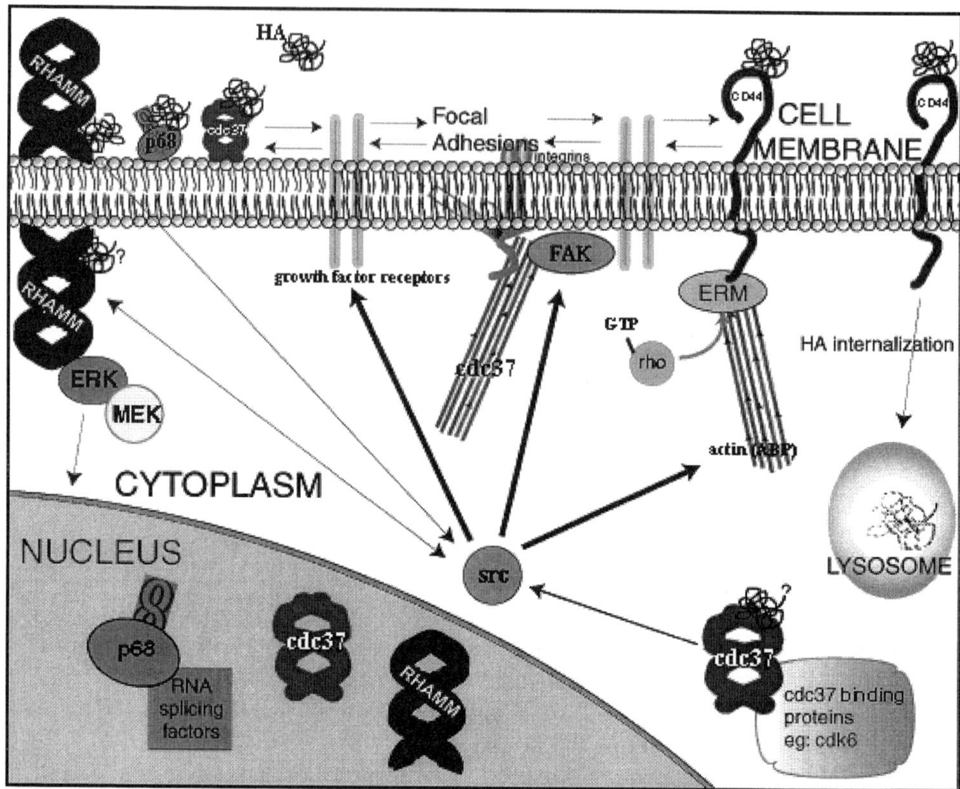

Figure 4 The cellular hyaladherins and their regulation of signaling. Following HA
binding, signaling occurs through both cell surface hyaladherins (i.e., RHAMM, cdc37,
and CD44) and intracellular hyaladherins (i.e., see RHAMM and cdc37) via the activation
or recruitment of important actin-regulating enzymes (also see text). These kinases alter
actin polymerization in focal adhesion complexes and lamellae orientation/extension,
events that are required for motility, cell cycle progression, and responsiveness to growth
factors. Intracellular RHAMM and cdc37 bind directly to key signaling enzymes including
erk and cdk6. Interestingly, both RHAMM and cdc37 control src activation. Apart from
its well-studied nuclear substrates, erk phosphorylates and activates cytoskeletal proteins,
including microtubule-associated proteins and myosin light chain kinase, which are involved in cytoskeletal organization during motility, wound repair, and contraction. Although the nuclear functions of RHAMM and cdc37 are not yet understood, p68, which
shares 100% homology with the complement receptor gclqR, binds to RNA splicing factors, including SF2.

CD44 appears to modify signals available to the cell at least in part by regulating the structure of the actin cytoskeleton via interactions between the cytoplasmic domain of CD44 and actin-binding proteins. These interactions appear to be dynamically regulated and result from modifications of the CD44 intracellular domain, including alternate splicing of variant exons, protein kinase C (PKC)–mediated phosphorylation, acylation by acyl-transferase, palmitoylation, and GTP binding (reviewed in 80). Part of the ability of CD44 to regulate cell motility is due to its direct binding to ERM (ezrin, radixin, and moesin) proteins (106,107). ERM proteins are thought to control the distribution of other adhesion molecules on the cell surface and to link actin to the plasma membrane, especially in cell surface projections (108). Binding of CD44 to ERM occurs best in the presence of phosphatidylinositol 4,5-bisphosphate (PIP$_2$) (107). Hirao and colleagues (107) have provided strong evidence that CD44 functions within a signaling cascade downstream of Rho. Rho belongs to the family of small guanosine triphosphatases (GTPases), including ras, rac, and cdc42, that regulate important actin-related events (109–111). This group speculates that activated Rho causes an up-regulation of PIP-5 kinase leading to increased cell membrane–bound PIP$_2$ levels, which then promotes CD44–ERM complex formation. CD44 may further regulate the Rho-GDP dissociation inhibitor (GDI) as it tightly binds to the CD44–ERM complex (see Fig. 4) (107). It is presently unclear, however, whether Rho-GDI recruits Rho to the plasma membrane to be activated or sequestered (112,113).

III. RHAMM

RHAMM is member of a group of cell-associated hyaladherins that occur at several cellular loci and that perform multiple functions in regulating cell motility and cell cycle (Fig. 5) (114–121). For instance, cell surface forms of RHAMM are transiently expressed in most cells but are nevertheless key to regulating cell motility as determined by antibody-blocking experiments (27–29,89,115,122–128). Intracellular forms of this class of hyaladherins, including RHAMM, bind to and chaperone signaling molecules involved in regulating cell cycle and cell motility (see Fig. 4) (37,38,40,41,127). These types of hyaladherins may also perform functions within the nucleus. Such hyaladherins typically lack a link module for binding HA but rather utilize short sequences encoding basic amino acid motifs (see Fig. 2) (52), which are required for cell motility and proliferation (89,127). Even though they are present on the cell surface (28,37–39,89,127,128), this class of hyaladherins is also characterized by an absence of both signal sequences and transmembrane domains. Therefore, the molecular basis for their subcellular distribution is not yet clear. Based upon their modular and dynamic subcellular location and the unique mechanism by which they bind to HA, these

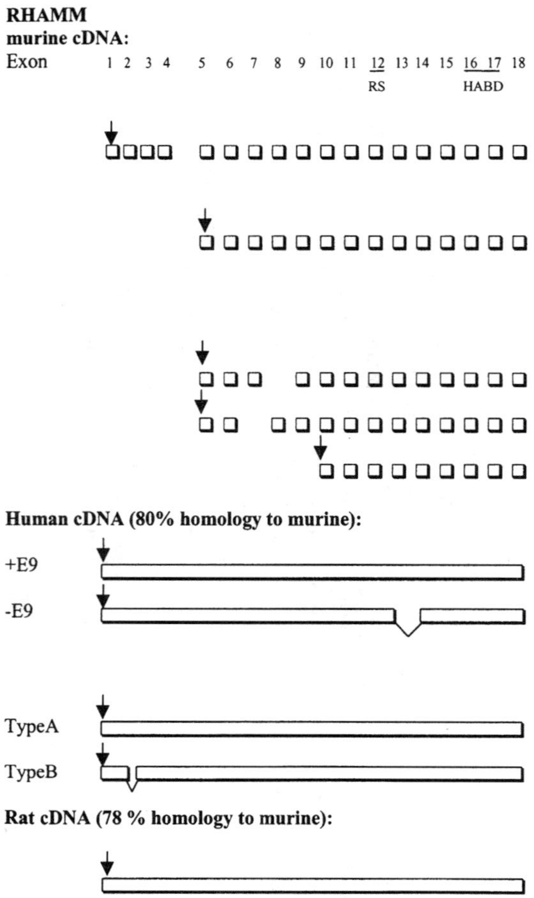

RHAMM
murine cDNA:

	Predicted Protein MW In Cell lysate:	Expression:	Location:	Physiological Role:
	85-95kD	- N.D.	- intracellular and cell surface?	- weakly transforming - does not rescue from apoptosis
	73kD	- appears shortly after plating in fibroblasts - after smooth muscle cell wounding - in H-*ras* transfected 10T1/2 cells - lung tissue after injury	- intracellular	- transforming - rescues from apoptosis
	70kD	- N.D.	- N.D.	- N.D.
	70kD	- N.D.	- N.D.	- N.D.
	58kD	- *ras*-transformed cells	- intracellular and cell surface?	- MT binding
	85-95kD	- human breast cancer tissue	- intracellular and extracellular	- overexpressed in subsets of primary breast cancer cells prognostic of poor outcome
	84kD	- } human breast cancer cell lines	- } intracellular	- N.D.
	82kD	- }	- }	- N.D.
	82kD	- smooth muscle cells	- cell surface	- involved in wounding response

proteins likely regulate cell motility and cell cycle in a manner that is fundamentally distinct from the more well-characterized HA receptor, CD44.

RHAMM was originally isolated from supernatant media of nonconfluent embryonic chick heart fibroblasts (119). Subsequently, it was found intracellularly and on the cell surface (41,89,125,126). It has emerged as a key regulator of HA-mediated motility and cytoskeletal remodeling (41). Since HA has been considered to act at the surface to regulate cell function, most studies have focused on the functions of surface-associated RHAMM, and this form of RHAMM has been shown to play a role in growth factor responses (127,128), motility (reviewed in 41,120,129), and cell cycle (121). Since, as noted above, RHAMM's location at the cell surface is often dynamic and transient, in particular decreasing rapidly after plating (127,130), it may function to initiate events relevant to cell motility, unlike CD44, which may sustain this cellular function. Several recent reports showing an absence of cell surface RHAMM (116,117,131,132) underscore the transient nature of this protein and emphasize the need for careful timed analyses to detect expression.

A. Structure

Two murine RHAMM cDNAs were originally isolated from fibroblasts (60,125), both of which contained in-frame start and upstream stop codons and, therefore, appeared to represent full-length cDNA (see Fig. 5). Later, a human RHAMM cDNA, which was longer than these murine RHAMM transcripts in its 5′ terminus, was isolated and has been designated the full-length RHAMM cDNA (61). The sequence of this human cDNA was recently confirmed (117) and a murine homologue of this RHAMM form has been reported (116), designated as IHABP. Sequence alignments and a recent database entry documenting an identical murine RHAMM cDNA confirm the identity of IHABP as RHAMM, a more appropriate name since it is now clear that there are many intracellular hyaladherins

---

Figure 5 The known exon structure of RHAMM complementary deoxyribonucleic acid (cDNA). Predicted RNA transcripts for mouse, rat, and human, based upon RT-PCR, primer extension, 5′ RACE, and isolation of full-length cDNA from expression libraries. Start codons are indicated by arrows. All isoforms contain HA-binding domains and at least one 20-amino-acid repeat sequence (RS). The murine cDNA and human RHAMM sequences share 85% identity. The murine and human isoforms show a variety of tissue distributions and their physiological roles are only beginning to be dissected (see text). *The exon structure of human and rat are unknown and available data in these species are based on cDNA isolation and RT-PCR.# The rat cDNA includes an additional unique 11-amino-acid sequence at its N-terminus that is present in human but has not yet been located in murine. This form is up-regulated in smooth muscle cells in vivo following wounding of arteries (Savani, personal communication, 1998).

(e.g., p68 and cdc37). The reported exon structure of the murine gene is incomplete and that of the human has not yet been published (see Fig. 5).

Evidence is accumulating for the existence of multiple RHAMM isoforms, consistent with reports of several full-length cDNAs encoded within the RHAMM gene. This includes the presence of multiple RNA transcripts (60,117,118) (see Fig. 5) detected via primer extension, 5′ RACE, and RT-PCR of poly A mRNA populations isolated from 3T3 cells (60,89), and the occurrence of several protein bands of molecular weight (MW) predicted by the above RNA transcripts, as detected in Western analysis using both monoclonal and polyclonal anti–murine RHAMM antibodies (41,116,117). These results suggest that RHAMM, like CD44, is subject to extensive alternative splicing (see Fig. 5). The subcellular location and function of each of the isoforms are only beginning to be dissected. For instance, the sequence of the cell surface form of RHAMM remains inconclusive (see Fig. 5), although antibody analysis indicates that it encodes exons 3, 4, 6, 7, 9, and 10 and HA-binding domains (60,89,127,128,133) and that these sequences are required for regulating cell motility.

B. RHAMM and Signaling

Surface RHAMM regulates signals generated by both HA (41,119,120) and growth factors, such as platelet-derived growth factor (PDGF) (127) and transforming growth factor-β (TGFβ) (128). Structure/function analysis of murine RHAMM using exon-specific antibodies suggests that exons 3, 4, 8, 9, 10, and 11 (using the murine nomenclature) (60) are required for cell surface RHAMM to regulate cell cycle and cell motility (60,89,118,127). The ability of HA to signal motility via RHAMM implies that the HA-binding domains are also necessary for signal transduction (see Fig. 5). Several additional studies also suggest that intracellular forms of RHAMM (see Fig. 5) control cell signaling pathways, with structure/function studies in particular indicating a key role for both the HA-binding domains and for exon 4 in controlling cell motility and cell proliferation via an association with signaling molecules such as erk1 (127).

Signals from HA–cell surface RHAMM interactions are associated with activation of src (134), focal adhesion turnover (126), and a reduction in the tyrosine phosphorylation focal adhesion kinase (FAK) (89). RHAMM-mediated activation of src is required for HA–RHAMM-regulated fibroblast motility, and both locomotion of these cells and activation of src by HA can be blocked with anti-exon 9/10 RHAMM antibodies (134). However, cells transfected with either a constitutively active form of src or v-src no longer require cell surface RHAMM (as detected by antibody blocking) for signaling motility, indicating that src is downstream of cell surface RHAMM (see Fig. 4). Nevertheless, v-src–induced disassembly of focal adhesions cannot occur in the absence of cellular expression of RHAMM (134). This, although not confirmed experimentally, is most easily interpreted by proposing that intracellular isoforms of RHAMM are required for src-generated effects on the cytoskeleton (see Fig. 4) and is consistent with the ability of a RHAMM isoform to coimmunoprecipitate with src (134).

Turnover of focal adhesions effected by RHAMM–HA interactions is accompanied by dephosphorylation of FAK, possibly as a result of activation of a phosphatase and/or redistribution of src. Interestingly, overexpression of an intracellular form of RHAMM, v4, that is transforming and that interacts with erk, modifies the pattern of protein tyrosine phosphorylation of src substrates, including focal adhesion kinase, cortactin, and cas (133). These modifications may be directly responsible for the ability of src, HA, and RHAMM to collectively regulate focal adhesion turnover and actin disassembly that appear to be key to permitting cell motility and to regulating growth factor responses (133,134). It appears likely that both cell surface and intracellular forms of RHAMM are required for src-controlled cytoskeletal modifications and an interplay between isoforms may exist (see Fig. 4). The mechanisms by which either a cell surface or intracellular RHAMM transmits and modifies such signals and whether other kinases that RHAMM interacts with, such as erk, are also involved in RHAMM-regulated cytoskeletal changes await further characterization.

In addition to its effect on src signaling, RHAMM isoforms encoding exon 4 (see Fig. 5), appear under certain conditions (e.g., subconfluence) to control the erk kinase cascade through ras (127). Mutations of intracellular RHAMM isoforms block signaling through ras (89) and activation of erk (127). Specifically, RHAMMv4 (73 kDa) (see Fig. 5) interacts with erk-1 kinase and its upstream activator MEK in ras- or RHAMM-transformed cells (124), and its overexpression constitutively activates this cascade. Thus, at least one form of RHAMM, in a manner possibly analogous to cdc37 (38,135), directly associates with kinases that regulate transformation, proliferation, and motility (127). Importantly, a RHAMM isoform of the same molecular weight predicted by the RHAMMv4 cDNA (e.g., 70–73 kDa) is uniquely up-regulated after wounding of smooth muscle cell monolayers (28). Furthermore, manipulation of RHAMMv4 expression or function alters the ability of PDGF, a key growth factor in response-to-injury processes to activate signaling cascades (127) and modify actin assembly (126,133). The role of erk in these functions remains to be investigated.

IV.   ROLE OF HYALADHERINS IN WOUND RESPONSES

A.   CD44 and Response to Injury

In healthy skin, CD44 is found on keratinocytes, hair follicle cells, eccrine sweat gland cells, and on dendritic cells in the dermis (78,136). CD44 and HA are present within the epithelial cell layer, but are most pronounced around keratinocytes during wound healing (12). Basal keratinocytes show the highest levels of CD44 expression within the stratified epithelium (137).

CD44 levels are significantly increased in damaged epithelium of asthmatic patients (138), as well as in alveolar macrophages during bleomycin-induced lung injury (131). During acute lung injury, fibroblasts express the 85-kDa isoform most intensely in filopodia and lamellipodia, and blocking antibody studies show this isoform is required for invasion into the provisional fibrin matrix of the wound (139). CD44 is also detected in type II pneumocytes in alveolar epithelium following lung injury (140). A CD44-related chondroitin sulfate proteoglycan is required for endothelial migration into this early wound matrix (68), and CD44 is up-regulated in motoneurons following nerve injury (141), in tubular epithelium of injured kidneys (142), in vascular smooth muscle cells in a rat carotid artery balloon injury model (143), and in epithelial and stromal cells of healing corneal epithelial wounds (144). Correlating with an absence of scar formation, a 56-kDa CD44 isoform is four times higher in fetal versus adult healed tissue (2). Although wound repair was not specifically examined, CD44 knockout mice demonstrated on abnormal distribution of hyaloid progenitors, indicating a defect in migration of these cells from the bone marrow that could influence repair of this tissue (145).

Direct evidence for a role of CD44 in wound repair is provided by experiments in which transgenic mice were created using CD44 antisense constructs. Animals showed abnormal accumulation of HA in the superficial dermis and a decrease in keratinocyte proliferation in response to carcinogens, as well as to epidermal growth factor (EGF) and fibroblast growth factor (FGF) (137). Skin elasticity was diminished, reepithelialization was delayed by 4 to 7 days and an abnormal contraction of the wound margin occurred (137). Inflammatory response was also delayed as measured by an absence of polymorphonuclear cells following TPA application compared with control mice. These results confirm a role for CD44 in HA metabolism and in keratinocyte proliferation/migration during wound repair that is consistent with in vitro data in previous sections of this review.

B. RHAMM and Wound Repair

A number of observations have also implicated RHAMM in wound repair. Synthetic peptides with varying affinities for HA that mimic RHAMM HA-binding domains competitively inhibit HA-directed cell locomotion (27,52) and wound contraction (Fig. 6C). Further, anti-RHAMM antisera inhibit smooth muscle cell locomotion in response to injury (28). In several injury models, cell surface RHAMM and HA are overexpressed in macrophages (Fig. 7B) (27,146), fibroblasts (147), keratinocyte (27), and smooth muscle cells (28) (Fig. 7A). However, several other reports have noted an absence of cell surface RHAMM on mono-

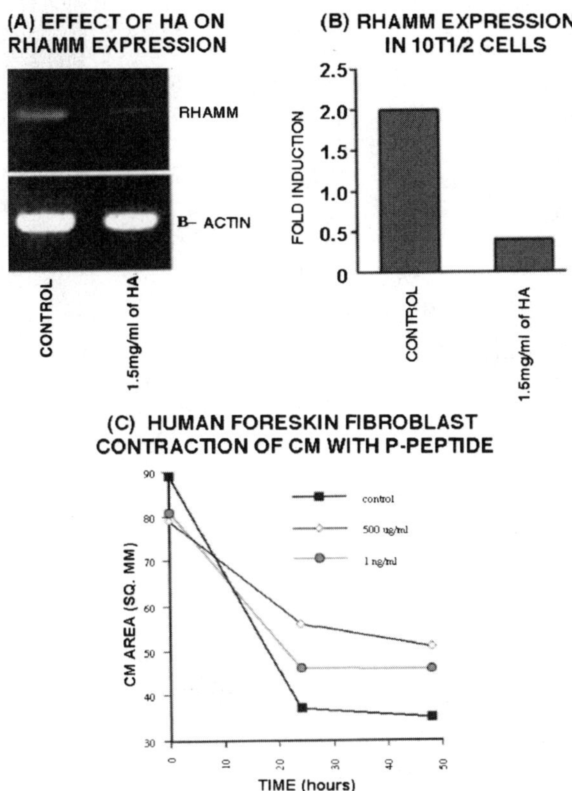

Figure 6 RT-PCR of RHAMM messenger RNA in fibroblasts in the presence or absence of HA (1.5mg/ml). RHAMM mRNA is significantly down-regulated (A) 5-fold as shown by densitometric analyses (B). (C) Contraction assay of human foreskin fibroblast on collagen matrix (CM) is significantly inhibited ($P < 0.001$, Student t-test) in the presence of an HA-binding peptide (p-peptide) similar to the RHAMM HA binding motif.

cytes (132) and alveolar macrophages responding to injury (146). Our studies (e.g., note Fig. 7B) reported a more acutely timed analysis that showed a transient expression of RHAMM on activated macrophages within the first several hours after injury, which the previous studies did not include, therefore likely missing detecting the transient nature of cell surface RHAMM. The ability of anti-RHAMM antibody to block TGF-β (128) and PDGF-BB–stimulated cell migration (Savani, personal communication, 1998), further suggests that growth factor signaling, particularly important to wound repair, may, at least in part, be dependent on RHAMM–HA interactions. It is interesting that generally, but not always, elevated cell surface RHAMM correlates with enhanced motility (e.g., see Fig.

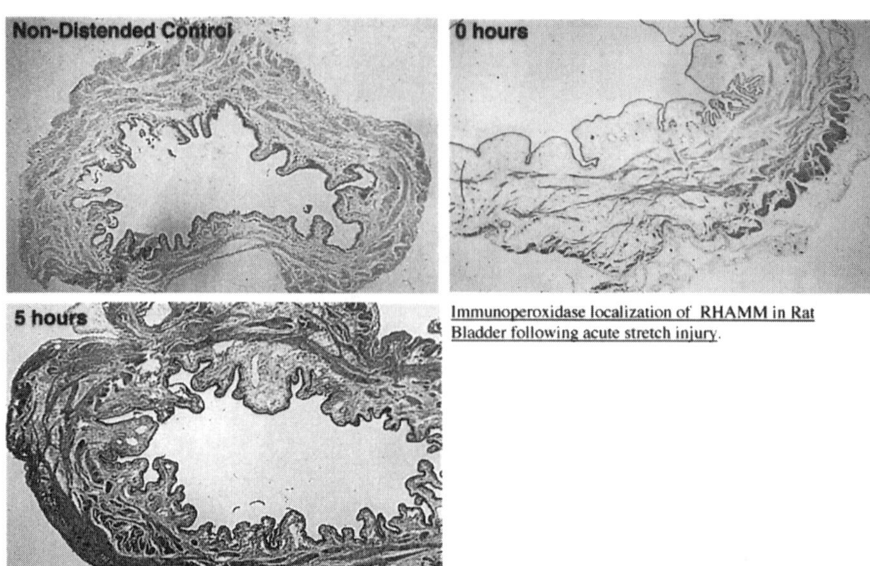

Figure 7A Immunoperoxidase localization of RHAMM in rat bladder following acute stretch injury. Bladders were distended with sterile saline to 40 cm H_2O for 15 minutes. Gross bleeding was noted in saline confirming injury. Bladders were harvested 0 to 48 hr after stretch injury. Controls are catheterized only. All sections (including control) probed with primary (Z2, anti-RHAMM) and secondary (goat anti-rabbit IgG) Ab. Note distension, thinning of epithelium, edema spaces, and fracture of muscle bundles immediately following injury at 0 hr. Intense RHAMM immunolocalization is noted by 5 hr. RHAMM expression returned to nondistended control levels by 24 hr (data not shown). (Magnification, 10×.) (From Ref. 150.)

7B). However, even in cases in which the level of cell surface RHAMM expression does not correlate with rapidity of cell motility (148) (Wang et al, personal communication, 1998), anti-RHAMM antibodies block cell motility as long as RHAMM is expressed at the cell surface.

Interestingly, the expression of both RHAMM and CD44 are up-regulated in fetal excision wounds, and this enhanced expression correlates with decreased HA content in the wound and with subsequent development of fibroplasia (147,13). It has also been reported that wound hyaluronidase is found in the cytoplasm of wounded fibroblasts. Therefore, it is possible that wound HA is rapidly internalized in fibrosing wounds, a process that is regulated by cell surface transgenic receptors, at least CD44 (65,66). Consistent with this possibility, mice that do not express CD44 accumulate HA within the matrix (137).

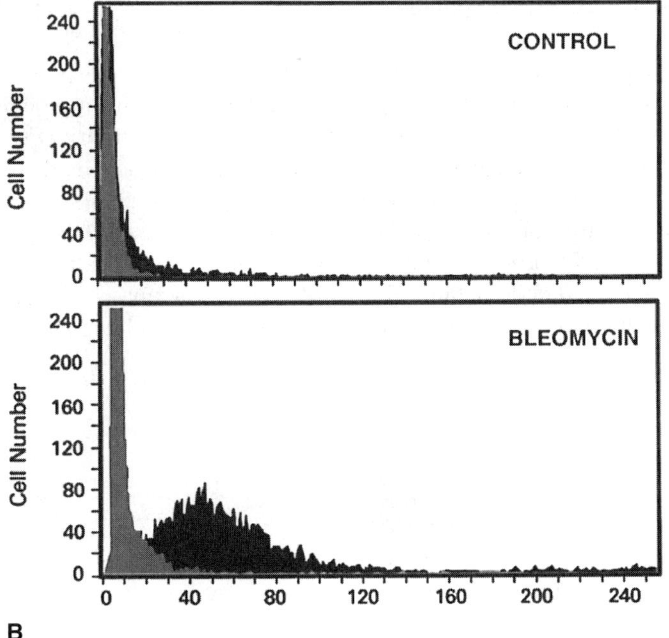

B

Figure 7B Increased cell surface expression of RHAMM in macrophages responding to lung injury. Rat alveolar macrophages were isolated by bronchoalveolar lavage 4 days after either intratracheal saline or bleomycin. Cell surface RHAMM expression was determined by flow cytometry. Lung injury was associated with an increased cell surface expression of RHAMM. Nonimmune IgG was used as a control (n = 3/group). Similar results were obtained in macrophages isolated 7 days after injury. (Data from Ref. 146.)

Addition of HA to cultures has recently been reported to down-regulate RHAMM in myocardiocytes (148) and we note a similar effect in skin fibroblasts (see Fig. 6A). We consider it possible, therefore, that RHAMM and other hyaladherins that also contain RHAMM-like HA-binding domains may be suppressed in fetal tissues containing a high level of HA, and that this suppression may contribute to the lack of fibrosis and contraction of fetal skin wounds. Indeed, the ability of peptides that mimic HA-binding domains of these hyaladherins to block contraction of collagen gels by fibroblast in vitro is consistent with this possibility (see Fig. 6C). This effect is also consistent with our observation that RHAMM can control activation of erk (127), a kinase implicated in the regulation of myosin light chain kinase (MLCK), which controls myosin contraction (149). However, further work is necessary to establish whether RHAMM/cdc37/p68 play a direct role in fibrosis and contraction of wounds.

V. SUMMARY AND CONCLUSIONS

The interaction of HA with hyaladherins appears to be key to tissue response-to-injury. The data presented in this review provide the framework for a model for the role of RHAMM, CD44, and HA in the tissue response to injury (Fig. 8). Tissue injury results in the local release of growth factors, which increase HA production, possibly initiate production of small HA fragments, and increase or initiate HA-binding ability of receptors' HA-receptor expression. CD44–HA interactions are proposed to promote monocyte activation and to localize inflammatory cells to activated endothelium. RHAMM–HA interactions may also contribute to the regulation of transmigration of these activated and adherent cells

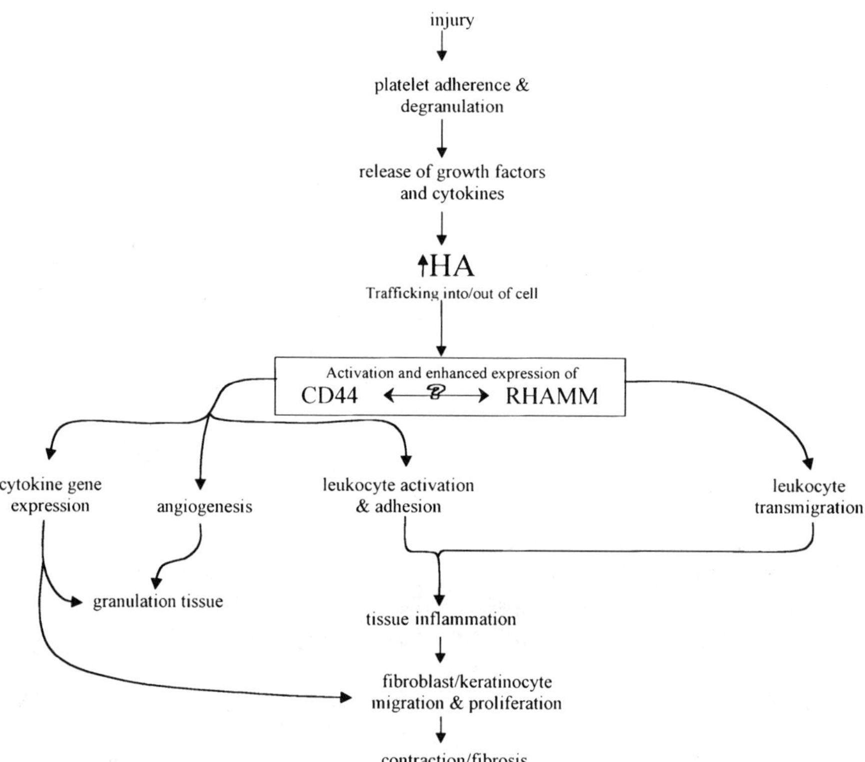

Figure 8 Overview of proposed multifunctional biological roles of the hyaladherins. Following HA up-regulation after injury, CD44 and RHAMM receptors display changes in key cell types causing enhanced motility and proliferation, etc., necessary and critical for wound healing.

into injured areas. Granulation tissue, consisting of newly formed blood vessels and a provisional matrix, is the consequence of the release of growth factors and cytokines, the expression of which is increased under the influence of HA fragments on monocyte-derived tissue macrophages. Growth factors recruit myofibroblasts to effect wound contraction and produce collagen for final healing of the wound. Internalization of HA by CD44, and possibly RHAMM, removes the influence of HA. We propose that high levels of HA that persist in early-gestation fetal skin wounds for as yet unknown reasons may down-regulate receptors such as RHAMM, resulting in reduced collagen production and wound contraction. This effect is predicted to be related to the ability of RHAMM to regulate erk kinase activity, which in turn controls myosin contraction.

Interference with the binding of HA to its receptors therefore holds promise as further novel targets to modify the response to injury and potentially reduce scar formation. While unlikely to be the sole requirement for scarless healing, these new therapies would greatly enhance the effort to reduce the adverse effects of wound repair.

REFERENCES

1. Nikkari ST, Jarvelainen HT, Wight TN, Ferguson M, Clowes AW. Smooth muscle cell expression of extracellular matrix genes after arterial injury. Am J Pathol 1994; 144:1348–1356.
2. Alaish SM, Yager D, Diegelmann RF, Cohen IK. Biology of fetal wound healing: hyaluronate receptor expression in fetal fibroblasts. J Pediatr Surg 1994; 29:1040–1043.
3. Haynes JH, Johnson DE, Mast BA, Diegelmann RF, Salzberg DA, Cohen IK, Krummel TM. Platelet-derived growth factor induces fetal wound fibrosis. J Pediatr Surg 1994; 29:1405–1408.
4. Longaker MT, Adzick NS, Hall JL, Stair SE, Crombleholme TM, Duncan BW, Bradley SM, Harrison MR, Stern R. Studies in fetal wound healing. VII. Fetal wound healing may be modulated by hyaluronic acid stimulating activity in amniotic fluid. J Pediatr Surg 1990; 25:430–433.
5. Mast BA, Haynes JH, Krummel TM, Diegelmann RF, Cohen IK. In vivo degradation of fetal wound hyaluronic acid results in increased fibroplasia, collagen deposition, and neovascularization. Plast Reconstr Surg 1992; 89:503–509.
6. Waldenstrom A, Martinussen HJ, Gerdin B, Hallgren R. Accumulation of hyaluronan and tissue edema in experimental myocardial infarction. J Clin Invest 1991; 88:1622–1628.
7. Hällgren R, Gerdin B, Tengblad A, Tufveson G. Accumulation of hyaluronan (hyaluronic acid) in myocardial interstitial tissue parallels development of transplantation edema in heart allografts in rats. J Clin Invest 1990; 85:668–673.
8. Hällgren R, Samuelsson T, Laurent TC, Modig J. Accumulation of hyaluronan

(hyaluronic acid) in the lung in adult respiratory distress syndrome. Am Rev Respir Dis 1989; 139:682–687.

9. Bray BA, Sampson PM, Osman M, Giandomenico A, Turino GM. Early changes in lung tissue hyaluronan (hyaluronic acid) and hyaluronidase in bleomycin-induced alveolitis in hamsters. Am Rev Respir Dis 1991; 143:284–288.

10. Nettelbladt O, Bergh J, Schenholm M, Tengblad A, Hallgren R. Accumulation of hyaluronic acid in the alveolar interstitial tissue in bleomycin-induced alveolitis. Am Rev Respir Dis 1989; 139:759–762.

11. Wells AF, Larsson E, Tengblad A, Fellstrom B, Tufveson G, Klareskog L, Laurent TC. The localization of hyaluronan in normal and rejected human kidneys. Transplantation 1990; 50:240–243.

12. Oksala O, Salo T, Tammi R, Hakkinen L, Jalkanen M, Inki P, Larjava H. Expression of proteoglycans and hyaluronan during wound healing. J Histochem Cytochem 1995; 43:125–135.

13. Ruggiero SL, Bertolami CN, Bronson RE, Damiani PJ. Hyaluronidase activity of rabbit skin wound granulation tissue fibroblasts. J Dent Res 1987; 66:1287–1287.

14. Iocono JA, Ehrlich HP, Keefer KA, Krummel TM. Hyaluronan induces scarless repair in mouse limb organ culture. J Pediatr Surg 1998; 33:564–567.

15. Mast BA, Diegelmann RF, Krummel TM, Cohen IK. Hyaluronic acid modulates proliferation, collagen and protein synthesis of cultured fetal fibroblasts. Matrix 1993; 13:441–446.

16. Yang Y, Ge S. [Effect of hyaluronic acid-stimulating factor on scar formation in wound healing process of deep partial thickness burns]. Chung Hua Cheng Hsing Shao Shang Wai Ko Tsa Chih 1995; 11:339–342.

17. Hellstrom S, Laurent C. Hyaluronan and healing of tympanic membrane perforations: an experimental study. Acta Otolaryngol (Stockholm) 1987; 442(suppl.): 54–61.

18. Chung JH, Fagerholm P, Lindstrom B. Hyaluronate in healing of corneal alkali wound in the rabbit. Exp Eye Res 1989; 48:569–576.

19. Ellis IR, Schor SL. Differential effects of TGF-beta 1 on hyaluronan sythesis by fetal and adult skin fibroblasts: implications for cell migration and wound healing. Exp Cell Res 1996; 228:326–333.

20. Toole BP. Developmental role of hyaluronate. Connect Tissue Res 1982; 10:93–100.

21. Wight TN, Kinsella MG, Qwarnstrom EE. The role of proteoglycans in cell adhesion, migration and proliferation. Curr Opin Cell Biol 1992; 4:793–801.

22. Rooney P, Kumar S. Inverse relationship between hyaluronan and collagens in development and angiogenesis. Differentiation 1993; 54:1–9.

23. Riessen R, Wight TN, Pastore C, Henley C, Isner JM. Distribution of hyaluronan during extracellular matrix remodeling in human restenotic arteries and balloon-injured rat carotid arteries Circulation 1996; 93:1141–1147.

24. Noble PW, Lake FR, Hension PM, Riches DW. Hyaluronate activation of CD44 induces insulin-like growth factor-1 expression by a tumor necrosis factor-alpha-dependent mechanism in murine macrophages. J Clin Invest 1993; 91:2368–2377.

25. DeGrendele HC, Estess P, Picker LJ, Siegelman MH. CD44 and its ligand hyaluronate mediate rolling under physiologic flow: a novel lymphocyte-endothelial cell primary adhesion pathway. J Exp Med 1996; 183:1119–1130.

26. Mohamadzadeh M, DeGrendele H, Arizpe H, Estess P, Siegelman M. Proinflammatory stimuli regulate endothelial hyaluronan expression and CD44/HA-dependent primary adhesion. J Clin Invest 1998; 101:97–108.

27. Savani RC, Khalil N, Turley EA. Hyaluronan receptor antagonists alter skin inflammation and fibrosis following injury. Proc West Pharmacol Soc 1995; 38:131–136.

28. Savani RC, Wang C, Yang B, Zhang S, Kinsella M, Wight TN, Stern R, Nance DM, Turley EA. Migration of bovine aortic smooth muscle cells following wounding injury. The role of hyaluronan and RHAMM. J Clin Invest 1995; 95:1158–1168.

29. Boudreau N, Turley E, Rabinovitch M. Fibronectin, hyaluronan and a hyaluronan binding protein contribute to increased ductus arteriosus smooth muscle cell migration. Dev Biol 1991; 143:235–247.

30. West DC, Kumar S. The effect of hyaluronate and its oligosaccharides on endothelial cell proliferation and monolayer integrity. Exp Cell Res 1989; 183:179–196.

31. McKee CM, Penno MB, Cowman M, Burdick MD, Strieter RM, Bao C, Noble PW. Hyaluronan (HA) fragments induce chemokine gene expression in alveolar macrophages. The role of HA size and CD44. J Clin Invest 1996; 98:2403–2413.

32. Kobayashi H, Terao T. Hyaluronic acid-specific regulation of cytokines by human uterine fibroblasts. Am J Physiol 1997; 273:C1151–C1159.

33. Akatsuka M, Yamamoto Y, Tobetto K, Yasui K, Ando T. Suppressive effects of hyaluronic acid on elastase release from rat peritoneal leucocytes. J Pharm Pharmacol 1993; 45:110–114.

34. Tamoto K, Nochi H, Tada M, Shimada S, Mori Y, Kataoka S, Suzuki Y, Nakamura T. High-molecular-weight hyaluronic acids inhibit chemotaxis and phagocytosis but not lysosomal enzyme release induced by receptor-mediated stimulations in guinea pig phagocytes. Microbiol Immunol 1994; 38:73–80.

35. Noble PW, McKee CM, Cowman M, Shin HS. Hyaluronan fragments activate an NF-kappa B/I-kappa B alpha autoregulatory loop in murine macrophages. J Exp Med 1996; 183:2373–2378.

36. Toole BP. Hyaluronan and its binding proteins, the hyaladherins. Curr Opin Cell Biol 1990; 2:839–844.

37. Grammatikakis N, Grammatikakis A, Yoneda M, Banerjee SD, Toole BP. A novel glycosaminoglycan-binding protein is the vertebrate homologue of the cell cycle control protein, cdc37. J Biol Chem 1995; 270:16198–16205.

38. Kimura Y, Rutherford SL, Miyata Y, Yahara I, Freeman BC, Yue L, Morimoto RI, Lindquist S. Cdc37 is a molecular chaperone with specific functions in signal transduction. Genes Dev 1997; 11:1775–1785.

39. Das S, Deb TB, Kumar R, Datta K. Multifunctional activities of human fibroblast 34-kDa hyaluronic acid-binding protein. Gene 1997; 190:223–225.

40. Deb TB, Datta K. Molecular cloning of human fibroblast hyaluronic acid-binding protein confirms its identity with P-32, a protein co-purified with splicing factor

SF2. Hyaluronic acid-binding protein as P-32 protein, co-purified with splicing factor SF2. J Biol Chem 1996; 271:2206–2212.

41. Entwistle J, Hall CL, Turley EA. HA receptors: regulators of signalling to the cytoskeleton [review]. J Cell Biochem 1996; 61:569–577.

42. Frost SJ, Kindberg GM, Oka JA, Weigel PH. Rat hepatocyte hyaluronan/glycosaminoglycan binding proteins: evidence for distinct divalent cation-independent and divalent cation-dependent activities. Biochem Biophys Res Commun 1992; 189: 1591–1597.

43. Underhill CB, Green SJ, Comoglio PM, Tarone G. The hyaluronate receptor is identical to a glycoprotein of Mr 85,000 (gp85) as shown by a monoclonal antibody that interferes with binding activity. J Biol Chem 1987; 262:13142–13146.

44. Aruffo A, Stamenkovic I, Melnick M, Underhill CB, Seed B. CD44 is the principal cell surface receptor for hyaluronate. Cell 1990; 61:1303–1313.

45. Zimmermann DR, Ruoslahti E. Multiple domains of the large fibroblast proteoglycan, versican. EMBO J 1989; 8:2975–2981.

46. Neame PJ, Barry FP. The link proteins. Experientia 1993; 49:393–402.

47. Hardingham TE, Fosang AJ, Dudhia J. The structure, function and turnover of aggrecan, the large aggregating proteoglycan from cartilage. Eur J Clin Chem Clin Biochem 1994; 32:249–257.

48. Milev P, Maurel P, Chiba A, Mevissen M, Popp S, Yamaguchi Y, Margolis RK, Margolis RU. Differential regulation of expression of hyaluronan-binding proteoglycans in developing brain: aggrecan, versican, neurocan, and brevican. Biochem Biophys Res Commun 1998; 247:207–212.

49. Sandson J, Hamerman D, Schwick G. Altered properties of pathological hyaluronate due to a bound inter-alpha trypsin inhibitor. Trans Assoc Am Physicians 1965; 78:304–313.

50. Zhao M, Yoneda M, Ohashi Y, Kurono S, Iwata H, Ohnuki Y, Kimata K. Evidence for the covalent binding of SHAP, heavy chains of inter-alpha-trypsin inhibitor, to hyaluronan. J Biol Chem 1995; 270:26657–26663.

51. Kohda D, Morton CJ, Parkar AA, Hatanda H, Inagaki FM, Campbell ID, Day AJ. Solution structure of the link module: a hyaluronan-binding domain involved in extracelluar matrix stability and cell migration. Cell 1996; 86:767–775.

52. Yang B, Yang BL, Savani RC, Turley EA. Identification of a common hyaluronan binding motif in the hyaluronan binding proteins RHAMM, CD44, and link protein. EMBO J 1994; 13:286–294.

53. Spicer AP, Roller ML, Camper SA, McPherson JD, Wasmuth JJ, Hakim S, Wang C, Turley EA, McDonald JA. The human and mouse receptors for hyaluronan-mediated motility, RHAMM, genes (HMMR) map to human chromosome 5q33.2-qter and mouse chromosome 11. Genomics 1995; 30:115–117.

54. Goodfellow PN, Banting G, Wiles MV, Tunnacliffe A, Parkar M, Solomon E, Dalchau R, Fabre JW. The gene, MIC4, which controls expression of the antigen defined by monoclonal antibody F10.44.2, is on human chromosome 11. Eur J Immunol 1982; 12:659–663.

55. Screaton GR, Bell MV, Jackson DG, Cornelis FB, Gerth U, Bell JI. Genomic structure of DNA encoding the lymphocyte homing receptor CD44 reveals at least 12 alternatively spliced exons. Proc Natl Acad Sci USA 1992; 89:12160–12164.

56. Ponta H, Wainwright D, Herrlich P. The CD44 protein family. Int J Biochem Cell Biol 1998; 30:299–305.

57. Gunthert U, Hofmann M, Rudy W, Reber S, Zoller M, Haubmann I, Matzku S, Wenzel A, Ponta H, Herrlich P. A new variant of glycoprotein CD44 confers metastatic potential to rat carcinoma cells. Cell 1991; 65:13–24.

58. Ghaffari S, Dougherty GJ, Lansdorp PM, Eaves AC, Eaves CJ. Differentiation-associated changes in CD44 isoform expression during normal hematopoiesis and their alteration in chronic myeloid leukemia. Blood 1995; 86:2976–2985.

59. Dalchau R, Kirkley J, Fabre JW. Monoclonal antibody to a human leukocyte-specific membrane glycoprotein probably homologous to the leukocyte-common (L-C) antigen of the rat. Eur J Immunol 1980; 10:737–744.

60. Entwistle J, Zhang S, Yang B, Wong C, Li Q, Hall CL, Mowat M, Greenberg AH, Turley EA. Characterization of the murine gene encoding the hyaluronan receptor RHAMM. Gene 1995; 163:233–238.

61. Wang C, Entwistle J, Hou G, Li Q, Turley EA. The characterization of a human RHAMM cDNA: conservation of the hyaluronan-binding domains. Gene 1996; 174:299–306.

62. Mackay CR, Maddox JF, Wijffels GL, Mackay IR, Walker ID. Characterization of a 95,000 molecule on sheep leucocytes homologous to murine Pgp-1 and human CD44. Immunology 1988; 65:93–99.

63. Goldstein LA, Zhou DF, Picker LJ, Minty CN, Bargatze RF, Ding JF, Butcher EC. A human lymphocyte homing receptor, the hermes antigen, is related to cartilage proteoglycan core and link proteins. Cell 1989; 56:1063–1072.

64. Lesley J, Hyman R, Kincade PW. CD44 and its interaction with extracellular matrix [review]. Adv Immunol 1993; 54:271–335.

65. Culty M, Nguyen HA, Underhill CB. The hyaluronan receptor (CD44) participates in the uptake and degradation of hyaluronan. J Cell Biol 1992; 116:1055–1062.

66. Hua Q, Knudson CB, Knudson W. Internalization of hyaluronan by chondrocytes occurs via receptor-mediated endocytosis. J Cell Sci 1993; 365–375.

67. Ayroldi E, Cannarile L, Migliorati G, Bartoli A, Nicoletti I, Riccardi C. CD44 (Pgp-1) inhibits CD3 and dexamethasone-induced apoptosis. Blood 1995; 86: 2672–2678.

68. Henke C, Bitterman P, Roongta U, Ingbar D, Polunovsky V. Induction of fibroblast apoptosis by anti-CD44 antibody: implications for the treatment of fibroproliferative lung disease. Am J Pathol 1996; 149:1639–1650.

69. Hamann KJ, Dowling TL, Neeley SP, Grant JA, Leff AR. Hyaluronic acid enhances cell proliferation during eosinopoiesis through the CD44 surface antigen. J Immunol 1995; 154:4073–4080.

70. Wayner EA, Carter WG. Identification of multiple cell adhesion receptors for collagen and fibronectin in human fibrosarcoma cells possessing unique alpha and common beta subunits. J Cell Biol 1987; 105:1873–1884.

71. Jalkanen S, Jalkanen M. Lymphocyte CD44 binds the COOH-terminal heparin-binding domain of fibronectin. J Cell Biol 1992; 116:817–825.

72. Radotra B, McCormick D, Crockard A. CD44 plays a role in adhesive interactions between glioma cells and extracellular matrix components. Neuropathol Appl Neurobiol 1994; 20:399–405.

73. Naujokas MF, Morin M, Anderson MS, Peterson M, Miller J. The chondroitin sulfate form of invariant chain can enhance stimulation of T cell responses through interaction with CD44. Cell 1993; 74:257–268.

74. Picker LJ, Nakache M, Butcher EC. Monoclonal antibodies to human lymphocyte homing receptors define a novel class of adhesion molecules on diverse cell types. J Cell Biol 1989; 109:927–937.

75. Toyama SN, Sorimachi H, Tobita Y, Kitamura F, Yagita H, Suzuki K, Miyasaka M. A novel ligand for CD44 is serglycin, a hematopoietic cell lineage-specific proteoglycan. Possible involvement in lymphoid cell adherence and activation. J Biol Chem 1995; 270:7437–7444.

76. Weber GF, Ashkar S, Glimcher MJ, Cantor H. Receptor-ligand interaction between CD44 and osteopontin (Eta-1). Science 1996; 271:509–512.

77. Mackay CR, Terpe HJ, Stauder R, Marston WL, Stark H, Gunthert U. Expression and modulation of CD44 variant isoforms in humans. J Cell Biol 1994; 124:71–82.

78. Tammi R, Ripellino JA, Margolis RU, Tammi M. Localization of epidermal hyaluronic acid using the hyaluronate binding region of cartilage proteoglycan as a specific probe. J Invest Dermatol 1988; 90:412–414.

79. Tuhkanen AL, Tammi M, Tammi R. CD44 substituted with heparan sulfate and endo-beta-galactosidase-sensitive oligosaccharides: a major proteoglycan in adult human epidermis. J Invest Dermatol 1997; 109:213–218.

80. Naor D, Slonov RV, Ish-Shalom D. CD44: structure, function, and association with the malignant process [review]. Adv Cancer Res 1997; 71:241–319.

81. Tolg C, Hofmann M, Herrlich P, Ponta H. Splicing choice from ten variant exons establishes CD44 variability. Nucleic Acids Res 1993; 21:1225–1229.

82. Lokeshwar VB, Bourguignon LY. Post-translational protein modification and expression of ankyrin-binding site(s) in GP85 (Pgp-1/CD44) and its biosynthetic precursors during T-lymphoma membrane biosynthesis. J Biol Chem 1991; 266: 17983–17989.

83. Bartolazzi A, Nocks A, Aruffo A, Spring F, Stamenkovic I. Glycosylation of CD44 is implicated in CD44-mediated cell adhesion to hyaluronan. J Cell Biol 1996; 132: 1199–1208.

84. Dasgupta A, Takahashi K, Cutler M, Tanabe KK. O-linked glycosylation modifies CD44 adhesion to hyaluronate in colon carcinoma cells. Biochem Biophys Res Commun 1996; 227:110–117.

85. Bennett KL, Modrell B, Greenfield B, Bartolazzi A, Stamenkovic I, Peach R, Jackson DG, Spring F, Aruffo A. Regulation of CD44 binding to hyaluronan by glycosylation of variably spliced exons. J Cell Biol 1995; 1623–1633.

86. Jackson DG, Bell JI, Dickinson R, Timans J, Shields J, Whittle N. Proteoglycan forms of the lymphocyte homing receptor CD44 are alternatively spliced variants containing the v3 exon. J Cell Biol 1995; 128:673–685.

87. Sleeman JP, Kondo K, Moll J, Ponta H, Herrlich P. Variant exons v6 and v7 together expand the repertoire of glycosaminoglycans bound by CD44. J Biol Chem 1997; 272:31837–31844.

88. Bajorath J, Greenfield B, Munro SB, Day AJ, Aruffo A. Identification of CD44 residues important for hyaluronan binding and delineation of the binding site. J Biol Chem 1998; 273:338–343.

89. Hall CL, Yang B, Yang X, Zhang S, Turley M, Samuel S, Lange LA, Wang C, Curpen GD, Savani RC, Greenberg AH, Turley EA. Overexpression of the hyaluronan receptor RHAMM is transforming and is also required for H-*ras* transformation. Cell 1995; 82:19–26.

90. Hyman R, Lesley J, Schulte R. Somatic cell mutants distinguish CD44 expression and hyaluronic acid binding. Immunogenetics 1991; 33:392–395.

91. Sherman L, Sleeman J, Herrlich P, Ponta H. Hyaluronate receptors: key players in growth, differentiation, migration and tumor progression [review]. Curr Opin Cell Biol 1994; 6:726–733.

92. Zheng Z, Katoh S, He Q, Oritani K, Miyake K, Lesley J, Hyman R, Hamik A, Parkhouse RM, Farr AG, et al. Monoclonal antibodies to CD44 and their influence on hyaluronan recognition. J Cell Biol 1995; 130:485–495.

93. Lokeshwar VB, Fregien N, Bourguignon LY. Ankyrin-binding domain of CD44(GP85) is required for the expression of hyaluronic acid-mediated adhesion function. J Cell Biol 1994; 126:1099–1109.

94. Galandrini R, Albi N, Tripodi G, Zarcone D, Terenzi A, Moretta A, Grossi CE, Velardi A. Antibodies to CD44 trigger effector functions of human T cell clones. J Immunol 1993; 150:4225–4235.

95. Pericle F, Sconocchia G, Titus JA, Segal DM. CD44 is a cytotoxic triggering molecule on human polymorphonuclear cells. J Immunol 1996; 157:4657–4663.

96. Galandrini R, Piccoli M, Frati L, Santoni A. Tyrosine kinase-dependent activation of human NK cell functions upon triggering through CD44 receptor. Eur J Immunol 1996; 26:2807–2811.

97. Tan PH, Santos EB, Rossbach HC, Sandmaier BM. Enhancement of natural killer activity by an antibody to CD44. J Immunol 1993; 150:812–820.

98. Webb DSA, Shimizu Y, Van Seventer GA, Shaw S, Gerrard TL. LFA-3, CD44 and CD45: physiological triggers of human monocyte TNF and IL-1 release. Science 1990; 249:1295–1297.

99. Taher TE, Smit L, Griffioen AW, Schilder TE, Borst J, Pals ST. Signaling through CD44 is mediated by tyrosine kinases. Association with p56lck in T lymphocytes. J Biol Chem 1996; 271:2863–2867.

100. Ilangumaran S, Briol A, Hoessli DC. CD44 selectively associates with active Src family protein tyrosine kinases Lck and Fyn in glycosphingolipid-rich plasma membrane domains of human peripheral blood lymphocytes. Blood 1998; 91:3901–3908.

101. Funaro A, Spagnoli GC, Momo M, Knapp W, Malavasi F. Stimulation of T cells via CD44 requires leukocyte-function-associated antigen interactions and interleukin-2 production. Hum Immunol 1994; 40:267–278.

102. Sommer F, Huber M, Rollinghoff M, Lohoff M. CD44 plays a co-stimulatory role in murine T cell activation: ligation of CD44 selectively co-stimulates IL-2 production, but not proliferation in TCR-stimulated murine Th1 cells. Int Immunol 1995; 7:1779–1786.

103. Bourguignon LY, Lokeshwar VB, Chen X, Kerrick WG. Hyaluronic acid-induced lymphocyte signal transduction and HA receptor (GP85/CD44)-cytoskeleton interaction. J Immunol 1993; 151:6634–6644.

104. Guo YJ, MA J, Wong JH, Lin SC, Chang HC, Bigby M, Sy MS. Monoclonal anti-CD44 antibody acts in synergy with anti-CD2 but inhibits anti-CD3 or T cell recep-

tor-mediated signaling in murine T cell hybridomas. Cell Immunol 1993; 152:186–199.

105. Bourguignon LYW, Zhu H, Chu A, Iida N, Zhang L, Hung M-C. Interaction between the adhesion receptor, CD44, and the oncogene product, p185HER2, promotes human ovarian tumor cell activation. J Biol Chem 1997; 272:27913–27918.

106. Tsukita S, Oishi K, Sato N, Sagara J, Kawai A, Tsukita S. ERM family members as molecular linkers between the cell surface glycoprotein CD44 and actin-based cytoskeletons. J Cell Biol 1994; 126:391–401.

107. Hirao M, Sato N, Kondo T, Yonemura S, Monden M, Sasaki T, Takai Y, Tsukita S, Tsukita S. Regulation mechanism of ERM (ezrin/radixin/moesin) protein/plasma membrane association: possible involvement of phosphatidylinositol turnover and Rho-dependent signaling pathway. J Cell Biol 1996; 135:37–51.

108. Vaheri A, Carpen O, Heiska L, Helander TS, Jaaskelainen J, Majander NP, Sainio M, Timonen T, Turunen O. The ezrin protein family: membrane-cytoskeleton interactions and disease associations. Curr Opin Cell Biol 1997; 9:659–666.

109. Hotchin NA, Hall A. Regulation of the actin cytoskeleton, integrins and cell growth by the Rho family of small GTPases. Cancer Surv 1996; 27:311–322.

110. Takaishi K, Kikuchi A, Kuroda S, Kotani K, Sasaki T, Takai Y. Involvement of rho p21 and its inhibitory GDP/GTP exchange protein (rho GDI) in cell motility. Mol Cell Biol 1993; 13:72–79.

111. Nishiyama T, Sasaki T, Takaishi K, Kato M, Yaku H, Araki K, Matsuura Y, Takai Y. Rac p21 is involved in insulin-induced membrane ruffling and rho p21 is involved in hepatocyte growth factor- and 12-O-tetradecanoylphorbol-13-acetate (TPA)-induced membrane ruffling in KB cells. Mol Cell Biol 1994; 14:2447–2456.

112. Takai Y, Sasaki T, Tanaka K, Nakanishi H. Rho as a regulator of the cytoskeleton. Trends Biochem Sci 1995; 20:227–231.

113. Araki S, Kikuchi A, Hata Y, Isomura M, Takai Y. Regulation of reversible binding of smg p25A, a ras p21-like GTP-binding protein, to synaptic plasma membranes and vesicles by its specific regulatory protein, GDP dissociation inhibitor. J Biol Chem 1990; 265:13007–13015.

114. Harrison RE, Turley EA. The effects of RHAMM on microtubule organization and dynamics (abstr). Mol Bio Cell 1997; 8:164a.

115. Lin Z, Turley EA. RHAMM overexpression prevents apoptosis in detached cells via a N-cadherin and erk dependent mechanism. Mol Biol Cell (submitted) 1998.

116. Hofmann M, Fieber C, Assmann V, Gottlicher M, Sleeman J, Plug R, Howells N, von SO, Ponta H, Herrlich P. Identification of IHABP, a 95 kDa intracellular hyaluronate binding protein. J Cell Sci 1998; 111:1673–1684.

117. Assmann V, Marshall JF, Fieber C, Hofmann M, Hart IR. The human hyaluronan receptor RHAMM is expressed as an intracellular protein in breast cancer. J Cell Sci 1998; 111:1685–1694.

118. Wang C, Thor AD, Moore D2, Zhao Y, Kerschmann R, Stern R, Watson PH, Turley EA. The overexpression of RHAMM, a hyaluronan-binding protein that regulates ras signaling, correlates with overexpression of mitogen-activated protein kinase and is a significant parameter in breast cancer progression. Clin Cancer Res 1998; 4:567–576.

119. Turley EA. Purification of a hyaluronate-binding protein fraction that modifies cell social behavior. Biochem Biophys Res Commun 1982; 108:1016–1024.

120. Toole BP. Hyaluronan in morphogenesis [review]. J Intern Med 1997; 242:35–40.

121. Mohapatra S, Yang X, Wright JA, Turley EA, Greenberg AH. Soluble hyaluronan receptor RHAMM induces mitotic arrest by suppressing cdc-2 and cyclin B1 expression. J Exp Med 1996; 183:1663–1668.

122. Turley EA, Hossain MZ, Sorokan T, Jordan LM, Nagy JI. Astrocyte and microglial motility in vitro is functionally dependent on the hyaluronan receptor RHAMM. Glia 1994; 12:68–80.

123. Nagy JI, Hacking J, Frankenstein UN, Turley EA. Requirement of the hyaluronan receptor RHAMM in neurite extension and motility as demonstrated in primary neurons and neuronal cell lines. J Neurosci 1995; 241–252.

124. Pilarski LM, Masellis SA, Belch AR, Yang B, Savani RC, Turley EA. RHAMM, a receptor for hyaluronan-mediated motility, on normal human lymphocytes, thymocytes and malignant B cells: a mediator in B cell malignancy? Leuk Lymphoma 1994; 14:363–374.

125. Hardwick C, Hoare K, Owens R, Hohn HP, Hook M, Moore D, Cripps V, Austen L, Nance DM, Turley EA. Molecular cloning of a novel hyaluronan receptor that mediates tumor cell motility. J Cell Biol 1992; 117:1343–1350. [Published erratum appears in J Cell Biol 1992; 118:753.]

126. Hall CL, Wang C, Lange LA, Turley EA. Hyaluronan and the hyaluronan receptor RHAMM promote focal adhesion turnover and transient tyrosine kinase activity. J Cell Biol 1994; 126:575–588.

127. Zhang S, Chang MC, Zylka D, Turley S, Harrison R, Turley EA. The hyaluronan receptor RHAMM regulates extracellular-regulated kinase. J Biol Chem 1998; 273: 11342–11348.

128. Samuel SK, Hurta RAR, Spearman MA, Wright JA, Turley EA, Greenberg AH. TGF-β1 stimulation of cell locomotion utilizes the hyaluronan receptor RHAMM and hyaluronan. J Cell Biol 1993; 123:749–758.

129. Delpech B, Girard N, Bertrand P, Courel MN, Chauzy C, Delpech A. Hyaluronan: fundamental principles and applications in cancer [review]. J Intern Med 1997; 242:41–48.

130. Turley E, Auersperg N. A hyaluronate binding protein transiently codistributes with p21k-ras in cultured cell lines. Exp Cell Res 1989; 182:340–348.

131. Teder P, Heldin P. Mechanism of impaired local hyaluronan turnover in bleomycin-induced lung injury in rat. Am J Respir Cell Mol Biol 1997; 17:376–385.

132. Weiss JM, Renkl AC, Ahrens T, Moll J, Mai BH, Denfeld RW, Schopf E, Ponta H, Herrlich P, Simon JC. Activation-dependent modulation of hyaluronate-receptor expression and of hyaluronate-avidity by human monocytes. J Invest Dermatol 1998; 111:227–232.

133. Chang CYM, Harrison R, Li A, Yang X, McCarthy JB, Turley EA. Fibronectin-RHAMM interactions regulate cell motility. FASEB J 1997; A1095:1397.

134. Hall CL, Lange LA, Prober DA, Turley EA. pp60$^{c\text{-src}}$ is required for cell locomotion regulated by the hyaluronan receptor RHAMM. Oncogene 1996; 13:2213–2224.

135. Silverstein AM, Grammatikakis N, Cochran BH, Chinkers M, Pratt WB. p50(cdc37) binds directly to the catalytic domain of raf as well as to a site on hsp90

that is topologically adjacent to the tetratricopeptide repeat binding site. J Biol Chem 1998; 273:20090–20095.

136. Yasaka N, Furue M, Tamaki K. CD44 expression in normal human skin and skin tumors. J Dermatol 1995; 22:88–94.

137. Kaya G, Rodriguez I, Jorcano JL, Vassalli P, Stamenkovic I. Selective suppression of CD44 in keratinocytes of mice bearing an antisense CD44 transgene driven by a tissue-specific promoter disrupts hyaluronate metabolism in the skin and impairs keratinocyte proliferation. Genes Dev 1997; 11:996–1007.

138. Lackie PM, Baker JE, Gunthert U, Holgate ST. Expression of CD44 isoforms is increased in the airway epithelium of asthmatic subjects. Am J Respir Cell Mol Biol 1997; 16:14–22.

139. Svee K, White J, Vaillant P, Jessurun J, Roongta U, Krumwiede M, Johnson D, Henke C. Acute lung injury fibroblast migration and invasion of a fibrin matrix is mediated by CD44. J Clin Invest 1996; 98:1713–1727.

140. Kasper M, Haroske G. Alterations in the alveolar epithelium after injury leading to pulmonary fibrosis. Histol Histopathol 1996; 11:463–483.

141. Jones LL, Kreutzberg GW, Raivich G. Regulation of CD44 in the regenerating mouse facial motor nucleus. Eur J Neurosci 1997; 9:1854–1863.

142. Sibalic V, Fan X, Loffing J, Wuthrich RP. Upregulated renal tubular CD44, hyaluronan, and osteopontin in kdkd mice with interstitial nephritis. Nephrol Dial Transplant 1997; 12:1344–1353.

143. Jain M, Lee W-S, Kashiki S, Foster LC, Tsai J-C, Lee M-E, Haber E. Role of CD44 in the reaction of vascular smooth muscle cells to arterial wall injury. J Clin Invest 1996; 97:596–603.

144. Asari A, Morita M, Sekiguchi T, Okamura K, Horie K, Miyauchi S. Hyaluronan, CD44 and fibronectin in rabbit corneal epithelial wound healing. Jpn J Ophthalmol 1996; 40:18–25.

145. Schmits R, Filmus J, Gerwin N, Senaldi G, Kiefer F, Kundig T, Wakeham A, Shahinian A, Catzavelos C, Rak J, Furlonger C, Zakarian A, Simard JJ, Ohashi PS, Paige CJ, Gutierrez RJ, Mak TW. CD44 regulates hematopoietic progenitor distribution, granuloma formation, and tumorigenicity. Blood 1997; 90:2217–2233.

146. Savani RC, Hou G, Liu P, Wang C, Simons FE, Grimm PC, Stern R, Greenberg AH, Khalil N. A role for hyaluronan in bleomycin-induced pulmonary inflammation. Am J Resp Cell Mol Biol 2000.

147. Lovvorn HN3, Cass DL, Sylvester KG, Yang EY, Crombleholme TM, Adzick NS, Savani RC. Hyaluronan receptor expression increases in fetal excisional skin wounds and correlates with fibroplasia. J Pediatr Surg 1998; 33:1062–1069.

148. Iocono JA, Bisignani GJ, Krummel TM, Ehrlich HP. Inhibiting the differentiation of myocardiocytes by hyaluronic acid. J Surg Res 1998; 76:111–116.

149. Klemke RL, Cai S, Giannini AL, Gallagher PJ, de LP, Cheresh DA. Regulation of cell motility by mitogen-activated protein kinase. J Cell Biol 1997; 137:481–492.

150. Bagli DJ. J Urology 162:832–840.

7
Hyaluronan: Aiming for Perfect Skin Regeneration

Endre A. Balazs and Nancy E. Larsen
Biomatrix, Inc., Ridgefield, New Jersey

I. INTRODUCTION

Hyaluronan (HA) is a naturally occurring polysaccharide with a large unbranched structure composed of repeating disaccharides of *N*-acetylglucosamine and β-glucuronic acid (1). Hyaluronan is present in all vertebrate tissues and body fluids, though it is most abundant in the skin (2). More than 50% of the total HA in the body is found in the skin (2,3), where it is essential to the stabilization and maintenance of the intercellular matrix and to various cell functions. The levels of HA in the skin change dramatically when the tissue structure is disrupted by injury and it is the first glycosaminoglycan synthesized following injury (4). Dramatic changes in HA also occur during development, aging, and pathological conditions (5). Therefore, it is reasonable to conclude that hyaluronan is of critical importance to the functional well-being of normal physiological processes.

It is well established that fetal healing, which occurs in an HA-rich environment, is scarless and represents a regeneration-like repair (6). Many investigators have suggested that exogenous hyaluronan may be therapeutically useful in wound repair (7–14). Numerous studies have been conducted in order to test this hypothesis. The results of these studies are often conflicting, perhaps due to the variability in the hyaluronan preparations used (purity, rheological properties, molecular weight, concentration, etc.) and the conditions of evaluation (continuous/noncontinuous presence of hyaluronan, occlusive/nonocclusive environment, etc.). However, some observations are striking and indicate that, under appropriate conditions using suitable hyaluronan, it appears that healing is enhanced and scarring reduced or eliminated (8–12,15).

143

In this chapter, the role of exogenous HA in wound healing and tissue repair is discussed. The properties of hyaluronan and the conditions under which it is applied will be examined in consideration of the desired biological outcome—perfect skin regeneration.

II. HYALURONAN AND SKIN

A. Structure and Molecular Weight

Hyaluronan has a very large average molecular weight (4–5×10^6) and is made up of repeating dimers of β-glucuronic acid and *N*-acetylglucosamine (Fig. 1) which form linear, unbranched polyanionic HA chains. The HA molecular chains form highly hydrated random coils, which entangle and interpenetrate each other at a relatively low concentration (16–21), producing highly elastoviscous solutions. Hyaluronan has the same chemical composition and molecular structure in all species and in all tissues. Therefore, in its highly purified form, it is not foreign to the human body (22,23).

B. Concentration in the Skin

The dermis contains more than half of the total HA in the body (2). The HA in the intercellular matrix is present at a relatively high concentration, 1 to 2 mg/ml, a concentration at which there is significant entanglement and exclusion of large particles. The concentration range of hyaluronan in all connective tissues is 0.1 to 10 mg/ml (3).

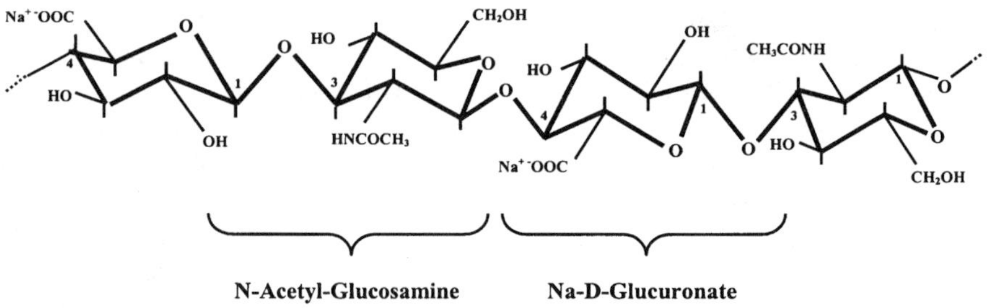

Figure 1 The tetrasaccharide segment of a sodium hyaluronan chain. The two monosaccharides *N*-acetyl-D-glucosamine and Na-D-glucuronate are linked together with a β $1 \rightarrow 4$ glucoside bond. The resulting disaccharides are linked together with β $1 \rightarrow 3$ glucoside bonds, forming a long unbranched chain.

C. Turnover of Hyaluronan in the Skin

In the 1950s, Schiller et al. measured the rate of synthesis of HA in the skin using [^{14}C]-acetate. The estimated turnover rate was 1.9 to 3.7 days in rabbit skin (24) and 2.6 to 4.5 days in rat skin (25–28). In the 1960s, Hardingham (29) obtained similar results in rat skin using [^{14}C]-glucose. Exogenous [^{3}H]-HA injected into the skin produced values that indicated a more rapid turnover than measured by Schiller; however, the values are consistent with the existence of two pools of HA in the skin, a large pool of free (>75%) and a small pool of bound HA (HA in the pericellular coats, fibroblasts and other interstitial structures). The HA in the large, free pool is removed and degraded by the local lymph nodes and the liver. The half-life of HA in the skin is normally 2 to 4 days, with the free pool turning over with a half-life of 8 to 16 hr.

The mechanism of removal of hyaluronan from skin was elucidated by Laurent et al. (30) using [^{125}I]-HA. The radiolabeled HA was injected subcutaneously in rabbits and the label was determined in skin, local lymph nodes, and the liver. They observed that 10 to 25% of HA breakdown took place locally in the skin, while the majority of breakdown occurred in the local lymph nodes and in the liver (30–32).

D. Functions of Hyaluronan

1. Structural Role

Hyaluronan in the skin has a protective, shock-absorbing, and structural stabilizing role in the extracellular matrix (ECM) of the skin (33). Hyaluronan fills the space between collagen fibrils and maintains the separation between fibers. In the human epidermis and dermis, hyaluronan density is highest in the middle spinous layer, lower in the basal layer, and absent in the granular and keratin layers (34). In the dermal layer, HA is identified between the collagen and elastin fibers (35). The tremendous water-retaining capacity of HA suggests that HA plays a role in maintaining the extracellular space, facilitating the transport of metabolites, and preserving tissue hydration (19,35).

2. Cellular Activities

a. General Cell Effects. The involvement of hyaluronan in cellular function was suggested long ago based on the ubiquitous presence of hyaluronan in the intercellular matrix and its accumulation during development, tissue repair, and tumorigensis. In the intercellular matrix, hyaluronan functions to regulate the movement, activity, and proliferation of white blood cells and cells of the lymphomyeloid system in connective tissue when they migrate to and from the lymph and blood vessels (36,37). In in vitro systems the chemotactic and random migration of white blood cells can be inhibited. This activity is dependent on the concentration of hyaluronan (Fig 2). The phagocytic activity of mononuclear phagocytes is also inhibited by even a relatively low concentration of hyaluronan (≤0.05 mg/ml) (38).

Migration and phagocytic effects of HA are dependent on the viscosity of the HA solution, and the effect is reversible. The viscous HA medium apparently stabilizes the membrane of these cells, which affects other biochemical events (i.e., release of prostaglandins, enzymes). This effect is a biomechanical effect on cell function since other viscous, biocompatible substances, such as gelatin and DNA, produce similar effects. As a primary component of the extracellular matrix, however, HA exerts biomechanical regulation over processes such as inflammation through its ability to modify the activity of cells involved in the inflammatory response.

b.   Molecular Sieve Effects.   The molecular network of hyaluronan functions as a charged molecular sieve and regulates the movement of solutes, metabolites, and other molecules in the extracellular space (21,33). The HA molecular network is able to exclude large molecules, such as fibrinogen and other proteins.

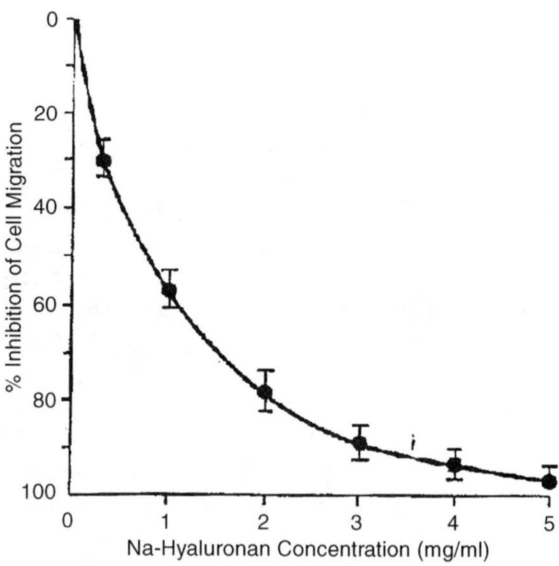

Figure 2   The effect of sodium hyaluronan solutions on migration of leukocytes (molecular weight ≅ 3 million).

The molecular sieve effect can have a dramatic restrictive effect on the formation of chemotactic gradients (39). Steric hindrance by the HA matrix may alter the chemotactic gradient and thereby influence the magnitude and nature of the inflammatory response.

c.   Role of Cell-Associated Receptors.   In the early 1990s, receptors for hyaluronan were cloned (CD44, RHAMM), permitting direct assessment of the role of these receptors in specific cell functions, such as adhesion, mobility, and proliferation. Specific antibodies, synthetic peptides, and genetic manipulation were developed that allowed receptor function to be blocked and the effects of this abrogation examined (40). In tumorigenesis studies, the CD44 receptor has been shown to promote proliferation and metastasis of tumor cells, and this activity is dependent on the HA-binding capacity of the cells. It also has been suggested that HA receptors are important in the repair process (41) and inflammation (42). The presence of HA receptors in skin epithelium (43–45), neutrophils (46), macrophages (47), activated T cells (48), and fibroblasts (41,42,49) has been demonstrated. Also reported is the presence of increased CD44 and RHAMM expression in fibroblasts of hypertrophic scars (41), in macrophages in inflamed skin (50), and in keratinocytes responding to local injury (40). Since these cells are essential to the skin repair process and are likely to be responsive to HA (because of the presence of receptors), it is likely that modulating their response to HA alters the inflammatory and fibrotic responses.

In a later section, results from in vitro and in vivo studies relating to the wound repair process are presented. The role of HA receptors in these processes is discussed.

E.   Effect of Aging

With increasing age, the quality of the human connective tissue deteriorates and this deterioration is most obvious in the skin. It has been suggested that the changes observed in aged skin, such as decreased turgidity, reduced support for microvessels, wrinkling, and altered elasticity, maybe the result of changes in the levels of HA in the dermis. Meyer and Stern (51) studied the pattern of extractability and content of HA as a function of aging. It was observed that with increasing age, there was a steady decline in the HA content of the upper epidermis, and a consistent rise in the HA content in the basal layer of the epidermis and in the upper portion of the papillary dermis. In aged senile skin, HA was absent from the epidermis but still present in the upper dermis (51). It was observed that neither the total concentration nor the polymer size of HA in the skin changed with increased age. However, there were differences in extractability as a function of age. It is theorized that the level of bound HA increases with increasing age and that this change may be related to the gross changes observed in aged skin.

Other investigators have reported that the HA content of skin decreases with increasing age (52,53); however, differences in extractability may account for these observations.

III. HYALURONAN IN WOUND REPAIR

A. Wound Repair Process

Skin repair in the adult following injury proceeds through four overlapping phases: homeostasis, inflammation, proliferation, and remodeling (54). At the time of injury, homeostatic mechanisms, including vasoconstriction, platelet aggregation, and fibrin deposition, are initiated to control local bleeding. The fibrin matrix acts as a scaffold on which inflammatory cells enter the wound (54,55). The inflammatory changes, which occur over a period of 12 to 72 hr, include accumulation of neutrophils at 12 to 24 hr, followed by macrophage infiltration at 48 to 72 hr. A dramatic increase in HA and fibronectin occurs at the same time as the macrophage infiltration is observed. Macrophages secrete various growth factors that enhance fibroplasia (56,57) and stimulate the influx of fibroblasts into the wound, where they are stimulated to proliferate and produce collagen. As fibroblast activity continues, the initial fibrin matrix is replaced by collagen. Remodeling of the wound matrix continues for years after injury due to the continuous synthesis and degradation of collagen. In adult healing, a collagenous scar is formed, which lacks the ordered structure of normal skin.

In contrast, repair of early-gestation fetal skin occurs in the absence of acute inflammation, without excessive fibroblast infiltration, and without massive collagen deposition. The healed wound resembles normal skin and, hence, reflects a regenerative-like process. Fetal skin repair occurs in the presence of abundant HA throughout the repair process (weeks), whereas in adult skin repair, HA levels peak at 2 to 4 days and then fall rapidly. Experimental studies have produced results that indicate that HA is critical to the ability of fetal wounds to heal by regeneration. In one study, application of *Streptomyces* hyaluronidase in fetal rabbit wounds (to reduce the HA content of the wound) resulted in increased fibroplasia, collagen deposition, and capillary formation (58). The results demonstrate that HA affects the cellular and matrix events in fetal healing and suggest that HA plays an important role in the process of fetal regeneration (58,59).

It is notable that only fetal skin and fetal bony tissue heal without scar formation; fetal wounds in muscles, tendons, and the gastrointestinal tract heal by fibrosis and contraction, as in the adult (60).

B. Exogenous Hyaluronan and Wound Repair (Adult)

1. Cutaneous Studies—In Vivo

In the early 1970s it was observed that application of high-molecular-weight ($>1 \times 10^6$ MW), purified HA to surgical incisions, which included controlled abrasion to the muscular fascia in rabbits, primates, and guinea pigs, decreased granulation tissue and fibrosis in 32 of 39 animals (7). In 32 animals, the subcutaneous scar on the HA-treated side was notably smoother, with less connective tissue reaction. Each animal served as its own control; identical surgical incisions and procedures were performed at two parallel sites on the body with only one side treated with HA. The investigators suggested that HA reduced the fibrotic reaction in wounds because of its physical property of viscoelasticity, which may enable it to provide a barrier-type effect to the factors and cells involved in tissue ingrowth and also to the effect of HA on cells of the inflammatory process.

The effects of ultrapure hyaluronan of different molecular weights ($>1 \times 10^6$, 100,000, and 10,000) were evaluated in a full-thickness (2 cm^2) wound healing model in female, large white pigs (61). Two hundred micrograms of each HA preparation (in 0.2 ml) was applied to each wound and the wound covered with a vapor-permeable dressing (Cutifilm). The model corresponds closely to the "wet" wound healing model (62). The results indicated that parameters of wound repair—wound contraction, angiogenesis, and wound strength (breaking strength)—were affected differently by HA of different molecular weights. High-molecular-weight HA enhanced the rate of early wound contraction; breaking strength at 21 days was reduced by high- and intermediate-molecular-weight hyaluronan. Angiogenesis was measured using a scanning laser (Doppler technique) and showed depression by high- and intermediate-molecular-weight hyaluronan on day 3, but all preparations of HA caused elevated blood flow on day 7. Histological differences due to treatment were not detected. In this study, as in others cited, the amount of hyaluronan applied to the wound is relatively small (200 µg/2 cm^2, applied as a dilute solution with a concentration of 1 mg/ml). All wounds produced extremely well-organized granulation tissue, indicative of the "normal" nature of these wounds and the difficulty in demonstrating improvement in wounds that heal "normally" (63).

In a different type of study using superficial wounds in normal and diabetic rat epithelium, Abatangelo et al. (8) observed that application of 2% HA (sterile, extracted from rooster comb tissue, Fidia), 2 ml applied every 8 hours, enhanced epithelium migration and differentiation, ultimately accelerating wound healing. The investigators observed a reduction in tissue fibrosis in HA-treated wounds. The dermal thickness of wound areas was measured at 24-hr intervals and was found to be consistently greater in HA-treated animals. Similarly, the epithelial cellularity (vertical cell counts through regenerated epithelial sheets) was increased in HA-treated wounds. The effects in diabetic and normal rats were similar; however, in diabetic rats, HA treatment had a more pronounced effect. The HA effect in diabetic rats may be related to the finding that markedly decreased HA levels are found in the skin of alloxan-diabetic rats (64,65). In diabetic rats, the HA-deficient extracellular matrix may be inadequate to support efficient cell migration and activity. The results are consistent with the regulatory function of the extracellular matrix and the ability of the HA component to influence cell behavior and reactivity.

In contrast, Bettinger et al. (66) reported in 1996 that HA (1.5% concentration, $<1 \times 10^6$ MW) applied to skin graft donor sites (partial-thickness wound) in human volunteers did not accelerate wound healing and there was no difference in the gross appearance of the resultant scar at 6 weeks and 3 months. However, in this study the test articles (1.5% HA and 1.5% glycerin, 0.5 ml per $1 \times 1 \times 0.16''$ wound site) were covered with an occlusive dressing (Tegaderm). Factors that may have affected the outcome of this study include the occlusive environment of the wound site (due to the application of Tegaderm occlusive dressing), the low molecular weight of the HA preparation, and the relatively small amount of HA applied to the wound site.

In clinical studies, cutaneous ulcers in human volunteers were treated topically with exogenous HA (MW $\cong 1 \times 10^6$). HA was found to have a beneficial effect in that healing was enhanced, based on clinical and histological studies, and was judged to be better than with conventional treatments (67–71).

2. Organ Culture

In 1998, Iocono et al. (15) used cultured mouse limbs harvested from time-dated pregnant CD-1 mice on gestational day 18 (term, 20 days). Each limb was wounded using a 1-mm microscapel (through/through stab wound) and the wound was closed with a single nylon suture before amputation and placement in organ culture. Half the cultures received HA applied directly to the wound site (4 mg/ml, final concentration 0.4 mg/ml), while the remainder received culture medium without HA. On day 7 the limbs were harvested and evaluated histologically by two observers unaware of the treatment regimen. The tissue sections were graded for healing by scarring, with scarring defined by the presence of thick, parallel collagen bundles beneath the epidermis under polarized light. In HA-treated organ culture limb wounds, the collagen fiber bundles had a basketweave pattern that was indistinguishable from unwounded dermis, while in control wounds, the collagen fiber bundles were in parallel arrays perpendicular to the incision, consistent with scar formation. The investigators concluded that direct repeated application of HA to wounds in limb explants promoted scarless repair and proposed that maintaining elevated levels of HA in adult wounds may decrease or eliminate scarring (15).

3. Tympanic Membrane

In the 1980s, studies in human volunteers with perforated tympanic membranes of the middle ear revealed that treatment with highly purified, 1%, high-molecular-weight HA (Healon®) resulted in more rapid healing with less scar formation (9). In tympanic membranes treated with 1% HA, the structural quality was improved, and as early as 2 weeks after closure, the tympanic membrane scar was partly transparent. Histological analysis revealed improved structural organization as compared with controls, with HA-treated tympanic membranes notably thinner and with a well-restored connective tissue layer with few fibroblasts and collagen fibers oriented parallel to the epithelial surface.

The investigators theorized that in the HA-enriched environment, cell motility was enhanced and that perhaps the prolonged presence of HA at the wound site was similar to the conditions in the fetal skin wound in which HA levels remain high for prolonged period of time throughout the healing process (6).

4.　Hamster Cheek Pouch Biopsy Model

The effect of HA on wound healing in the hamster cheek pouch model was evaluated (10). In this model, a 2-mm diameter hole was cut through the entire tissue with a biopsy punch. The wound was patched with a pellet of absorbable gelatin sponge (Gelfoam®) soaked either in water or HA solution (1.6 mg/ml, in water). The HA used in this study was highly purified and of high molecular weight (2–4 $\times$ 10^{6}MW). Sponges (control and HA-soaked) were reapplied at 1, 3, 5, and 7 days postinjury. Fluorescein isothiocyanate dextran was injected intravenously for quantitation of macromolecular permeability at 2-day intervals (intravital microscopy). In control wounds at early time points, the repair site was surrounded by widespread extravasation of the fluorescent tracer, an index of inflammation. In HA-treated animals, there was a 66% reduction in the area of extravasation of the fluorescent tracer. Histological differences were not remarkable. Wound size decreased almost twice as fast in HA-treated animals compared with controls. Healing required 16 or more days in the control group but averaged fewer than 9 days in the presence of HA.

The effects of HA in this model are difficult to attribute simply to the physical properties of the HA used, since a significant dilution (1.6 mg/ml) produced only a slightly elastoviscous solution. The investigators suggested that HA may have enhanced healing through its interaction with inflammatory cells and as part of a process in which cell proliferation, migration, and differentiation are modulated. The role of HA in maintenance of tissue hydration, which is well known to have a beneficial effect on healing, may also participate in the mechanism of HA acceleration of healing in this model. In addition, the use of a support matrix (Gelfoam) localizes the HA to the site of injury. Therefore, even at this low concentration of HA, there may have been sufficient prolonged contact with the wound site to produce desirable biological effects.

5.　HA Receptor Studies (CD44, RHAMM)

To evaluate the potential effects of HA, Savani et al. (40) developed synthetic peptides that have various HA-binding capacities. Peptides were evaluated for their effects on fibroblast locomotion and neutrophil and macrophage chemotaxis. Synthetic peptides with strong HA-binding capacity significantly inhibited fibroblast locomotion and chemotaxis of neutrophils and macrophages, while control peptides, consisting of the same amino acids arranged randomly, had no effect.

A rat pouch biopsy in vivo model was used to evaluate the in vivo effect of HA-binding peptides (receptor antagonists). Scrambled peptide was used as a control. In addition, expression of the HA receptor RHAMM was measured during skin repair, and was found to increase in migrating epithelial cells closing the wound, in macrophages accumulating at the wound site 2 days after injury, and in fibroblasts at later stages of repair. Application of peptide antagonists appears to decrease macrophage accumulation at the wound site at 24 hr; at 4 weeks there was decreased collagen alignment and wound contracture. The investigators suggested that HA receptor interactions are critical to the process of inflammation, and subsequent fibrosis, and the HA-binding peptides may provide a means of influencing the inflammatory process. These findings are interesting and may be considered consistent with the observations from many studies regarding the effects of HA in wound repair, specifically in the ability of HA to modify inflammatory processes and fibrosis (7,33,37,38,72). The precise actions of the synthetic peptide cannot be determined from the information provided in the report. During in vitro cell culture studies, in which very little HA would be present, the addition of the peptide had a rather dramatic effect, unlikely to be due solely to the interruption of HA receptor binding. In addition, the effect may indicate that the peptide itself interacts with the receptor, providing actions similar to those of HA. Since an HA control was not included in the studies, it is not possible to conclude that results would have been similar in the presence of supplemental HA and/or peptide. The use of synthetic peptides as a means of controlling inflammation and fibrosis is an interesting research tool for the elucidation of these processes. However, the potential undesirable immunological and biological effects of introducing exogenous foreign peptide substances to an active wound site must be considered and assessed more fully prior to practical, clinical use.

6. Artificial Skin

Collagen-based artificial skin (Terudermis®) was soaked in 0.3% HA (Seikagaku) in phosphate-buffered saline and grafted into skin defects in rats. Control grafts were soaked in normal saline solution. Full-thickness wounds were made on the right and left sides of the back (1.5 × 1.5 cm) on either side of the spine. On each rat the wound on the left was covered with a control graft and the wound on the right was covered with an HA-treated graft. Tissues were harvested at 7 and 14 days for histological analysis. In the presence of HA, there was greater cellular tuft infiltration and an increased number of capillaries in the graft as compared with the control (73).

The results indicated that HA imbibed into an artificial skin induced more connective tissue and blood vessel formation than in artificial skin alone. This was a beneficial effect in that an accelerated ingrowth of granulation tissue provided a more suitable graft bed for the subsequent split-thickness skin graft that must be applied. The graft bed is essential to the survival of the grafted skin, and therefore a dense network of capillaries and fibroblasts in the graft bed is of great advantage. The mechanism of the observed response in this model is not known; however, the presence of a high concentration of low-molecular-weight HA at the site may affect angiogenic activity as HA degradation products have been implicated as important regulatory molecules that control cellular functions involved in new blood vessel formation in the healing wound (59,74).

7. Effect of Hyaluronan on Collagen Matrix Contracture

Scar contraction is the process by which the area of lost tissue in open wounds is concentrically decreased, facilitating repair of wounds in which tissue loss is substantial. However, prevention of scar contraction is desirable in order to reduce scarring. It has been proposed that a primary effect of HA on tissue repair is to prevent overcontraction and formation of scarring (75). The effect of HA on inhibition of wound contraction was demonstrated in an in vitro floating collagen fibrillar matrix (CFM) contraction model. Contraction by fibroblasts was significantly reduced when concentrations of HA (>1mg/ml, MW $1–2 \times 10^6$) were present in the media. Low concentrations of HA did not produce this effect, nor did chondroitin sulfate. The investigators theorized that high concentrations of HA may serve as a barrier to interrupt the communication between fibroblasts and collagen, or as a matrix that facilitates fibroblast migration and thereby decreases CFM contraction. The investigators also stated that viscosity alone is not a major factor in inhibiting CFM contraction; however, the effect of low-viscosity, high-concentration HA (low MW) preparations was not evaluated. Therefore, it is difficult to conclude that viscosity is not important since this conclusion was based only on results from testing with carboxymethylcellulose (CMC) and NOCC (*N,o*-carboxymethylchitosan), and not on results generated using a low-viscosity HA preparation. If the low-viscosity HA produced the desired effect, only then could one conclude that viscosity is not important.

IV. SUMMARY AND CONCLUSIONS

The effects of topical exogenous HA on the healing of dermal wounds have been investigated by many independent investigators in recent years. Most researchers have found that HA provides a beneficial effect with regard to the quality of tissue repair scar formation (8–12,15). The results indicate that the greatest benefit is achieved using highly purified, high-molecular-weight HA at a concentration >1 mg/ml and under conditions in which the HA is maintained at the wound site on a continuous basis for a prolonged period of time. In studies in which HA failed to promote or enhance the wound repair process, the conditions under which testing was conducted were suboptimal in that the HA preparation was inadequate (concentration, molecular weight, viscoelasticity, purity), the HA was not maintained at the wound site, or another condition was present that adversely affected the wound repair activities, for example, the use of an occlusive secondary dressing (66).

The purity of exogenous HA is critical in order to limit contaminating substances, such as proteins, endotoxin, etc., which may be inflammatory in nature and may produce undesirable biological effects. When placed into a wound bed, impure HA may lead to a protracted inflammatory phase, which is associated with increased tissue damage and fibrosis. Molecular weight and viscoelasticity are important to the formation of a viscoelastic barrier and to the maintenance of continuous and prolonged contact with the injured tissue surface. Low-molecular-weight and/or very dilute HA preparations rapidly diffuse from the injured site, although in some model systems this condition is overcome through artificial means, such as in organ culture and biopsy models.

HA is unlikely to be the sole factor in regulating wound repair; however, compelling features of the biological effects of HA suggest that its presence may be a key factor. For example, no other natural or synthetic polymer exhibits the multiple and diverse effects attributed to HA. In addition, HA modulates inflammation through its effect on polymorphonuclear cells, macrophages, lymphomyeloid migration, chemotacic gradients, phagocytosis, generation of free radicals by polymorphonuclear cells (PMN), and, finally, as a high-capacity scavenger for free radicals. Each of these activities is pertinent when one considers that a protracted inflammatory response has been implicated in the development of fibrotic tissue and excessive collagen deposition (76,77).

Also, in adult wound healing, the inflammatory phase is substantial, protracted, and accompanied by the presence of elevated enzyme levels, proteolytic degradation, and subsequent loss of fibrinolytic activity. Loss of fibrinolytic activity results in accumulation of fibrin (instead of its removal), which leads to excessive collagen deposition. It may be envisioned that by maintaining HA at the wound site there is enhanced modulation of inflammation and fibrinolytic activity is preserved; fibrin does not accumulate and excessive collagen deposition does not occur.

Evolution, perhaps, is responsible for the current state of adult wound repair, in which a robust inflammatory phase has evolved that optimizes the conditions for an excessive but effective response, and one in which the chances for successful repair, i.e., wound closure, are optimized. The decline in HA content after only a few days in adult wounds facilitates the development of a marked acute inflammatory response that not only removes bacteria and foreign matter, but also creates a situation of elevated cytokine levels, high proteolytic activity, and elevated growth factor and free radical levels.

It has been proposed that HA–fibrinogen interaction or binding plays a key structural role in the organization of the fibrin matrix. This interaction may facilitate cell infiltration and migration into the matrix (55,78) and may influence the collagen matrix that forms. Scientific evidence is not described which supports the proposed mechanism; however, it has been established that there is a specific binding interaction between HA and fibrinogen (79,80).

A procoagulant effect of HA on fibrin formation has also been proposed (78). However, the results from coagulation and fibrin(ogen) studies do not support such a procoagulant effect (80). In fact, the presence of HA (0.5–1 mg/ml) was found to reduce the rate of fibrin gel formation. Under the same conditions, when the absorbance at 450 nm is measured, there is an observed increase in the rate and magnitude of absorbance. However, the same effect is observed when other viscous natural polymers, such as DNA, are present with the fibrinogen during fibrin formation.

The optical density results suggest that the presence of HA has a physical effect on the fibrin matrix that forms. Since HA has the capacity to interact with, and bind to, the fibrinogen molecule, it may be through this mechanism that HA influences, or perhaps limits, fibrin formation.

It is important to note once again that there are marked differences between adult and fetal skin wound healing, and many of these differences could be affected by the continuous presence of HA at the wound sites, as presented in Table 1.

Table 1 Differences Between Adult and Fetal Healing

	Adult	Fetal	Role of HA
Fluid environment	No	Yes	Hydration
Sterile environment	No	Yes	Barrier matrix
Acute inflammation	Yes	No	Chemotactic gradient, lymphomyeloid cell migration, free radical scavenger
Scab formation	Yes	No	Fibrinogen/HA interaction
Speed to closure	Slower	Faster	Epithelial migration
Epithelialization	Slower	Faster	Epithelial migration
Underlying cell growth	Absent	Present	Inflammatory cell movement, fluid environment
Matrix deposition	Slower	Faster	HA/fibrinogen interaction
Scar formation	Yes	No	HA/fibrinogen interaction

Source: Ref. 81.

The results from studies conducted under highly controlled conditions, such as in organ culture and biopsy models, support a pivotal role for HA in bringing about more normal skin regeneration.

It is the common goal of many investigators and physicians to have the ability to positively influence the outcome of adult skin tissue repair in the clinical setting. Most importantly, they wish to balance the normal biological activities of repair with those conditions that promote regeneration and reduced scar or scarless repair. Indeed, the application of exogenous HA will be critical to the achievement of this goal: normal skin regeneration in the adult wound.

REFERENCES

1. Meyer K. Chemical structure of hyaluronic acid. Fed Proc 1958; 17:1075–1077.
2. Reed RK, Lilja K, Laurent TC. Hyaluronan in the rat with special reference to the skin. Acta Physiol Scand 1988; 134:405–411.
3. Laurent TC, Fraser JRE. Hyaluronan. FASEB J 1992; 6:2397–2406.
4. Bently JP. Mucopolysaccharide synthesis in wound healing. In: Dunphy JE, Van Winkle Jr. W, eds. Repair and Regeneration. New York: McGraw-Hill, 1968:151–160.
5. Juhlin L. Hyaluronan in skin. J Int Med 1997; 242:61–66.
6. Longaker MT, Chiu ES, Adzick NS, Stern M, Harrison MR, Stern R. Studies in fetal wound healing. V. A prolonged presence of hyaluronic acid characterizes fetal wound fluid. Ann Sug 1991; 213:292–296.
7. Rydell N. Decreased granulation tissue reaction after installment of hyaluronic acid. Acta Orthop Scand 1970; 41:307–311.
8. Abatangelo G, Martelli M, Vecchia P. Healing of hyaluronic acid-enriched wounds: histological observations. J Surg Res 1983; 35:410–416.
9. Hellstrom S, Laurent C. Hyaluronan and healing of tympanic membrane perforations. An experimental study. Acta Otolaryngol (Stockh) 1987; 442:54–61.
10. King SR, Hickerson WL, Proctor KG, Newsome AM. Beneficial actions of exogenous hyaluronic acid on wound healing. Surgery 1991; 109:76–84.
11. Mast BA, Flood LC, Haynes JH. Hyaluronic acid is a major component of the matrix of the fetal rabbit skin and wounds: implications for healing by regeneration. Matrix 1991; 11:63–68.
12. Longaker MT, Whitby DJ, Jennings RW. Adult skin in the fetal environment heals with scar formation. Surg Forum 1990; 41:639–641.
13. Balazs EA, Band PA, Denlinger JL, Goldman AI, Larsen NE, Leshchiner EA, Leshchiner A, Morales B. Matrix engineering. Blood Coag Fibrinol 1991; 2:173–178.
14. Balazs EA, Denlinger JL. Clinical uses of hyaluronan. In: Evered D, Whelan J, eds. The Biology of Hyaluronan. New York: John Wiley, 1989:265–280.
15. Iocono J, Ehrlich HP, Keefer KA, Krummel TM. Hyaluronan induces scarless repair in mouse limb organ culture. J Pediatr Surg 1998; 33:564–567.
16. Balazs EA. Physical chemistry of hyaluronic acid. Fed Proc 1958; 17:1086–1093.

17. Balazs EA. Sediment volume and viscoelastic behavior of hyaluronic acid solutions. Fed Proc 1966; 25:1817–1822.

18. Gibbs DA, Merrill EW, Smith KA, Balazs EA. Rheology of hyaluronic acid. Biopolymers 1968; 6:777–791.

19. Balazs EA, Gibbs DA. The rheological properties and biological function of hyaluronic acid. In: Chemistry and Molecular Biology of the Intercellular Matrix. New York: Academy, 1970:1241–1253.

20. Dea IC, Moorhouse R, Rees DA, Arnott S, Guss JM, Balazs EA. Hyaluronic acid: a novel, double helical molecule. Science 1973; 179:560–562.

21. Comper WD, Laurent TC. Physiological function of connective tissue polysaccharides. Physiol Rev 1978; 58:255–315.

22. Richter W. Non-immunogenicity of purified hyaluronic acid preparations tested by passive cutaneous anaphylaxis. Int Arch Allergy Appl Immunol 1974; 47:211–217.

23. Richter W, Ryde E, Zetterström EO. Non-immunogenicity of purified sodium hyaluronate preparations in man. Int Arch Allergy Appl Immunol 1979; 59:45–48.

24. Schiller S, Mathews MB, Goldfaber L, Ludowieg J, Dorfman A. The metabolism of mucopolysaccharides in animals. II. Studies in skin utilizing labeled acetate. J Biol Chem 1955; 212:531–535.

25. Schiller S, Mathews MB, Cifonelli JA, Dorfman A. The metabolism of mucopolysaccharides in animals. III. Further studies on skin utilizing C^{14}glucose, C^{14} acetate, and S^{32}sodium sulfate. J Biol Chem 1956; 218:139–145.

26. Schiller S, Dorfman A. The metabolism of mucopolysaccharides in animals. IV. The influence of insulin. J Biol Chem 1957; 218:139–145.

27. Schiller S, Dorfman A. The metabolism of mucopolysaccharides in animals: the effect of cortisone and hydrocortisone on rat skin. Endocrinology 1957; 60:376–381.

28. Schiller S, Slover GA, Dorfman A. Effect of the thyroid gland on metabolism of acid mucopolysaccharides in skin. Biochim Biophys Acta 1962; 58:27–33.

29. Hardingham TE, Phelps CF. The tissue content and turnover rates of intermediates in the biosynthesis of glycosaminoglycans in young rat skin. Biochem J 1968; 108: 9–16.

30. Laurent UBG, Dahl LB, Reed RK. Catabolism of hyaluronan in rabbit skin takes place locally, in lymph nodes and liver. Exp Physiol 1991; 76:695–703.

31. Laurent TC, Fraser JRE. The properties and turnover of hyaluronan. In: Functions of the Proteoglycans. Chichester: Wiley, 1986:9–29.

32. Fraser JRE, Laurent TC, Engström-Laurent A, Laurent UGB. Elimination of hyaluronic acid from the blood stream in the human. Clin Exp Pharmacol Physiol 1984; 11:17–25.

33. Balazs EA, Denlinger JL. Clinical uses of hyaluronan. In: Evered D, Whelan J, eds. The Biology of Hyaluronan. New York: John Wiley, 1989: 265–280.

34. Tammi R, Ripellino JA, Margolis RU, Tammi M. Localization of epidermal hyaluronic acid using the hyaluronate binding region of cartilage proteoglycan as a specific probe. J Invest Dermatol 1988; 90:412–414.

35. Ghersetich I, Lotti T, Campanile G, Grappone C, Dini G. Hyaluronic acid in cutaneous intrinsic aging. Int J Dermatol 1994; 33:119–122.

36. Darzynkiewicz Z, Balazs EA. Effect of connective tissue intercellular matrix on

lymphocyte stimulation. I. Suppression of lymphocyte stimulation by hyaluronic acid. Exp Cell Res 1971; 66:113–123.

37. Balazs EA, Darzynkiewicz Z. The effect of hyaluronic acid on fibroblasts, mononuclear phagocytes and lymphocytes. In: Kulonen E, Pikkarainen J, eds. Biology of the Fibroblast. London: Academic, 1973:237–252.

38. Forrester JV, Balazs EA. Inhibition of phagocytosis by high molecular weight hyaluronate. Immunology 1980; 40:435–446.

39. Forrester JV, Wilkinson PC. Inhibition of leukocyte locomotion by hyaluronic acid. J Cell Sci 1981; 44:315–331.

40. Savani RC, Khalil N, Turley EA. Hyaluronan receptor antagonists alter skin inflammation and fibrosis following injury. West Pharmacol Soc 1995; 38:131–136.

41. Messadi DV, Bertolami CN. CD44 and hyaluronan expression in human cutaneous scar fibroblasts. Am J Pathol 1993; 142:1041–1049.

42. Toole BP. Hyaluronan and its binding proteins, the hyaladherins. Curr Opin Cell Biol 1990; 2:839–844.

43. Wang C, Tammi M, Tammi R. Distribution of hyaluronan and its CD44 receptor in the epithelia of human skin appendages. Histochemistry 1992; 98:105–112.

44. Alho AM, Underhill CB. The hyaluronate receptor is preferentially expressed on proliferating epithelial cells. J Cell Biol 1989; 108:1557–1565.

45. Green SJ, Tarone G, Underhill CB. Distribution of hyaluronate and hyaluronate receptors in the adult lung. J Cell Sci 1988; 90:145–156.

46. Bazil V, Horejsi V. Shedding of the CD44 adhesion molecule from leukocytes induced by anti-CD44 monoclonal antibody simulating the effect of a natural receptor ligand. J Immunol 1992; 149:747–753.

47. Underhill CB, Nguyen HA, Shizari M, Culty M. CD44 positive macrophages take up hyaluronan during lung development. Dev Biol 1993; 155:324–336.

48. Pilarski LA, Miszta H, Turley EA. Regulated expression of a receptor for hyaluronan-mediated motility on human thymocytes and T cells. J Immunol 1993; 150: 4292–4302.

49. Sherman L, Sleeman J, Herrlich P, Ponta H. Hyaluronate receptors: key players in growth, differentiation, migration and tumor progression. Curr Opin Cell Biol 1994; 6:726–733.

50. Penneys NS. CD44 expression in normal and inflamed skin. J Cutaneous Pathol 1993; 20:250–253.

51. Meyer LJ, Stern R. Age-dependent changes of hyaluronan in human skin. J Invest Derm 1994; 102:385–389.

52. Longas MO, Russell CS, He XY. Evidence for structural changes in dermatan sulfate and hyaluronic acid with aging. Carbohydr Res 1987; 159:127–136.

53. Fleischmajer R, Perlish JS, Bashey RI. Human dermal glycosaminoglycans and aging. Biochim Biophys Acta 1972; 279:265–275.

54. Schilling JA. Wound Healing. Surg Clin North Am 1976; 56:869–874.

55. Weigel PH, Fuller GM, LeBouef RD. A model for the role of hyaluronic acid and fibrin in the early events during the inflammatory response and wound healing. J Theor Biol 1986; 119:219–234.

56. Leibovich DS, Ross R. The role of the macrophage in wound repair. A study with hydrocortisone and antimacrophage serum. Am J Pathol 1975; 78:71–100.

57. Diegelmann RF, Cohen IK, Kaplan AM. The role of macrophages in wound repair. A review. Plast Reconstr Surg 1981; 68:107–113.

58. Mast BA, Haynes JH, Krummel TM, Diegelmann RF, Cohen IK. In vivo degradation of fetal wound hyaluronic acid results in increased fibroplasia, collagen deposition and neurovascularization. Plast Reconstr Surg 1992; 89:503–509.

59. West DC, Kumar S. The effect of hyaluronate and its oligosaccharides on endothelial cell proliferation and monolayer integrity. Exp Cell Res 1989; 183:179–196.

60. Laurent C. The action of hyaluronan on repair processes in the middle ear. In: Laurent TC, ed. The Chemistry, Biology and Medical Applications of Hyaluronan and Its Derivatives. London: Portland, 1998:283–289.

61. Arnold F, Jia C, He C, Cherry GW, Carbow B, Meyer-Ingold W, Bader D, West DC. Hyaluronan, hetergeneity, and healing: the effects of ultrapure hyaluronan of defined molecular size on the repair of full-thickness pig skin wounds. Wound Repair Regen 1995; 3:299–310.

62. Breuing K, Eriksson E, Liu P, Miller D. Healing of partial thickness porcine wounds in a liquid environment. J Surg Res 1991; 52:50–58.

63. Arnold F, West DC. Angiogenesis in wound healing. Pharmacol Ther 1992; 52: 407–422.

64. Schiller J, Dorfman A. The distribution of acid mucopolysaccharides in skin of diabetic rats. Biochim Biophys Acta 1963; 78:371.

65. Schiller J, Dorfman A. The metabolism of mucopolysaccharides in animals. The influence of insulin. J Biol Chem 1957; 227:625.

66. Bettinger DA, Mast B, Gore D. Hyaluronic acid impedes reepithelialization of skin graft donor sites. J Burn Care Rehab 1996; 17:302–304.

67. Passarini B, Tosti A, Fanti PA, Varotti C. [Effect of hyaluronic acid on the reparative process of non-healing ulcers. Comparative study]. G Ital Dermatol Venereol 1982; 117:27–30 [Italian].

68. Torregrossa F, Caroti A. [Clinical verification of the use of topical hyaluronic acid under non-adhesive gauze in the therapy of torpid ulcers]. G Ital Dermatol Venereol 1983; 118:41–44 [Italian].

69. Venturini D. [Clinical observations on the use of hyaluronic acid in dermatologic therapy]. G Ital Dermatol Venereol 1985; 120:5–10 [Italian].

70. Celleno L, Piperno S, Bracaglia R. [Clinico-experimental studies on the use of hyaluronic acid in skin healing processes]. G Ital Dermatol Venereol 1985; 120:47–56 [Italian].

71. Retanda G. [Hyaluronic acid in the process of reparation of cutaneous ulcers. Clinical experience]. G Ital Dermatol Venereol 1985; 120:71–75 [Italian].

72. Rydell N, Balazs EA. Effect of intra-articular injection of hyaluronic acid on the clinical symptoms of osteoarthritis and on granulation tissue formation. Clin Orthop 1971; 80:25–32.

73. Murashita T, Nakayoma T, Hirano T, Ohashi S. Acceleration of granulation tissue ingrowth by hyaluronic acid in artificial skin. Br J Plast Surg 1996; 49:58–63.

74. West DC, Hampson IN, Arnold F, Kumar S. Angiogenesis induced by degradation products of hyaluronic acid. Science 1985; 228:1324–1326.

75. Huang-Lee LLH, Wu JH, Nimni ME. Effects of hyaluronan on collagen fibrillar matrix contraction by fibroblasts. J Biomed Mater Res 1994; 28:123–132.

76. Schultz GS. Comparative tissue repair. The 3rd International Congress on Pelvic Surgery and Adhesion Prevention, San Diego, CA, Feb 29-Mar 2, 1996.

77. Frantz FW, Bettinger DA, Haynes JH, Johnson DE, Harney KM, Dalton HP, Yager DR, Diegelman RF, Cohen IK. Biology of fetal repair: the presence of bacteria in fetal wounds induces an adult-like healing response. J Pediatr Surg 1993; 28:428–434.

78. Weigel PH, Frost SJ, LeBoeuf RD, McGary CT. The specific interaction between fibrin(ogen) and hyaluronan: possible consequences in haemostasis, inflammation and wound healing. In: Evered D, Whelan J, eds. The Biology of Hyaluronan. New York: John Wiley, 1989:248–264.

79. LeBoeuf RD, Raja RH, Fuller GM, Weigel PH. Human fibrinogen specifically binds hyaluronic acid. J Biol Chem 1986; 261:12586–12592.

80. Larsen NE. Management of adhesion formation and soft tissue augmentation with viscoelastics: hyaluronan derivatives. In: Laurent TC, ed. The Chemistry, Biology and Medical Applications of Hyaluronan and its Derivatives. London: Portland, 1998:267–282.

81. Crombleholme TM. Response of fetal tissue to wounding. 3rd International Congress on Pelvic Surgery and Adhesion Prevention, San Diego, CA, Feb 29–Mar 2, 1996.

8

Molecular Mechanisms in Keloid Biology

William J. H. Kim and Howard Levinson
New York University Medical Center, New York, New York

George K. Gittes and Michael T. Longaker
New York University School of Medicine, New York, New York

I. INTRODUCTION

Keloids represent a pathological response to cutaneous injury creating disfiguring scars with no known satisfactory treatment. They are unique to humans and are characterized by an overabundant extracellular matrix (ECM) deposition, especially collagen (1). Clinically, the lesions characteristically extend beyond the boundaries of the original wound and are seen predominantly in darker-pigmented individuals, including African-Americans, Hispanics, and Asians (2). Keloids are benign skin ''tumors'' that can be caused by even minor skin injury, such as ear piercing. In general, excessive or pathological scar formation after trauma or surgery can have devastating consequences, such as body disfigurement and organ dysfunction. The exact pathogenic mechanisms underlying keloids continue to be elusive, though much of the research focus has recently been aimed at the biomolecular pathways responsible for excessive ECM accumulation. In this review, we discuss previous keloid research as well as focus attention on more recent progress made in the understanding of molecular mechanisms of keloid formation. These recent studies are aimed at providing a basis for the development of more effective keloid treatments.

II. ETIOLOGY OF KELOIDS

The term keloid is derived from the Greek *"khele,"* for crab claw (3). Keloids appear with equal frequency in males and females and may occur at any age, but they most often appear between the ages of 10 and 30 (4). They are typically raised, firm masses of hyperplastic connective tissue and fibroblasts.

Many potential pathways have been invoked as important in the pathogenesis of keloids. For example, the presence of numerous mast cells in keloids suggests a role of mast cells in keloid pathogenesis. Elevated mast cell histamine may be a contributing factor to the abnormal cell growth observed in keloid (5). Interestingly, histamine has been found to up-regulate procollagen type I production in keloid fibroblasts (6,7). Hormone overproduction states, such as hypersecretion of estrogen, hyperthyroidism, or adrenocortical hypersecretion, have all been associated with keloids (8). In addition, keloid fibroblasts exposed to tamoxifen (an estrogen antagonist) have decreased transforming growth factor-β (TGF-β) levels, decreased proliferation, and decreased collagen production (9).

An immune response may also be involved in keloid pathogenesis. Rossi et al. (10) reported that serum levels of immunoglobulin G (IgG), immunoglobulin M (IgM) and complement C3 and C4 were all normal in keloid patients. However, the extractable IgG from keloid tissue was significantly increased compared with that found in normal skin and normal scar controls, suggesting a localized immune response to the keloid. Class I human leukocyte antigen (HLA-A and -B) profiles did not show significant differences between keloid patients and controls. In contrast, class II (HLA-DR and -DQ) histocompatibility analyses in keloid patients showed a prevalence of HLA-DR5 and -DQw3 in keloid patients (10). Finally, higher incidence of circulating IgG complement has also been reported in keloid patients (11,12).

To our knowledge, keloids have never been reported in albino humans. Both autosomal dominant and autosomal recessive genetic inheritance patterns have been suggested for keloid patients, but the conflicting nature of reports make conclusions difficult (4,13). Keloid formation is often related to traumatic injury, but not every injury results in a keloid in patients who have formed keloids in the past. Local skin factors are believed to contribute to keloid formation. Increased skin tension, motion in the wound, dermal allergens, and infection have all been implicated in keloid formation (4,8). Keloids transplanted to an area of low skin tension have been shown to resolve spontaneously (14). Within a given keloid there may be regional variations in microenvironment. For example, the center of a keloid is relatively acellular compared with the periphery of the lesion.

III. CLINICAL CHARACTERISTICS AND TREATMENTS

Clinically, keloids appear as a scar that grows beyond the confines of the original wound and rarely regresses over time. Keloids may arise immediately after injury or years later. They have a propensity to form in melanocyte-rich regions such as the face, neck, deltoid, presternal area and ear lobes. In rare instances, they have also been reported to appear on the cornea (15,16). Malignant degeneration is rare and poorly documented at best (4). Patients often seek treatment for relief from pruritus, pain, mass effect, or for aesthetic reasons. In the past, several drugs have been investigated for the purpose of inhibiting collagen synthesis and accelerating the removal of excessive collagen deposited in keloids. Historically, these drugs have included collagen cross-linking inhibitors (β-aminoproprionitrile fumarate [BAPN] and penicillamine), antimicrotubular agents (colchicine), and corticosteroids. Alternative treatments with calcium channel blockers, radiation, laser, cryotherapy, chemotherapy, pressure therapy, and Silastic gel sheeting as yet all have unsatisfactory outcomes (8,17–21). Recurrence and side effects limit the utility of all of these treatments. Calcium channel blockers work by altering cell morphology and inhibiting the incorporation of proline into collagen (22,23). Typical keloid treatment currently consists of intralesional corticosteroid injections, used individually or in combination with surgery. Unfortunately, these lesions are often refractory to all therapy, underscoring the need for further research.

Keloids are frequently compared with hypertrophic scars. Their gross appearance is similar, although keloids grow beyond wound margins and rarely resolve (24). However, the two lesions are histologically distinct. Contrary to the orderly appearance of collagen fibers in normal skin or the fine, randomly organized fibers of hypertrophic scars, keloids have stretched collagen fibers aligned in the epidermal plane (25). The abundant collagen fibrils are thick, tightly packed, acellular structures in the deep dermal portion of the keloid. Keloid collagen does, however, appear to be of the same molecular type as collagen in normal skin (26). Keloids contain relatively few cells at their center and no myofibroblasts (27). In contrast, hypertrophic scars have connective tissue in nodular structures containing α-smooth muscle actin–positive fibroblasts with small blood vessels and fine, randomly oriented collagen fibrils (1). Keloids appear to be made up of a heterogenous population of cells that behave differently depending on their location. For example, cellular growth properties and production of collagen I vary among regions within a keloid (28).

IV. EXTRACELLULAR MATRIX REMODELING AND SYNTHESIS IN KELOID FIBROBLASTS

Tissue repair is accomplished through a complex cascade of events involving various cell types, extracellular matrix components, cytokines, and other soluble factors (29). A cascade of repair events begins with the formation of a fibrin-rich blood clot and ends with the restructuring of newly synthesized scar tissue. Several vital sequential stages have been identified in the repair process, namely inflammation, fibroplasia, granulation tissue, and scar maturation. Keloid fibroblasts show an elevated gene expression for collagen, fibronectin, elastin, and proteoglycan in vitro (30,31). Compared with normal dermal fibroblasts, keloid fibroblasts show an aberrant response to metabolic modulators, implicating their possible role in the pathogenesis of keloids (32).

In vitro studies have aided in the identification and characterization of many of the factors that play a role in wound healing. For example, keloid fibroblast gene expression may be altered greatly by interaction with the surrounding ECM. Many of these cell–ECM interactions are mediated through cell adhesion receptors called integrins (33). Integrin expression is regulated by cytokines in an autocrine and paracrine manner.

Proteolytic degradation of ECM is also an essential control point in tissue repair and remodeling. The serine proteases, including plasminogen activator (PA) and matrix metalloproteinases (MMPs), are ECM-degrading enzymes that provide a lytic cascade for ECM remodeling (34–36). The major function of PA is conversion of plasminogen into plasmin. Plasmin is a fibrinolytic enzyme that degrades ECM proteins and also converts procollagenase into its active collagenase form (37). Thus, PA initiates the proteolytic cascade. In turn, plasmin activates TGF-β by releasing it from its latency-associated peptide (38). TGF-β then acts on its target molecules regulating plasminogen activator inhibitor-1 (PAI-1), MMPs, tissue inhibitor of metalloproteinase-1 (TIMP-1), and genes encoding ECM components and their integrin receptors (39).

Controversy still exists as to whether keloids have increased collagen production, decreased degradation, or both. Prolyl hydroxylase, the rate-limiting enzyme in collagen synthesis, is up-regulated in keloids (3). Measurement of radioactive ^{14}C incorporation into hydroxyproline indicates an initial up-regulation of collagen synthesis in keloid followed by a return to baseline over two years (40). Increased PAI-1 expression at both the mRNA and protein levels is seen in keloid fibroblasts (41). Increased PAI-1 reduces plasmin-stimulated collagenase production and plasmin activity (42). As a result, keloid fibroblasts exhibit a decreased capacity for fibrinolysis and fibrin clot degradation (41). Although poorly understood, the elevated levels of PAI-1 by keloid fibroblasts may have significant consequences for the repair steps that follow fibrin clot dissolution.

The growth rate of keloid fibroblasts has also been studied. Higher numbers of proliferating fibroblasts are detected at the periphery of keloid lesions (28). Of interest, the center of keloids lack proliferating cells (43). Finally, multiple growth curves produced from in vitro cultures showed no difference between normal and keloid fibroblast growth kinetics (44).

V. TRANSFORMING GROWTH FACTOR-β SIGNAL TRANSDUCTION IN KELOIDS

Transforming growth factor-β has been implicated in the pathogenesis of keloids. TGF-β increases production of ECM elements, such as fibronectin and collagen, and up-regulates cellular expression of the matrix receptor integrins (39). Increased levels of TGF-β messenger ribonucleic acid (mRNA) and protein are associated with excessive collagen synthesis and ECM accumulation in keloids (45). Other studies have shown that keloid fibroblasts exhibit an altered response to the addition to exogenous TGF-β (46). It has been shown that keloids demonstrate an increase in synthesis of fibronectin, collagen, and DNA in response to TGF-β (31,46,47).

The three TGF-β isoforms identified in mammals (TGF-β1, -β2, and -β3) are thought to have different biological activities in wound healing (39). TGF-β1 and -β2 are believed to promote fibrosis and scar formation, while TGF-β3 has been shown to be both scar inducing and scar reducing in different situations (48,49). We recently found that TGF-β1 and -β2 proteins are highly expressed in keloid fibroblasts compared with normal human dermal fibroblasts. In contrast, the expression of TGF-β3 protein was comparable in both the normal and keloid cell lines (50).

The mechanism of TGF-β receptor signaling has been intensively studied to understand TGF-β–mediated cellular responses. TGF-β and its family members (activin and bone morphogenetic proteins) signal through heteromeric transmembrane serine/threonine kinases known as type I and type II receptors (51,52). Upon binding by TGF-β ligand, the activated type II receptor recruits type I receptor and phosphorylates the type I receptor. Numerous type I–like receptor proteins have been identified and the biological response to TGF-β in a given cell type appears to be defined by the particular type I receptor engaged in the complex. Receptor activation leads to phosphorylation of receptor-associated TAK1-binding proteins, which activate the TAK1 kinase cascade, or SMADs, a set of evolutionarily conserved proteins that translocate to the nucleus to activate transcription (51,53). TGF-β stimulates the synthesis of numerous ECM components (39). Keloid fibroblasts respond to TGF-β by further increasing their already augmented rate of collagen synthesis, a phenomenon not detected in fibroblasts from normal scar (31,47,54). The altered responses of keloid fibroblasts to TGF-β might reflect a change that occurs either at the receptor level or during postreceptor signaling (54).

Many groups are actively pursuing antagonists to TGF-β that regulate the phenotypes of connective tissue cells during repair. The clinical purpose of this work is to regulate excessive cell proliferation, as well as the synthesis and contraction of ECM during wound repair by scar fibroblasts. Approaches taken to antagonize TGF-β–stimulated fibrosis include the use of neutralizing anti–TGF-β antibodies, the use of naturally occurring TGF-β–binding proteoglycan decorin, and the use of mannose 6-phosphate, an antagonist of TGF-β activation (48,55,56).

VI. OTHER GROWTH FACTORS AND CYTOKINES IN KELOIDS

In addition to TGF-β, several cytokines and growth factors have been implicated in the pathogenesis of keloids, including epidermal growth factor (EGF), fibroblast growth factor (FGF), and platelet-derived growth factor (PDGF) (2,57). The release and activation of growth factors during the inflammatory phase of healing is a prerequisite for subsequent processes, including angiogenesis, reepithelialization, recruitment and proliferation of fibroblasts, and matrix deposition (58–60). Angiogenesis is stimulated by chemoattractants and mitogens, such as heparin, FGF, interleukin-8 (IL-8), and insulin-like growth factor-1 (IGF-1) (61). Wound reepithelialization occurs following the migration of epithelial cells from the wound margin and epidermal appendages. This process is enhanced by EGF, TGF-α, and IGF-1 (60,62).

Fibroblast recruitment, proliferation, and production of ECM are strongly influenced by the profibrotic growth factors PDGF, IGF-1, and TGF-β, as well as FGF-2 (39). These profibrotic growth factors up-regulate ECM protein production, increase the rate of proliferation and/or migration of fibroblasts, and inhibit the production of proteases required to maintain the balance between ECM production and degradation (2). Platelet-derived growth factor and connective tissue growth factor have been implicated in the biology underlying fibrosis, and are targets for therapeutic inhibition of fibrosis (63). Cytokines such as interleukin-1, tumor necrosis factor -α, and interferon-γ and -α, which all suppress the synthesis of collagen, have been used as antifibrotic agents in vitro and clinically (7,64).

Despite the recent advancement in therapeutic designs for fibroproliferative disorders, additional studies are still required to establish efficacy, timing, and optimal dosages of these potential agents for clinical application. Further studies are required to investigate the endogenous temporal and spatial expression of these agents during normal wound repair in order to understand the mechanisms regulating normal healing with a goal to manipulate pathological scarring.

VII. FUTURE DIRECTIONS

The difficulty in the treatment of keloids arises from the complexity of the molecular and cellular biology of keloids. The potential mechanisms in keloid formation are summarized in Figure 1. Increased understanding at each level of pathogenesis may lead to the development of new therapies. Control of profibrotic growth factor effects by monoclonal antibody techniques, growth factor receptor antagonists, and through the development of antisense oligonucleotide and gene therapies offers substantial potential. Further appreciation of the immunological response to injury and the regulation of wound healing by the immune system may allow specific growth factor therapy to down-regulate profibrotic signals. Finally, with intense pursuit of skin replacements and the enhanced understanding of the role of the dermis in regulating scar contracture and hypertrophy, skin replacement or wound tissue engineering may provide new therapies.

The complex nature of the repair process and the lack of proper in vitro and in vivo animals models for scar formation have hindered progress in revealing the mechanisms underlying pathological scar formation. Recent in vitro culture studies allow for a defined system with well-defined parameters (cell type, cell number, matrix type and concentration). These in vitro systems are well suited for some creative designs to investigate the mechanisms underlying both normal and abnormal healing processes.

Transgenic and knockout animals also provide a new approach to the investigation of gene function in vivo (60). For example, definitive proof of the involvement of plasmin in wound repair is provided by plasminogen-deficient mice (65). These mice exhibit severely impaired healing of skin wounds, abnor-

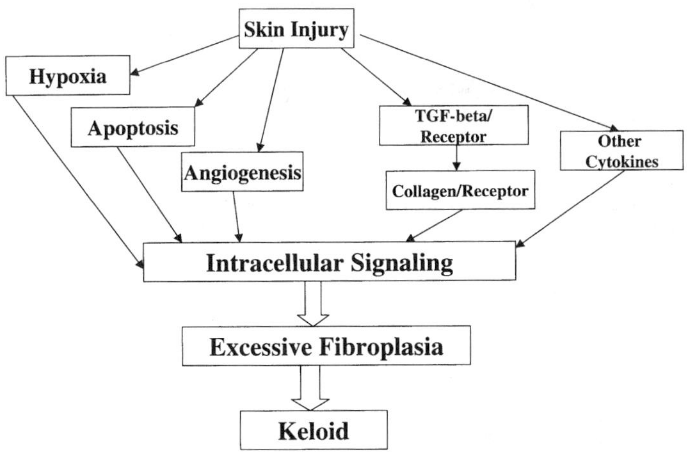

Figure 1 Theoretical model for molecular mechanisms in keloid. Upon injury, skin initiates cellular responses, such as hypoxia, apoptosis, angiogenesis, and cytokine-induced signaling, leading to excessive fibroplasia and eventually keloid formation.

mal keratinocyte migration, and protrusion of excessive granulation tissue in the middle of the wound, resembling a raised scar.

In this review, we discussed recent progress made in the understanding of molecular mechanisms of keloid scar formation. These ongoing studies will provide a basis for the development of more effective keloid treatments.

REFERENCES

1. Tredget EE, Nedelec B, Scott PG, Ghahary A. Hypertrophic scars, keloids, and contractures. The cellular and molecular basis for therapy. Surg Clin North Am 1997; 77(3):701–730.
2. Tuan TL, Nichter LS. The molecular basis of keloid and hypertrophic scar formation. Mol Med Today 1998; 4(1):19–24.
3. Ladin D. The art and science of wound care. Plast Reconstr Surg 1995; 96(3):748.
4. Murray JC, Pollack SV, Pinnell SR. Keloids: a review. J Am Acad Dermatol 1981; 4(4):461–470.
5. Russel JD, Russell SB, Trupin KM. The effect of histamine on the growth of cultured fibroblasts isolated from normal and keloid tissue. J Cell Physiol 1977; 93(3):389–393.
6. Kikuchi K, Kadono T, Takehara K. Effects of various growth factors and histamine on cultured keloid fibroblasts. Dermatology 1995; 190(1):4–8.
7. Tredget EE, Shankowsky HA, Pannu R, Nedelec B, Iwashina T, Ghahary A, Taerum TV, Scott PG. Transforming growth factor-beta in thermally injured patients with hypertrophic scars: effects of interferon alpha-2b. Plast Reconstr Surg 1998; 102(5): 1317–1328; discussion 1329–1330.
8. Oluwasanmi JO. Keloids in the African. Clin Plast Surg. 1974; 1(1):179–195.
9. Chau D, Mancoll JS, Lee S, Zhao J, Phillips LG, Gittes GK, Longaker MT. Tamoxifen downregulates TGF-beta production in keloid fibroblasts. Ann Plast Surg 1998; 40(5):490–493.
10. Rossi A, Bozzi M. HLA and keloids: antigenic frequency and therapeutic response. G Ital Dermatol Venereol 1989; 124(7–8):341–344.
11. Kazeem AA. The immunological aspects of keloid tumor formation. J Surg Oncol 1988; 38(1):16–18.
12. Bloch EF, Hall MG Jr, Denson MJ, Slay-Solomon V. General immune reactivity in keloid patients. Plast Reconstr Surg 1984; 73(3):448–451.
13. Omo-Dare P. Genetic studies on keloid. J Natl Med Assoc 1975; 67(6):428–432.
14. Calnan JS, Copenhagen HJ. Autotransplantation of keloid in man. Br J Surg 1967; 54(5):330–335.
15. Shoukrey NM, Tabbara KF. Ultrastructural study of a corneal keloid. Eye 1993; 7(pt 3):379–387.
16. Lahav M, Cadet JC, Chirambo M, Rehani U, Ishii Y. Corneal keloids—a histopathological study. Graefes Arch Clin Exp Ophthalmol 1982; 218(5):256–261.

17. Banfalvi T, Boer A, Remenar E, Oberna F. Treatment of keloids (review of the literature, therapeutic suggestions). Orv Hetil 1996; 137(34):1861–1864.

18. Hirshowitz B, Lindenbaum E, Har-Shai Y, Feitelberg L, Tendler M, Katz D. Static-electric field induction by a silicone cushion for the treatment of hypertrophic and keloid scars. Plast Reconstr Surg 1998; 101(5): 1173–1183.

19. Lawrence WT. Treatment of earlobe keloids with surgery plus adjuvant intralesional verapamil and pressure earrings. Ann Plast Surg 1996; 37(2):167–169.

20. Clavere P, Bedane C, Bonnetblanc JM, Bonnafoux-Clavere A, Rousseau J. Postoperative interstitial radiotherapy of keloids by iridium 192: a retrospective study of 46 treated scars. Dermatology 1997; 195(4):349–352.

21. Alster TS, Nanni CA. Pulsed dye laser treatment of hypertrophic burn scars. Plast Reconstr Surg 1998; 102(6):2190–2195.

22. Doong H, Dissanayake S, Gowrishankar TR, LaBarbera MC, Lee RC. The 1996 Lindberg Award. Calcium antagonists alter cell shape and induce procollagenase synthesis in keloid and normal human dermal fibroblasts. J Burn Care Rehabil 1996; 17(6 Pt 1):497–514.

23. Lee RC, Ping JA. Calcium antagonists retard extracellular matrix production in connective tissue equivalent. J Surg Res 1990; 49(5):463–466.

24. Nemeth AJ. Keloids and hypertrophic scars. J Dermatol Surg Oncol 1993; 19(8): 738–746.

25. Kelly AP. Keloids. Dermatol Clin 1988; 6(3):413–424.

26. Clore JN, Cohen IK, Diegelmann RF. Quantitative assay of types I and III collagen synthesized by keloid biopsies and fibroblasts. Biochim Biophys Acta 1979; 586(2): 384–390.

27. Ehrlich HP, Desmouliere A, Diegelmann RF, Cohen IK, Compton CC, Garner WL, Kapanci Y, Gabbiani G. Morphological and immunochemical differences between keloid and hypertrophic scar. Am J Pathol 1994; 145(1):105–113.

28. Appleton I, Brown NJ, Willoughby DA. Apoptosis, necrosis, and proliferation: possible implications in the etiology of keloids. Am J Pathol 1996; 149(5):1441–1447.

29. Werb Z. ECM and cell surface proteolysis: regulating cellular ecology. Cell 1997; 91(4):439–442.

30. Kischer CW, Wagner HN Jr, Pindur J, Holubec H, Jones M, Ulreich JB, Scuderi P. Increased fibronectin production by cell lines from hypertrophic scar and keloid. Connect Tissue Res 1989; 23(4):279–288.

31. Babu M, Diegelmann R, Oliver N. Fibronectin is overproduced by keloid fibroblasts during abnormal wound healing. Mol Cell Biol 1989; 9(4):1642–1650.

32. Friedman DW, Boyd CD, Mackenzie JW, Norton P, Olson RM, Deak SB. Regulation of collagen gene expression in keloids and hypertrophic scars. J Surg Res 1993; 55(2):214–222.

33. Hynes RO. Integrins: versatility, modulation, and signaling in cell adhesion. Cell 1992; 69(1):11–25.

34. Lim YT, Sugiura Y, Laug WE, Sun B, Garcia A, DeClerck YA. Independent regulation of matrix metalloproteinases and plasminogen activators in human fibrosarcoma cells. J Cell Physiol 1996; 167(2):333–340.

35. Schnaper HW, Kopp JB, Poncelet AC, Hubchak SC, Stetler-Stevenson WG, Klotman PE, Kleinman HK. Increased expression of extracellular matrix proteins and

decreased expression of matrix proteases after serial passage of glomerular mesangial cells. J Cell Sci 1996; 109(pt 10):2521–2528.

36. Mignatti P, Rifkin DB. Plasminogen activators and matrix metalloproteinases in angiogenesis. Enzyme Protein 1996; 49(1–3):117–137.

37. Declerck P. Plasminogen activator-inhibitor 1: biochemical, structural and functional studies. Verh K Acad Geneeskd Belg 1993; 55(5):457–473.

38. Lyons RM, Gentry LE, Purchio AF, Moses HL. Mechanism of activation of latent recombinant transforming growth factor beta 1 by plasmin. J Cell Biol 1990; 110(4): 1361–1367.

39. Roberts AB. Molecular and cell biology of TGF-beta. Miner Electrolyte Metab 1998; 24(2–3):111–119.

40. Craig RD, Schofield JD, Jackson DS. Collagen biosynthesis in normal and hypertrophic scars and keloid as a function of the duration of the scar. Br J Surg 1975; 62(9): 741–744.

41. Tuan TL, Zhu JY, Sun B, Nichter LS, Nimni ME, Laug WE. Elevated levels of plasminogen activator inhibitor-1 may account for the altered fibrinolysis by keloid fibroblasts. J Invest Dermatol 1996; 106(5):1007–1011.

42. Montgomery AM, De Clerck YA, Langley KE, Reisfeld RA, Mueller BM. Melanoma-mediated dissolution of extracellular matrix: contribution of urokinase-dependent and metalloproteinase-dependent proteolytic pathways. Cancer Res 1993; 53(3):693–700.

43. Ladin DA, Hou Z, Patel D, McPhail M, Olson JC, Saed GM, Fivenson DP. p53 and apoptosis alterations in keloids and keloid fibroblasts. Wound Repair Regen 1998; 6(1):28–37.

44. Russell JD, Witt WS. Cell size and growth characteristics of cultured fibroblasts isolated from normal and keloid tissue. Plast Reconstr Surg 1976; 57(2):207–212.

45. Peltonen J, Hsiao LL, Jaakkola S, Sollberg S, Aumailley M, Timpl R, Chu ML, Uitto J. Activation of collagen gene expression in keloids: co-localization of type I and VI collagen and transforming growth factor-beta 1 mRNA. J Invest Dermatol 1991; 97(2):240–248.

46. Babu M, Diegelmann R, Oliver N. Keloid fibroblasts exhibit an altered response to TGF-beta. J Invest Dermatol 1992; 99(5):650–655.

47. Bettinger DA, Yager DR, Diegelmann RF, Cohen IK. The effect of TGF-beta on keloid fibroblast proliferation and collagen synthesis. Plast Reconstr Surg 1996; 98(5):827–833.

48. Shah M, Foreman DM, Ferguson MW. Neutralising antibody to TGF-beta 1,2 reduces cutaneous scarring in adult rodents. J Cell Sci 1994; 107(Pt 5): 1137–1157.

49. Shah M, Foreman DM, Ferguson MW. Neutralisation of TGF-beta 1 and TGF-beta 2 or exogenous addition of TGF-beta 3 to cutaneous rat wounds reduces scarring. J Cell Sci 1995; 108(Pt 3):985–1002.

50. Lee T, Chin G, Kim WJH, Gittes GK, Longaker MT. Differential expression of TGF-beta 1, beta 2 and beta 3 in keloid fibroblats. Ann Plast Surg 1999; 43(2):179–184.

51. Massague J. TGFbeta signaling: receptors, transducers, and Mad proteins. Cell 1996; 85(7):947–950.

52. Kim WJH, Gittes GK, Longaker MT. Signal transduction in wound pharmacology. Arch Pharmacol Res 1998; 21:487–495.
53. Derynck R. SMAD proteins and mammalian anatomy. Nature 1998; 393(6687): 737–739.
54. Younai S, Nichter LS, Wellisz T, Reinisch J, Nimni ME, Tuan TL. Modulation of collagen synthesis by transforming growth factor-beta in keloid and hypertrophic scar fibroblasts. Ann Plast Surg 1994; 33(2):148–151.
55. Dennis PA, Rifkin DB. Cellular activation of latent transforming growth factor beta requires binding to the cation-independent mannose 6-phosphate/insulin-like growth factor type II receptor. Proc Natl Acad Sci USA 1991; 88(2):580–584.
56. Border WA, Noble NA, Yamamoto T, Harper JR, Yamaguchi Y, Pierschbacher MD, Ruoslahti E. Natural inhibitor of transforming growth factor-beta protects against scarring in experimental kidney disease. Nature 1992; 360(6402):361–364.
57. Harper RA. Keloid fibroblasts in culture: abnormal growth behaviour and altered response to the epidermal growth factor. Cell Biol Int Rep 1989; 13(4):325–335.
58. O'Kane S, Ferguson MW. Transforming growth factor beta s and wound healing. Int J Biochem Cell Biol 1997; 29(1):63–78.
59. Skokan SJ, Davis RH. Principles of wound healing and growth factor considerations. J Am Podiatr Med Assoc 1993; 83(4):223–227.
60. Martin P. Wound healing—aiming for perfect skin regeneration. Science 1997; 276(5309):75–81.
61. Klagsbrun M. Angiogenic factors: regulators of blood supply-side biology. FGF, endothelial cell growth factors and angiogenesis: a Keystone symposium, Keystone, CO, USA, April 1–7, 1991. New Biol 1991; 3(8):745–749.
62. Cohen IK, Crossland MC, Garrett A, Diegelmann RF. Topical application of epidermal growth factor onto partial-thickness wounds in human volunteers does not enhance reepithelialization. Plast Reconstr Surg 1995; 96(2):251–254.
63. Igarashi A, Okochi H, Bradham DM, Grotendorst GR. Regulation of connective tissue growth factor gene expression in human skin fibroblasts and during wound repair. Mol Biol Cell 1993; 4(6):637–645.
64. Berman B, Duncan MR. Short-term keloid treatment in vivo with human interferon alfa-2b results in a selective and persistent normalization of keloidal fibroblast collagen, glycosaminoglycan, and collagenase production in vitro. J Am Acad Dermatol 1989; 21(4 Pt 1):694–702.
65. Romer J, Bugge TH, Pyke C, Lund LR, Flick MJ, Degen JL, Dano K. Impaired wound healing in mice with a disrupted plasminogen gene. Nat Med 1996; 2(3): 287–292.

9
Molecular and Cellular Biology of Dermal Fibroproliferative Disorders

Barbara S. Bauer, Edward E. Tredget, Paul G. Scott, and Aziz Ghahary
University of Alberta, Edmonton, Alberta, Canada

I. INTRODUCTION

A. Clinical Features

Hypertrophic scarring (HSc) and keloids are characterized as dermal fibroproliferative disorders, which also include liver cirrhosis and fibrosis, pulmonary fibrosis, atherosclerotic disease of vasculature, and multiorgan/tissue systemic diseases, such as progressive systemic sclerosis (scleroderma) and rheumatoid arthritis. Keloids can form following minor trauma to the skin, such as ear piercings or acne, whereas HSc scars usually form following injury to the deep dermis (1,2). The highest incidence of HSc occurs on body surfaces that are subject to high tension, such as the anterior chest, shoulders, flexor surfaces of the extremities, and the anterior neck (3). Hypertrophic scarring and keloids are characterized by excess extracellular matrix (ECM) deposition in the dermis and subcutaneous tissues and, unlike normal wound repair, which results in a fine-line scar, keloids and HSc form hard, elevated, red, and sometimes itchy scars that may cause pain, disfigurement, and contractures (Fig. 1).

It is important to distinguish HSc and keloids, as the treatments vary. The key differences are that HSc remains within the confines of the wound margin and eventually undergoes partial resolution spontaneously, whereas keloids are capable of invading surrounding tissue and usually require medical intervention, as they rarely regress spontaneously. There is believed to be a genetic (4,5) and racial predisposition for the development of keloids in darker-skinned races, as 15 to 20% of Blacks, Hispanics, and Asians are afflicted with the disorder. Children

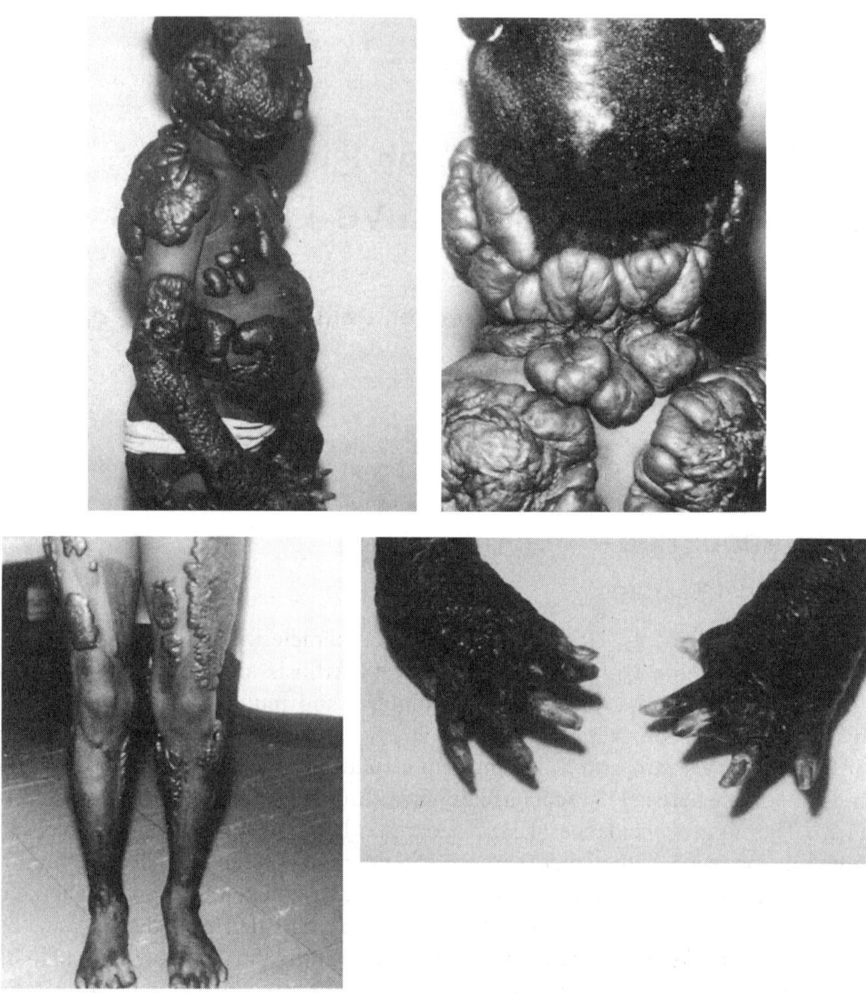

Figure 1 A 12-year-old black child with severe keloids following a scald injury (From Scott PG, Ghahary A, Chambers MM, Tredget EE. Biological basis of hypertrophic scarring. In: Malhotra S, ed. Advances in Structural Biology. Greenwich, Connecticut, JAI Press, 1994:157.)

entering puberty and pregnant women are reportedly more susceptible to increases in keloid size, which may be associated with changes in hormone levels.

B. Cellular Biology of Wound Healing

Immediately following injury, a number of sequenced events occur leading to the release of growth factors and cytokines, which mediate subsequent inflammation, cell proliferation, extracellular matrix deposition, contraction, and remodeling (Fig. 2). Hypertrophic scarring and keloids are the result of aberrations in the normal progression of healing leading to excessive extracellular matrix deposition and, often, the formation of contractures. Contractures are the pathological shortening of scar tissue, which result in cosmetic and functional deformity, as opposed to wound contraction in normal healing, which acts to reduce the wound surface area.

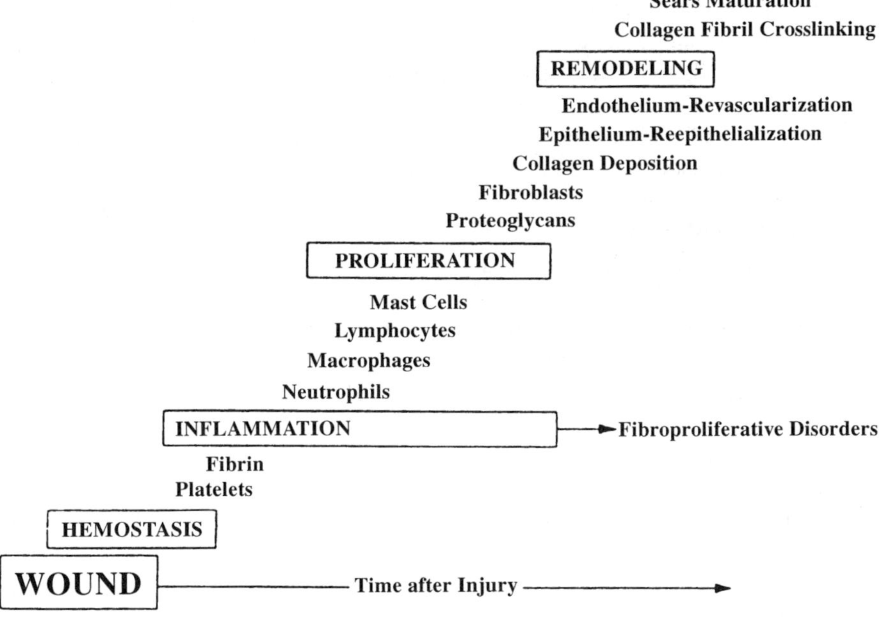

Figure 2 The phases of normal wound repair follow an orderly sequence of events that are regulated by the chronologic appearance of a number of different cell types over the course of healing. Prolonged activity or abnormal levels of fibrogenic cytokines released during the inflammatory phase may lead to fibroproliferative disorders (From Ref. 1.)

Wound healing involves a complex cascade of events in which alterations in key factors can have a great impact on the outcome of the scar. After wounding, platelets degranulate and the coagulation and complement pathways are activated to initiate the formation of a fibrin clot that acts as a mesh for the binding of inflammatory cells, fibroblasts, and growth factors (6). Platelets release many growth factors, which function as chemotactic agents for neutrophils, macrophages, epithelial cells, mast cells, endothelial cells, and fibroblasts. These include epidermal growth factor (EGF) (7), insulin-like growth factor-1 (IGF-1) (8), platelet-derived growth factor (PDGF) (9,10), and transforming growth factor-β (TGF-β) (11). Within 24 hr, neutrophils infiltrate the wound and phagocytose bacteria. Macrophages then infiltrate the wound to clear damaged host cells and debris and release chemotactic factors for fibroblasts, such as PDGF (12,13) and TGF-β1 (14). The PDGF released from platelets and macrophages leads to proliferation and migration of fibroblasts. This process is required for the formation for granulation tissue, which develops from the connective tissue in the damaged area and consists mainly of small vessels, inflammatory cells, fibroblasts, myofibroblasts and ECM proteins (15). Basic fibroblast growth factor (bFGF) and vascular endothelial growth factor (VEGF) promote angiogenesis by stimulating endothelial cell proliferation leading to the formation of capillary tubes. Basic FGF is released by damaged endothelial cells and macrophages (16) and stimulates endothelial cells to release plasminogen activator and procollagenase (17). Plasminogen activator converts plasminogen to plasmin and procollagenase to collagenase, both of which function to digest the basement membrane. Heparin released from mast cells also acts as a chemoattractant for endothelial cells, which are able to migrate to the wound due to the disruption of the basement membrane.

The transformation of granulation tissue into a mature scar requires a balance between matrix biosynthesis and degradation. The degradation of extracellular matrix occurs through the action of collagenases, proteoglycanases, and other proteases released from mast cells, macrophages, endothelial cells and fibroblasts. Extracellular matrix biosythesis is mainly the function of dermal fibroblasts, which produce collagens, fibronectin, proteoglycans, and other components. A disruption of this balance by either an excess in ECM synthesis or a deficiency in degradation or remodeling may result in the formation of keloids or HSc (18,19) (Fig. 3).

The development of HSc appears to occur following a prolonged period of inflammation. Prolongation of the inflammatory stage of wound healing due to infection or an extremely large or deep wound leads to an exaggerated response by inflammatory cells and a subsequent excess of cytokine release, such as TGF-β and IGF-1, which are fibrogenic cytokines. It has been shown that wounds that do not heal within three weeks have a higher probability of HSc formation (20). Keloid formation appears to have a strong genetic predisposition. Oluwasanmi (21) found increased plasma cells and gammaglobulin deposition in Africans and

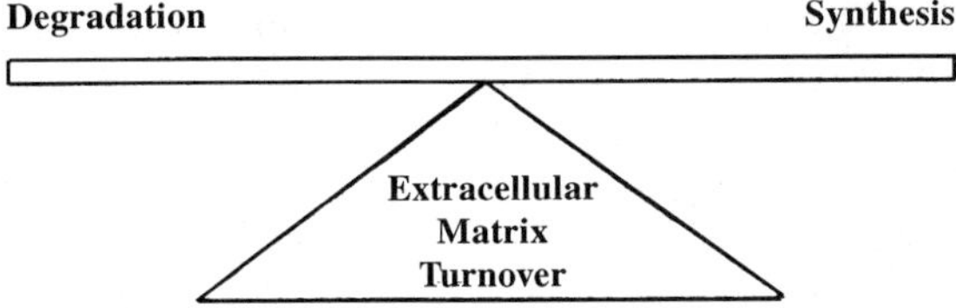

Figure 3 Regeneration of extracellular matrix homeostasis requires a dynamic balance between synthesis and degradation to achieve optimal wound healing (From Ref. 1.)

hypothesized that the activity of the immune system may regulate the production of connective tissue during the repair process. Cohen et al. (22) studied keloids and demonstrated an increase in tissue immunoglobulin G (IgG), which indicates that there is an immunological aspect to keloid formation. However, it was not determined what the IgG was directed toward. In these keloid patients, there was no difference in serum IgG or complement levels compared with normal subjects. Cohen et al. also reported that there was no correlation between HLA phenotype and keloid formation.

II. CELLULAR FACTORS

A. Fibroblasts and Myofibroblasts

Fibroblasts are the most common cell type found in HSc (23,24). During wound healing, some fibroblasts undergo morphological and biochemical changes such that they have phenotypic characteristics of both fibroblasts and smooth muscle cells. When treated with smooth muscle stimulants, strips of granulation tissue containing these differentiated cells contracted (25). These cells were subsequently called myofibroblasts to reflect contractile activity of this cell type (reviewed in 26). Gabbiani et al. (27) described the morphological changes that occurred in the fibroblast following wounding. These changes include the formation of stress fibers or microfilaments, nuclear indentations which are often found in contractile cells (28–30), and peripheral attachment sites. Darby et al. (31) demonstrated the gradual evolution of fibroblasts into myofibroblasts using α-smooth muscle actin as a marker. Alpha-smooth muscle actin (α-SMA), an actin isoform found in contractile vascular smooth muscle, is expressed by almost all myofibroblast populations in vivo (32).

There has been some debate over the type of cellular motility involved in wound contraction. It has been proposed that myofibroblasts are responsible for wound contraction (33–36) due to the presence of stress fibers rich in actin. Myofibroblasts are interconnected via gap junctions and adhere to the ECM via the fibronexus (37). It was suggested that in granular tissue, many myofibroblasts act as a contractile unit and pull on the connective tissue. Alternatively, single fibroblasts may be capable of reorganizing connective tissue during cell locomotion via tractional forces rather than contractile forces (38,39). It has been proposed that cellular filipodia elongate and retract using tractional forces, a movement resembling that of a tank tread. Attachment sites on fibroblasts have been reported by Izzard and Lochner (40) using interference reflection microscopy. They observed dark streaks where the ventral surface of fibroblasts came in close contract with a glass surface, and they called these streaks focal contacts. Using time-lapsed cinematography, it was shown that the focal contacts remained stationary and, as the cell moved forward, new focal contacts formed at the leading edge and preexisting contacts occupied increasingly posterior positions. These focal contacts have since been equated with adhesions (41). The tractional strength of the fibroblast exceeded that required for locomotion of the cell, leading Harris et al. (39) to suggest that this process is also involved in rearranging the collagen network from a random one into straight bundles. These workers also noted that stress fibers were not required for this process to occur. Herman et al. (42) reported that cellular motility is not usually associated with stress fibers containing actin and myosin but, instead, motility occurred when the proteins were diffused and presumably disassembled. They suggested that these stress fibers anchor the cell to the substrate, as many stress fibers terminate on attachment plaques (40,43) and contraction only occurs after the attachment plaque is released (44,45). Interestingly, when wound contraction is strongest, few stress fibers are expressed. Contraction of fibroblast-populated collagen lattices (FPCL) showed that fibroblasts were most contractile at 48 hr, when they had few stress fibers, whereas at 96 hr, when contraction was minimal, stress fibers were strongly expressed (46). Doillon et al. (47) used a rat model to demonstrate that actin-rich fibroblasts are not directly involved in wound contraction since they are maximally expressed at 15 days after wounding, which corresponds to contraction stability. Alignment of actin filaments in the fibroblasts with new collagen bundles was observed, which indicated strong adhesions between the fibroblasts and the ECM, thereby facilitating collagen rearrangement. Darby et al. (31) reported that in a rat wound model, stress fibers or microfilaments containing α-SMA appeared on day 6, while wound contraction was linear beginning on day 4. This study also found that the expression of α-SMA was maximal at day 15, at which point it gradually decreased and was absent by day 30. From days 20 to 25, apoptotic bodies were noted. Almost certainly, fibroblasts have contractile properties and are involved in wound contraction. However, it has been suggested that α-SMA expression corresponds to the end of the migration phase of the myofibroblasts, which are then terminally differentiated (48).

Darby et al. (31) and Desmoulière and Gabbiani (48) have shown that the number of myofibroblasts undergoing apoptosis increases as the wound closes, resulting in a decrease in cellularity as healing progresses. Basic fibroblast growth factor has been shown to accelerate healing (16) and induce apoptosis in cultured chick embryonic neural retina cells (49), and in oligodendrocytes (50). Basic FGF released from platelets is mitogenic toward fibroblasts, decreases the ability of fibroblasts to contract collagen fibers (51), and induces apoptosis of myofibroblasts. Fibroblasts from rat palatal mucosa were transformed into myofibroblasts with TGF-β treatment in vitro in growth-arrested conditions (low serum) (52) and showed a higher level of apoptosis following bFGF treatment. It has been proposed that when granulation tissue cells are not removed, there remains a high degree of cellularity and a subsequent increase in HSc and keloid formation (53). Fibroblasts from hypertrophic scars have shown higher basal levels of contraction in fibrin matrix gels than fibroblasts from keloids and normal dermis, which may be due in part to the autocrine effect of TGF-β1 (54) or an increased sensitivity of the fibroblasts to TGF-β1. The extracellular matrix has also been implicated in the phenotypic changes of fibroblasts into myofibroblasts (55). Mechanical tension in the absence of wounding has been shown to induce the myofibroblasts' phenotype, while in wounding alone few myofibroblasts were present. In a wound environment, this tension may be provided by the shear force caused by fibroblast migration (38).

B. Mast Cells

Mast cells are reported to be 4-fold higher in HSc than normal skin and 1.5 times as many as in mature scar (56). Mast cells appear as collagen synthesis begins in granulation tissue (57). Histamine release from these cells may contribute to the formation of HSc through vasodilatory effects, which increase the leakage of plasma proteins into the region (58). Mast cells may also contribute to fibrosis by releasing chymase, which has been shown to release the fibrogenic growth factor transforming growth factor-β1, in its inactive or latent form, from the extracellular matrix (59). Smith et al. (60) proposed that histamine and heparin from mast cells may lead to the development of keloids and HSc by increasing the rate of collagen production (61–63). They reported a statistically significant increase in these fibrotic conditions in those individuals suffering from atopic allergies.

III. EXTRACELLULAR MATRIX ABNORMALITIES

A. Collagen

The major classes of extracellular matrix components are collagens, elastic fibers, noncollagenous glycoproteins, such as fibronectin, and various proteoglycans. Collagen fibrils and fibers provide tensile strength to connective tissues and an increase in collagen content is usually considered the hallmark of fibrosis. It is worth noting however, that in a hypertrophic scar the proportion of collagen on a dry-weight basis is about 30% lower than in normal dermis or mature scar (64). This is because of the larger increases in other extracellular matrix components, such as fibronectin and the proteoglycans (see below). Nevertheless, the absolute amount of collagen (expressed per unit surface area) is elevated because of the grossly thickened dermis. In some regions of postburn hypertrophic scars, much of the collagen is organized not (as in normal dermis) into fibers and fiber bundles running parallel to the tissue surface, but into thin fibrils, which can be seen in the electron microscope to be irregular in outline and widely separated by interfibrillar matrix (24). In the light microscope, these areas of the scar appear rather fine-textured, with the fibroblasts arranged in ''whorls'' or ''nodules.''

The most abundant form of collagen in the skin is type I, with smaller amounts (10–15% in adults) of type III, a collagen that is characteristically a higher proportion of the total in fetal tissues and in early wounds (see Chapter 5).

Type V is another fibril-forming collagen known to be present in small amounts in skin (65) but which may account for up to 10% of the collagen in hypertrophic scars (66). Immunohistochemistry has been used to localize type V collagen to basement membranes or to the immediately subjacent connective tissue (67,68), so that its elevation in hypertrophic scars may reflect the increased vascularity. However, it is also a component (along with types I and III collagens) of heterotypic fibrils in many tissues, including skin, and, like type III collagen, it reduces the diameters of copolymeric fibrils formed in vitro (69,70). Its location within the hypertrophic scars has apparently not been defined.

Expression of messenger ribonucleic acid (mRNA) for type VI collagen is elevated in keloids compared with normal dermis (71). The type VI collagen monomer consists of a short, triple-helical domain flanked by two large globular domains. It assembles into dimers and tetramers that link end-to-end to form thin, beaded filaments (72). These filaments are organized into a meshwork oriented approximately perpendicular to the major fibrils in dermis and other connective tissues and are especially prominent in neurofibromatous lesions in the skin (73). It may be speculated that type VI collagen comprises the interfibrillar filaments that are prominent in hypertrophic scars (74).

Collagen fibers in keloids are thicker and are more abundant than are found in HSc and tend to form acellular nodules in the deep dermis. Hypertrophic scarring also forms nodules or whorls of collagen with fewer distinct collagen fibers and fiber bundles; however, they usually contain islands of α-SMA staining myofibroblasts (75). Another characteristic of HSc is that there is a lack of epithelial ridges and increased thickness of dermis and epidermis (24). The orientation of the wound may be important in the formation of HSc. Skin tension and collagen organization are directional, and wounds that are oriented in the relaxed skin tension lines are protected from stress by collagen fibers and thus form normal mature scars (76).

B. Glycosaminoglycans and Proteoglycans

Proteoglycans (PGs) are complex macromolecules in which specific glycosaminoglycan (GAG) chains are attached to a protein core. Glycosaminoglycans contain sulfate and carboxylate residues and are therefore highly polyanionic; the predominant GAGs in normal skin are dermatan sulfate (DS) and hyaluronic acid (HA), with smaller amounts of chondroitin sulfate (CS) (77). Chondroitin 4-sulfate is present in very small amounts in normal skin in contrast to HSc in which it is readily demonstrated, especially in the nodules (78) (see Chapter 1).

C. Fibronectin

Fibronectin is a glycoprotein that functions in the adhesion of cells and macromolecules to the ECM (79). Because of its specific functional domains and cell-binding sites, fibronectin is able to interact with a variety of cell types and function as a chemotactic agent for inflammatory cells, a scaffold for fibroblast migration and ECM deposition, and a regulator of cell growth and gene expression. Fibronectin has been reported to bind TGF-β (80), and an increase in fibronectin has been measured in HSc (81). The ability of fibronectin to induce cell migration and ECM synthesis suggests that its persistence may be involved in the development of fibrosis.

D. Elastin

In normal skin, a random organization of collagen and a network of elastin give skin its strength, elasticity, and flexibility. In contrast, mature scars have large parallel-organized collagen bundles and a scattered elastin network (82). It has been suggested that there is a temporary absence of elastin from hypertrophic scars, which contributes to their hardness and inelasticity. De Vries et al. (83) used a human punch biopsy wound model and found that elastin-coated native collagen matrices made from insoluble collagen fibers stimulated the formation of ECM consisting of mature collagen fibers, reduced fibroblast and myofibroblast accumulation, and resulted in minimal wound contraction (84). In contrast, matrices coated with hyaluronic acid and fibronectin stimulated wound contraction.

It has been suggested that fragments of altered elastin fibers in injured tissue may be partially responsible for the chronic inflammatory response of immature HSc, and the altered fibers may interfere with the production of new elastin fibers (85). As the scar matures, elastic fibers return (24). Compton et al. (86) reported that elastin fibers are detected only years after wounding and that their appearance is one of the final events in healing.

IV. FIBROGENIC GROWTH FACTORS

Cells communicate with each other through the specific binding of cytokines and growth factors with protein receptors on their cell membranes. The functions of growth factors are diverse and include stimulation or inhibition of cell proliferation, differentiation, migration, or gene expression, depending on the cell type involved (87). Of the many growth factors and cytokines potentially involved in HSc and keloids, transforming growth factor-β is certainly one of the most complex and pleiotropic. Because of the many functions of this growth factor, its regulation is considered crucial in the control of normal wound healing.

A. Transforming Growth Factor-β1

Transforming growth factor-β belongs to a supergene family consisting of three groups, the TGF-βs, the activins, and the bone morphogenic proteins (BMPs). Five isoforms of TGF-β have been identified to date; TGF-β1, -β2, -β3, -β4, and -β5. Of these, TGF-β1, -β2, and -β3 are found in mammals (88). Transforming growth factor-β is released from platelets into the wound environment following injury and acts as a chemotactic agent for neutrophils, T lymphocytes, monocytes, and fibroblasts (88,89). Although TGF-β is essential for normal wound healing (90,91), overexpression or persistent expression of this growth factor may lead to fibrosis as seen in HSc and keloids.

Transforming growth factor-β1 is implicated in the formation of HSc and keloids because of its ability to elicit an overproduction of ECM proteins. This is achieved both by up-regulation of collagen synthesis and down-regulation of collagenase production (92,93). It has been reported that TGF-β1 mRNA expression is greater in postburn HSc relative to that of normal tissue obtained from the same patients (94). It has also been shown that TGF-β1 is capable of up-regulating its own receptor expression (95,96) and stimulating the differentiation of fibroblasts into myofibroblasts (97).

Transforming growth factor-β1 is secreted as a small latent complex (LTGF-β1) consisting of a 25-kDa dimeric mature protein and an N-terminal pro-protein called the latency-associated peptide (LAP) (98). Important features of the LAP are the presence of three N-linked oligosaccharides, two of which include mannose 6-phosphate (M6P) (99). In cells such as fibroblasts, platelets, and bone cells, the LTGF-β1 complex may form a large latent complex with latent TGF-β1 binding protein (LTBP), a 125- to 205-kDa glycoprotein that is required for the secretion and targeting of TGF-β1 in some cells (100). The binding of LTBP masks the M6P moieties on LAP and prevents the uptake of LTGF-β into lysosomes. After its release from degranulating platelets, TGF-β1 can exist as the small latent complex and be sequestered in the ECM (101), or as the large latent complex and either be released into the serum (88) or be bound to the ECM, where it can be released by proteolytic cleavage. It is generally believed that either a conformational change of the latent complex or dissociation of LAP is required for activation of TGF-β1 (102,103) as the TGF-β receptors do not recognize LTGF-β1 (104).

Wakefield et al. (105) studied the tissue distribution of both recombinant latent and active TGF-β1 in rats. Active TGF-β1 was shown to accumulate in the lungs, liver, and kidney, which is similar to the tissue distribution of α2-macroglobulin (106,107), which is a carrier molecule involved in the clearance of active TGF-β1. Conversely, latent TGF-β1 did not accumulate in any one organ, instead, it was present in low levels in all organs. The authors suggested that the LAP may extend the half-life of TGF-β1 in circulation by preventing it from complexing with α2-macroglobulin. Thus, while active TGF-β1 may act locally in an autocrine or paracrine fashion, latent TGF-β in circulation may have endocrine activity.

Dickson et al. (108) used [^{125}I]-TGF-β1 to demonstrate the distribution of administered active TGF-β in mice and rats. The investigators showed that the microvascular endothelium was the major site of TGF-β binding. In response to tissue injury, TGF-β up-regulates adhesion molecules and has chemotactic properties. However, it has previously been suggested that a major function of systemic TGF-β may be to reduce adhesiveness of endothelial cells for immune cells by inhibiting E-selectin expression (109–112). This function is perhaps best demonstrated by MRL/1pr mice, a murine autoimmune model used to study diseases such as systemic lupus erythematosus (SLE). In these mice, the TGF-β1 gene is disrupted and an inflammatory response results in death 2 to 3 weeks after birth (113,114). Whereas increased local production of TGF-β1 may result in fibrotic disorders by activating fibroblasts, endocrine TGF-β1 interacts mainly with endothelial cells (115) and, to a lesser degree, fibroblasts and macrophages (116,117). Chronic inflammation can lead to excessive systemic TGF-β as a control mechanism to dampen the immune response. Use of TGF-β as an immunosuppressant has been suggested; however, excessive TGF-β may lead to an unresponsive immune system, resulting in life-threatening bacterial infections. Elevated endocrine TGF-β has been noted in conditions that result in immunosuppression, such as SLE, human immunodeficiency virus (HIV), and arthritis (118–120).

The mechanisms by which TGF-β1 activation occurs in vivo have not been fully elucidated. Plasmin is capable of activating TGF-β1 by cleaving LAP (121–124). Plasmin is also the major fibrinolytic enzyme involved in wound healing and it is activated from its precursor form, plasminogen, by urokinase-type plasminogen activator (uPA) and tissue-type plasminogen activator (tPA). Activation of plasmin is inhibited by plasminogen activator inhibitor-1 (PAI-1). Transforming growth factor-β1 itself is capable of regulating plasmin activation, and thus, potentially at least, of controlling its own activation, by up-regulating PAI-1. Tuan et al. (125) reported a decrease in uPA and an increase in PAI-1 levels in keloid fibroblasts versus normal fibroblasts, suggesting a decrease in the role of keloid fibroblasts in fibrinolysis. This same pattern was shown after treating normal fibroblasts with TGF-β1. Another function of plasmin is the activation of matrix metalloproteases, such as collagenase, which is crucial in wound remodeling (126). Transforming growth factor-β1 also has a role in the regulation of matrix metalloproteinases by stimulating the synthesis of tissue inhibitor of metalloproteinases-1 (TIMP-1) (127) and inhibiting collagenase mRNA (93).

Mast cell chymase, in contrast to plasmin, is released as an active heparin-bound enzyme that is not easily inhibited by protease inhibitors (128–132). Chymase releases TGF-β1 as a large latent complex 10-fold more efficiently than plasmin, but is not directly involved in TGF-β1 activation. However, chymase does allow for exposure and subsequent activation of latent TGF-β by other factors.

The mannose 6-phosphate/insulin-like growth factor-2 (M6P/IGF-2) receptor may be involved in the activation of LTGF-β1. Dennis and Rifkin (133) have demonstrated the binding of the small latent complex to the M6P/IGF-2 receptor via the two mannose 6-phosphate moieties on the LAP. Exogenous M6P and anti-M6P receptor were able to inhibit the activation of LTGF-β1 in bovine aortic endothelial and smooth muscle cells in coculture. However, neither M6P nor anti-M6P had any effect on basal cell migration, the activity of exogenously added TGF-β1, the activation of LTGF-β1 by plasmin, or the release of LTGF-β1 from cells. Ghahary et al. (134) have studied the mechanism of TGF-β1 activation via the M6P/IGF-2 receptor in a coculture system, and found that latent TGF-β1 released from genetically modified keratinocytes is capable of increasing collagen expression from dermal fibroblasts. This effect was inhibited in a dose-dependent manner by the addition of mannose 6-phosphate. This study also suggested that activation of TGF-β1 is due to a conformational change rather than due to cleavage of LAP from mature TGF-β1. Isolated fibroblast cell membranes were incubated with either latent TGF-β1 or latent TGF-β1 and recombinant active TGF-β1. Using the mink lung epithelial cell growth inhibition assay, a standard assay for demonstrating TGF-β1 bioactivity, it was shown that after centrifugation, supernatants from latent TGF-β1 alone did not significantly inhibit cell growth compared with those incubated with active TGF-β1. These results suggest that interaction of latent TGF-β1 with the M6P/IGF-2 may not result in cleavage of LAP from mature TGF-β1. Although the precise mechanism by which M6P/IGF-2 receptors are involved in LTGF-β1 activation is unknown, activation does require PA and plasmin (123,135). It has been proposed that the effective concentrations of both enzyme and substrate are increased by binding to the cell surface, thus facilitating the activation and release of LTGF-β1.

In vitro studies have suggested a role for retinoids in the activation of TGF-β1 through their ability to increase plasminogen and plasmin levels and to increase the expression of cellular type II transglutaminase (136). Transglutaminase has been shown to be required for TGF-β1 activation, possibly by concentrating plasminogen activator to the extracellular matrix by cross-linking it to fibronectin (137). Thrombospondin is a glycoprotein that is also capable of activating both the large and small latent complexes of TGF-β but without proteolytic cleavage of LAP from TGF-β1. Instead, it may work by inducing a change in conformation (138). Similar to thrombospondin, it has been suggested that IgG may also be capable of activating TGF-β independent of proteases (139). Active TGF-β1 in MRL/1pr mice was found complexed to IgG in B cells and plasma cells. This complex was shown to strongly inhibit neutrophil function by inhibiting the adhesion and subsequent uptake of bacteria to activated neutrophils. The IgG–TGF-β complex was shown to be 500 times more potent than recombinant active TGF-β in suppressing neutrophil function. This may be due to a more efficient presentation of active TGF-β1 to neutrophil TGF-β receptors by IgG or because IgG functions as a carrier molecule, thus extending the half-life of active TGF-β in circulation (139).

Once TGF-β1 is activated, it is capable of binding to heteromeric receptor complexes consisting of type I (RI) and type II (RII) receptors. Each of these receptors possesses a different serine/threonine kinase and both receptors are required for signal transduction following TGF-β1 binding. Receptor type II is necessary for the recruitment and activation of RI (140), and RI is responsible for the propagation of the signal to downstream targets (141,142). In normal human skin, RI and RII are present in the epidermis, epidermal appendages, and in vascular cells. Schmid et al. (143) reported that in granulation tissue, the expression of both receptors increased and, as remodeling proceeded, the levels decreased. However, in HSc, the levels of both RI and RII remained high for up to 20 months after injury. It was proposed that the failure to clear high receptor-expressing fibroblasts during remodeling induced a positive feedback loop for the autoinduction of TGF-β1. TGF-β1 is capable of autoinducing TGF-β1 mRNA transcription via activation of the AP-1 complex consisting of *c-jun* and *c-fos* proto-oncogene proteins (144). High levels of the cytokine may thus persist long after the initiating stimulus and this may contribute to the development of fibroproliferative disorders.

The downstream molecules responsible for TGF-β1 signal transduction are able to produce diverse cellular responses following TGF-β1 binding to its receptor. Transforming growth factor-β1 is both a stimulatory and an inhibitory molecule. It is a chemoattractant for monocytes, neutrophils, and fibroblasts, and induces the release of interleukin-1 (IL-1), interleukin-6 (IL-6), tumor necrosis factor-α (TNF-α), and bFGF from these cells (127). The effect of TGF-β1 on target cells depends on many factors, including cell origin, the state of differentiation, local concentrations of activating and inhibiting molecules, and the presence of other growth factors and cytokines (127).

The half-life of active TGF-β is approximately 2 to 3 minutes and yet physiological levels are maintained at about 5 ng/ml in normal humans, which indicates that carrier proteins may be involved in transporting TGF-β in the plasma (145). Thrombospondin, IgG, or α2-macroglobulin may act as carrier molecules for latent TGF-β (105).

Once activated, regulation of TGF-β1 appears to occur by its binding molecules, such as the proteoglycan decorin, in the ECM and α2-macroglobulin in the circulation. Mast cells may enhance the levels of TGF-β1, as heparin is capable of releasing active TGF-β1 from α2-macroglobulin (146). It has been reported that patients with HSc and keloids have a statistically significant increase in allergy symptoms (60), which are often associated with an increase in IgE levels and mast cells counts (147). The decrease in decorin content in HSc (discussed above) may be in part due to TGF-β1. Scott et al. (148) used normal and HSc fibroblasts from the same patients to show that decorin synthesis was lower in HSc compared with normal fibroblasts, and following TGF-β1 treatment, decorin was further reduced in all 6 strains of HSc and in 5 of the 6 strains of normal fibroblasts. After removal of TGF-β1 and passaging cells, decorin synthesis was no longer suppressed. The decrease in decorin following TGF-β1 treatment is in agreement with the results of Kahari et al. (149) who treated normal human skin and gingival fibroblasts with TGF-β1. Proteoglycans may normally function to control cell proliferation by regulating growth factors, such as TGF-β1 and bFGF, in the ECM (150,151), or conversely, down-regulation of decorin expression in HSc by TGF-β1 may be associated with the increased cell numbers involved.

The localization of decorin, versican, biglycan, and TGF-β has been demonstrated in normal skin, mature scars, and HSc (152). In normal skin, decorin was present throughout the dermis, versican and biglycan were present in very low levels, and TGF-β1 was not detected. In HSc, decorin was present in the deep dermis and a narrow zone under the epidermis but was absent in the ultrastructural nodules typical of HSc, whereas TGF-β1 was localized to the nodules and the deep dermis. Scott et al. (152) proposed that the co-localization of TGF-β1 and decorin in the deep dermis may be important in the resolution of the scar, as staining for both was quite intense in this region in the mature scars.

B.   Insulin-Like Growth Factor-1

Insulin-like growth factor-1 is another growth factor that may promote excessive matrix deposition in HSc and keloids due to its mitogenic effects (153) and its ability to stimulate synthesis of certain PGs (154) and collagen by fibroblasts

(155). Insulin-like growth factors are expressed in most tissues at various stages in development and may function as autocrine, paracrine, or endocrine factors (156). In the uterus, IGF-1 is mainly regulated by estrogen (157). Estrogen is involved in the proliferation of many uterine cells, such as stromal and epithelial cells resulting in uterine growth (158). It has been shown that IGF-1 mRNA (159) and the IGF-1 receptor (160) expression are increased following estrogen treatment. Estrogen has also been shown to down-regulate insulin-like growth factor binding protein (IGFBP)-1, a binding protein capable of inhibiting the growth-promoting effects of IGF-1 (161). There may be an estrogen-responsive element in the IGF-1 gene, which interacts with an activated estrogen receptor. In rats, estrogen has been shown to inhibit the expression of IGF-1 mRNA in tissues such as kidney, lung, and liver (162). However, recent studies in humans and primates indicate that low doses of estrogen may stimulate growth in other tissues (163–165), perhaps through enhanced growth hormone secretion (166).

Insulin-like growth factor-1 in the serum is bound to specific binding proteins, which protect it from proteolytic degradation (167,168). Type III collagen and fibronectin are capable of binding IGFBP-3 and -5 (168), so that IGF-1 released from immune and epithelial cells may associate with the ECM. Insulin-like growth factor-1 may contribute to the development of HSc due to its ability to increase mRNAs for type I and type III procollagens and down-regulate collagenase activity (93,155). Ghahary et al. (155) have demonstrated an approximately 2-fold increase in IGF-1 mRNA in HSc compared with normal dermis from the same patients. Treating dermal fibroblasts with IGF-1 was associated with a 150% increase in pro-α1(I) mRNA and a 170% increase in pro-α1(III) mRNA.

Insulin-like growth factor-1 levels in HSc could be increased by the disruption of sweat and sebaceous glands following injury (169). In normal skin, IGF-1 is localized to the epithelial cells located in the superficial epidermal layer, sweat and sebaceous glands, and in the deep dermis. However, in HSc, these structures are disrupted. Reepithelialization is dependent upon deep dermal epithelial cells migrating from the residual sweat and sebaceous elements where they are able to secrete IGF-1 in the presence of dermal fibroblasts. As these cells contribute to reepithelialization and to the healing of sweat and sebaceous glands in the skin, the fibroblasts may no longer be exposed to IGF-1. This could facilitate the resolution of HSc. Interestingly, animals such as the rat, rabbit, mouse, and pig lack sweat glands similar to those seen in humans and do not develop keloids or HSc.

Insulin-like growth factor-1 may also be capable of inducing TGF-β1 expression in dermal fibroblasts, thus augmenting the fibrotic environment. These growth factors are coexpressed in several physiological and pathological conditions by different cell types, such as fibroblasts (170,171), platelets (8,172), and activated macrophages (172,173). Ghahary et al. (174) reported that treatment of fibroblasts with IGF-1 caused an increase in transcription of TGF-β and protein production, and this effect persisted for at least 48 hr after withdrawing IGF-1. It was proposed that IGF-1 may stimulate the expression of TGF-β1 mRNA in dermal fibroblasts through activation of the AP-1 complex. Transforming growth factor-β1 may then act as an autocrine factor and induce its own further expression.

V. EMERGING THERAPIES

Controlling excess ECM deposition appears to be key in preventing HSc and keloids. This could be achieved either by controlling the deposition of collagen or by increasing the activity of collagenase and thus promoting collagen degradation. Interferons have been shown to be potent antifibrotic factors and, recently, the peptide hormone relaxin has also been considered as a candidate for the management of fibroproliferative disorders.

A. Interferons

Interferon-α (IFN-α), -β, and -γ were originally identified on the basis of their antiviral activity. IFN-α and -β are produced by almost all nucleated cells and IFN-γ is produced by activated T lymphocytes. Interferons bind to high-affinity receptors, each of which is associated with two tyrosine kinases from the Janus family. These kinases phosphorylate cytoplasmic signal transduction proteins that are then capable of enhancing or inhibiting the transcription of various genes (175). All three interferons are capable of decreasing the synthesis of types I and III collagen (176,177), inhibiting fibroblast proliferation, and controlling cytoskeletal protein-mediated wound contraction. Interferon-α2b may also function to reduce wound cellularity in the later stages of healing by inducing apoptosis of fibroblasts (178). The effect of IFN-α2b in a model of wound contraction was demonstrated by Nedelec et al. (179), whereby collagen lattices were seeded with fibroblasts from matched tissue samples of human HSc and normal dermis. Treatment with IFN-α2b decreased the rate and degree of contraction by both normal and HSc fibroblasts. This process involved a lag phase, indicating that protein synthesis was required (180–182). Although others have reported an increased ability of HSc fibroblasts to contract these lattices compared with normal fibroblasts (183), Nedelec et al. (179) reported similar rates of contraction. The mechanism by which IFN-α2b inhibits contraction may be through reduction in mRNAs of β- and γ-actin, as actin filaments are required for fibroblast elongation and contraction (34,38,184,185). In addition to the reduction in actin mRNA, Nedelec et al. (179) also noted changes in the organization of microfilaments, the bipolar morphology characteristic of contractile cells was lost following IFN-α2b treatment.

Interferon-α2b may also modulate the effects of fibrogenic growth factors. Insulin-like growth factor-1 is expressed in higher levels in HSc than normal dermis (155), where it acts as a mitogen (186). Recently, it was shown that IFN-α2b suppresses the fibrogenic effects of IGF-1 (187). Human fibroblasts grown in culture were treated with IFN-α2b and IGF-1 and showed a 44% decrease in hydroxyproline (an index of collagen protein) and an approximately 4-fold increase in collagenase activity over cells treated with IGF-1 alone. An important distinction between IFN-α2b and IFN-γ is that IFN-α2b is capable of increasing expression of collagenase while IFN-γ decreases collagenase activity (188).

Interferons are also capable of inducing the production of nitric oxide (NO) by fibroblasts. Nitric oxide is an intracellular messenger molecule, which may have roles in immunoregulation and inflammation (189). Nitric oxide can be released from phagocytes, hepatocytes, and in cartilage (190,191). Its effects include prevention of platelet aggregation (192), inhibition of histamine release from mast cells (193), and increase in metalloproteinase activation. Metalloproteinases, such as collagenase and stromelysin, are synthesized as proenzymes and require activation in the ECM. Murrell et al. (194) showed that in the presence of inflammatory mediators, such as interleukin-1β and tumor necrosis factor-α, both nitric oxide synthase and metalloproteinase activity were increased in explants of bovine and human cartilage. It has been reported that fibroblasts from HSc produce less NO than those from normal dermis (195) and may, therefore, have a diminished ability to activate collagenase. Wang et al. (196) reported that fibroblasts from normal skin produced NO constitutively and after induction following exposure to IFN-γ and lipopolysaccharide. Nitric oxide is also a vasodilator and could cause an increase in blood flow and migration of cells to the site of injury.

The use of IFN-α2b in vivo has had promising results in fibroproliferative disorders. Berman and Flores (197) studied the recurrence rates of excised keloids treated with IFN-α2b and triamcinolone acetonide (TAC) injections. Surgical removal of keloids is normally associated with a recurrence rate of 45 to 100% (53,176). Berman and Flores reported a 51.2% recurrence of excised lesions with no treatment, 58.5% recurrence of TAC-treated lesions, and only an 18.7% recurrence of IFN-α2b–treated keloids. Since IFN-α and -β enhance keloid collagenase activity, intralesional injection of IFN-α2b may be capable of increasing collagen breakdown and reducing the size of nonexcised lesions (177). In fact, systemic injection of IFN-α2b may serve to compensate for an deficiency in keloid patients, as decreased levels of IFN-γ and IFN-α have been reported in circulating immune cells of these patients (198).

Interferon-γ is another promising antifibrogenic agent, as shown by its ability to decrease collagen deposition around subcutaneously implanted foreign bodies in mice (199). Harrop et al. (200) studied matched HSc and normal skin fibroblasts in vitro and reported that IFN-γ (1000 U/ml) reduced types I (55%) and III (36%) procollagen mRNA and collagen production (34%) in HSc cells, which were as sensitive to IFN-γ as the normal fibroblasts.

A clinical study using both IFN-α2b and IFN-γ has recently been reported by Tredget et al. (201). Patients with HSc were treated with subcutaneous IFN-α2b. Punch biopsies and blood samples were taken before, during and after treatment. Dermal fibroblasts were isolated from the explants. Interferon-α2b and -γ treatment of normal fibroblasts inhibited the proliferation of the cells in the absence of TGF-β1. Transforming growth factor-β1 treatment of both normal and HSc fibroblasts was found to increase proliferation and collagen production of both cell types in a dose-dependent manner that was antagonized by IFN-α2b and -γ when administered separately and in combination (a weak additive effect was noted). Both interferons also inhibited the amount of TGF-β1 mRNA and protein synthesized by both normal and HSc fibroblasts. Serum samples from the patients indicated higher levels of circulating TGF-β1 than a pool of normal individuals and treatment with IFN-α2b significantly reduced TGF-β1 levels from HSc patients into the normal range during and shortly after treatment. Interferon-α2b also decreased TGF-β1 mRNA in HSc tissue into the normal range within one month. Another clinical study involved administering recombinant IFN-α2b subcutaneously to nine patients with HSc (202). These patients initially had elevated serum TGF-β1 levels relative to normal controls, significantly elevated plasma N^τ-methylhistamine (the stable metabolite of histamine), and 2-fold increases in mast cell numbers in the resolving scar. With systemic IFN-α2b, N^τ-methylhistamine levels decreased to normal without significant changes in mast cell numbers, suggesting a reduction in mast cell degranulation. Mast cell chymase is capable of activating matrix-bound TGF-β1 (59), and histamine stimulates collagen synthesis and cross-linking (57,203).

B. Relaxin

Relaxin is a hormone of ovarian origin that is involved in pregnancy and parturition by inducing collagen remodeling by an unknown mechanism. Relaxin is a member of the same family as insulin and insulin-like growth factors (204). It is similar to the interferons in that it is capable of stimulating nitric oxide production (192).

Vasilenko et al. (205) demonstrated the growth-promoting effects of relaxin on the uterus, cervix, and vagina of rats and found that relaxin decreased total collagen and increased total glycosaminoglycans. The net result was an increased growth of the uterus, cervix, and vagina by increasing water content and tissue mass. A model proposed by the authors was that relaxin increases the distensibility of the collagen matrix of the uterus.

C. Anti–Transforming Growth Factor-β

Fetal wounds heal without scarring and have a lower inflammatory and cytokine response compared with adults (206,207). Administration of TGF-β to fetal wounds induces scarring (208). Suppression of TGF-β in adults by using antibodies, which target TGF-β has been proposed as a possible therapy to reduce scar formation. Shah et al. (209,210) used an adult rat dermal wound model to demonstrate that anti–TGF-β1,2 administration at the time of wounding or shortly after resulted in a dose-dependent reduction in scarring. The wounds treated with anti–TGF-β1,2 had fewer macrophages, monocytes, and blood vessels than control wounds. The anti–TGF-β1,2 wounds also had reduced type I and type III collagen and fibronectin levels, but retained the same tensile strength as controls. The similarity in wound strength in the anti–TGF-β1,2 wounds, despite the lower collagen content, was considered to be due to the regular arrangement of the fibrils in these wounds compared with abnormally oriented collagen fibrils in wounds treated with TGF-β–irrelevant antibody or no injection (209). The authors suggest that the reduction in TGF-β immediately after wounding helps prevent scarring by decreasing the recruitment of immune cells. It may also alter levels of PDGF, bFGF, as well as the autocrine induction of TGF-β. Early administration of anti–TGF-β may also decrease the synthesis of PAI-1 and increase the synthesis of plasminogen and plasmin, which aid in fibrinolysis as ECM production ensues. This may result in a more organized pattern of the ECM proteins.

D. Mannose 6-Phosphate

Another potential therapy for the prevention of fibroproliferative disorders is exogenous mannose 6-phosphate. As previously discussed, latent TGF-β binds to the M6P/IGF-2 receptor, and its activation is inhibited by the addition of M6P (99,133) or antibodies directed against this receptor (133). It has not been determined whether cell surface–associated plasmin alone activates latent TGF-β after it binds to the M6P/IGF-2 receptor (133), or whether latent TGF-β is internalized and the low pH in the endosomal compartment is responsible for activation (211). Although further investigation is required to determine potential side effects of administration, it is reasonable to consider M6P as a therapy for excessive scarring.

VI. GENE THERAPY

Current standard therapies for the treatment of HSc and keloids have had limited success. Surgical excision without adjuvant therapy is associated with a high rate of recurrence (53,176). HSc and keloids are the result of a variety of cellular and molecular processes that are disrupted. By understanding the growth factors and cellular processes involved, therapies can be designed that either provide factors that are diminished in the pathological condition or, conversely, provide factors to regulate wound healing and prevent excess scaring.

New recombinant deoxyribonucleic acid (DNA) technologies have increased the availability of growth factors and also furthered our understanding of their functions. Clinical application of growth factors has gained considerable interest. However, the use of recombinant proteins is limited because of their relative expense and often very short half-lives (105,212). The goal of gene therapy is to transfer the gene of interest into specific cells where it will direct the synthesis of recombinant protein. This form of therapy may have several advantages over the direct administration of recombinant proteins. Proteins made by the host may be more likely to be sustained at therapeutic concentrations and frequent injections would not be required. Gene delivery may be achieved either ex vivo or in vivo (213). Ex vivo gene therapy involves the isolation of cells from a biopsy before transplanting them back into the host. This technique is limited to those cells that are amenable to cell culture and transplantation but has the advantage that conditions of genetic modification can be controlled. The in vivo technique involves delivering the gene directly into the tissue. The potential disadvantage of this method is the accuracy required for targeting the appropriate tissue.

Although nonviral methods, such as liposomes and particle-mediated gene therapy, give lower transfer efficiencies than viral methods, these methods can yield positive results. Liposomes consist of one or more lipid bilayer membranes with fatty acid tails on the interior and hydrophilic heads facing exterior, exposed to the aqueous phase. These bilayers form aqueous compartments and the lipid composition and preparation technique determines the size and shape of the vesicle. Targeting of the liposome may be achieved by inserting monoclonal antibodies into the outer membrane (214,215). The skin is amendable to gene therapy because of its accessibility. Liposomes can deliver their contents to the skin either by dehydration of the liposome in the stratum corneum (216) or by penetration of the skin through hair follicles (217,218).

Early liposomes were made with phosphatidylserine, which has a net negative charge (219–221). For the lipid–DNA interaction to occur, DNA first had to be encapsulated by reverse phase evaporation using phosphatidylserine and cholesterol. A more efficient method of DNA incorporation was later developed by using cationic lipids, which interact with negatively charged strands of DNA. The complex is then taken into the target cell either by fusing with the plasma membrane (222–224) or through endocytosis, following which the DNA may escape from either early or late endosomes into the cytoplasm (224–226). Cationic lipids transfect different cell types with varying efficiencies and the level of toxicity may also vary with cell type (222,227–234). Cationic liposomes have been used to deliver plasmid DNA, RNA (235), and protein (236,237).

The advantages of lipofection are that the size of the gene to be delivered is not limited, it is easier to prepare and test compared with viral constructs and it is relatively nontoxic. However, this method is associated with a low frequency of stable transfection, 100 to 1000 times more DNA is required for liposomal delivery compared with adenoviral constructs (238). Thus far, liposomes are the only nonviral gene transfer method being tested in clinical trials.

Particle-mediated gene transfer uses microparticles, such as gold or tungsten, coated with DNA. The particles are then used to bombard the cells or tissue at a high force in order to penetrate the cell membrane and deliver the DNA to the cytoplasm. However, in addition to the possibility of damaging the cell membrane, the transferred genes are expressed transiently and the frequency of stable integration is low (239). The advantages of this method are its applicability to in vivo gene transfer, the capability of transferring large DNA molecules, and the ability to use it on a variety of cell types since the cell membrane is unable to act as a selective barrier.

Viral vectors provide the most efficient methods for gene transfer to date. Replication-deficient recombinant viral particles may be used for gene transfer into human cells. Retroviruses used for gene therapy are single-stranded RNA viruses approximately 8 kilo basepairs (kbp) in size. They are made replication deficient by deleting all viral sequences except those required for packaging RNA into the virion, integration of viral DNA into the genome, and expression of proviral encoded proteins (240–242). These deleted sequences are replaced with the desired gene (243). Packaging cells replace those functions that are deleted. The packaging cells shed the viral particles into the medium, which is then incubated with target cells. The virus adsorbs onto the target cell using specific receptors or enters via endocytosis (244). Once the viral envelope fuses with the target cell, viral RNA enters the cytosol where it is reverse-transcribed into double-stranded DNA before it is randomly integrated into the host cell genome (240,241,243). Retroviruses are capable of stable integration in a variety of cell types with minimal rearrangement; however, this method is limited as to the size of gene that can be transferred (less than 6 kbp). A further disadvantage of this method of gene transfer is that integration of most retroviruses (HIV being the exception) only occurs in dividing cells during nuclear breakdown (245,246). Integration is limited by the rate of intracellular decay of the retrovirus such that only viruses that enter cells shortly before division are able to integrate into the host genome. There is current research underway using a retroviral vector based on a lentivirus that is capable of integrating into the genome of nonproliferating cells (247). Other disadvantages include the possibility of insertional mutagenesis, possibly of a tumor suppressor gene, resulting in tumorigenesis. The retrovirus might also recombine with a replication-competent virus (248).

Recombinant adenoviruses are double-stranded, nonenveloped DNA viruses approximately 36 kbp in size. The use of adenoviral gene transfer is relatively safe following the deletion of genes required for replication and cellular transformation. Deletion of viral genes is also necessary to accommodate the gene of interest since the size of the viral genome cannot exceed 105% in order to be packaged into virion procapsid (249). New techniques are being developed whereby adenoviruses act as carriers for DNA (250). The adenovirus can attach and penetrate the cell via coated pits. Once inside the endocytic vesicles, the adenovirus causes lysis of the vesicle before degradation occurs. The advantage of this method of gene transfer is that larger DNA molecules may be used than if the DNA were inside the viral capsid. However, this method is less efficient than when the gene is inside the capsid and the complexes can aggregate, which may result in toxicity.

This form of gene delivery demonstrates a broad host range, the highest gene transfer efficiency in vivo, and these viruses can infect both dividing and nondividing cells with high efficiency. In contrast to retroviruses, which may cause insertional mutagenesis, adenoviral replication occurs outside the nucleus. However, possible disadvantages of this method include an inflammatory response to viral particles and the transient gene expression, which may be due to a dilution effect as cells divide, degradation of vector DNA, or to the immune response elicited by viral proteins (251,252). The inflammatory response presently prevents the repeated use of adenoviruses due to neutralizing antibodies and cellular immunity (253,254).

Although better gene transfer using viral methods can be obtained compared with nonviral methods, there are risks, including the potential of replication-competent viruses and, in the case of retroviruses, target cell transformation by insertional mutagenesis.

The effects of fibrogenic growth factors, such as TGF-β1, appear to be central in the development of HSc and keloids, so therapies directed toward decreasing bioactive levels of these growth factors or correcting the ECM defects manifested by them appear to be key in controlling these lesions.

By understanding the regulation of TGF-β1, it is possible to develop methods, such as the use of connective tissue growth factor antagonists, that minimize levels of active TGF-β1, but not to the point at which the required effects of TGF-β1 are also lost. Decorin is able to bind and neutralize TGF-β through its core protein (255). Isaka et al. (256) had shown that injection of recombinant decorin into rats with experimental glomerulonephritis was as effective as using anti–TGF-β1 antibodies in reducing ECM accumulation in the glomeruli. This same group later used muscle-based gene therapy using the rat skeletal muscle to produce the recombinant protein. It is known that decorin is a secreted protein that when injected is taken up by the liver, kidney, and lung (257). Decorin gene transfer was shown to decrease proteinuria in these rats, decrease glomerular

TGF-β1 mRNA expression 37% lower than control (pAct-CAT transfected), and decrease ECM accumulation. This reduction may be adequate in reducing fibrosis without an extreme reduction, which is pathological (258). This study demonstrated the ability to safely deliver a protein into the systemic circulation by injecting the DNA into skeletal muscle. The potential therapeutic effects of decorin lie not only in its ability to bind and neutralize TGF-β1 but also in its role in collagen fibril organization (148).

Another therapeutic agent for fibroproliferative disorders that is being studied is IFN-α2b. Interferons are cytokines with antiproliferative properties and it has been suggested that they would be successful in counteracting some of the process occurring in HSc and keloids. The interferons have been shown to decrease collagen synthesis and inhibit proliferation and chemotaxis of normal human fibroblasts (200,259–261). IFN-α2b may also be able suppress the effects of IGF-1 (discussed above). The effect of interferon-α2b was demonstrated by encapsulating it in liposomes and applying it topically to guinea pig wound to assess its effect on wound healing (262). A significant reduction in the rate of contraction was reported after 5 days, which continued up to 10 days. There was also a reduction in pro-α1(I) type I collagen and pro-α1(III) mRNA. Since dermal fibrotic conditions are associated with an excess of type I and type III collagen, this finding suggests that IFN-α2b may be a successful therapeutic agent.

IFN-α has recently been considered in cancer therapy due to its antiproliferative properties (263). In particular, IFN-α has been shown to inhibit chronic myelogenous leukemia (CML) bone marrow progenitor growth (264,265). The CML progenitor cells express higher levels of Fas receptor in the presence of IFN-α and this is thought to make them more susceptible to apoptosis. Therefore overexpression of IFN-α may inhibit CML growth but still allow normal cell growth. Adenovirus-mediated gene transfer was used to transfect IFN-α into normal human CD34$^+$ stem cells in vitro and the investigators found no suppression of cell growth or differentiation. This method of gene transfer may prove successful in wound healing models due to its lack of suppressive effects on normal cells and its transient expression.

REFERENCES

1. Tredget EE, Nedelec B, Scott PG, Ghahary A. Hypertrophic scars, keloids, and contractures: the cellular and molecular basis for therapy. Surg Clin N Am 1997; 77:701–730.
2. Tuan T, Nichter LS. The molecular basis of keloid and hypertrophic scar formation. Mol Med Today 1998; 19–24.
3. Cohen IK, McCoy BJ. The biology and control of surface overhealing. World J Surg 1980; 4:297–299.

4. Alhady SMA and Sivanantharajah K. Keloids in various races. Plast Reconstr Surg 1969; 44:564–566.

5. Omo-Dare P. Genetic studies on keloid. J Natl Med Assoc 1975; 67:428–432.

6. Wysocki AB, Grinnell F. Fibronectin profiles in normal and chronic wound fluid. Lab Invest 1990; 63:825–831.

7. Oka Y, Orth DN. Human plasma epidermal growth factor/β-urogastrone is associated with blood platelets. J Clin Invest 1983; 72:249–259.

8. Karey KP, Sirbasku DA. Human platelet-derived mitogens. II. Subcellular localization of insulin like growth factor-1 to the α-granule and release in response to thrombin. Blood 1989; 74:1093–1100.

9. Kohler N, Lipton A. Platelets as a source of fibroblast growth-promoting activity. Exp Cell Res 1974; 87:297–301.

10. Ross R, Glomset JA, Kariya B, Harker L. A platelet dependent serum factor that stimulates the proliferation of arterial smooth muscle cells in vitro. Proc Natl Acad Sci USA 1974; 71:1207–1210.

11. Assoian RK, Komoriya A, Meyers CA, Miller DM, Sporn MB. Transforming growth factor-β in human platelets. Identification of a major storage site, purification and characterization. J Biol Chem 1983; 258:7155–7160.

12. Grotendorst GR, Chang T, Seppa HE, Kleinman HK, Martin GR. Platelet-derived growth factor is a chemoattractant for vascular smooth muscle cells. J Cell Physiol 1983; 113:261–266.

13. Seppa H, Grotendorst GR, Seppa SI, Schiffman E, Martin GR. Platelet-derived growth factor is chemotactic for fibroblasts. J Cell Biol 1982; 92:584–588.

14. Roberts AB, Sporn MB, Assoian RK, Smith JM, Roche NS, Wakefield LM, Heine UJ, Liotta LA, Falanga V, Kehrl JH. Transforming growth factor type beta: rapid induction of fibrosis and angiogenesis in vivo and stimulation of collagen formation in vitro. Proc Natl Acad Sci USA 1986; 83:4167–4171.

15. Desmouliere A, Badid C, Bochaton-Pillat M-L, Gabbiani G. Apoptosis during wound healing, fibrocontractive diseases and vascular wall injury. Int J Biochem Cell Biol 1997; 29:19–30.

16. Abraham JA, Klagsbrun M. Modulation of wound repair by members of the fibroblast growth factor family. In: Clark RAF, ed. The Molecular and Cellular Biology of Wound Repair. New York: Plenum, 1996:195–248.

17. Clark RAF. Wound repair: overview and considerations. In: Clark RAF, ed. The Molecular and Cellular Biology of Wound Repair. New York: Plenum, 1996:275–298.

18. Nedelec B, Tredget EE, Ghahary A. The molecular biology of wound healing following thermal injury: the role of fibrogenic growth factors. In: Critical Care of the Burn Patient. Barcelona: Springer-Verlag, 1996.

19. Raghow R. The role of extracellular matrix in post inflammatory wound healing and fibrosis. FASEB J 1994; 8:823–831.

20. Deitch EA, Wheelahan TM, Rose MP, Clothier J, Cotter J. Hypertrophic burn scars: Analysis of variables. J Trauma 1983; 23:895–898.

21. Oluwasanmi JO. Keloids in the African. Clin Plast Surg 1974; 1:179–195.

22. Cohen IK, McCoy BJ, Mohanakumar T, Diegelmann RF. Immunoglobulin, com-

plement, and histocompatibility antigen studies in keloid patients. Plast Reconstr Surg 1979; 63:689–695.

23. Blackburn WR, Cosman B. Histologic basis of keloid and hypertrophic scar differentiation. Clinicopathologic correlations. Arch Pathol 1966; 82:65–71.

24. Linares HA, Kischer CW, Dobrkovsky M, Larson DL. The histiotypic organization of the hypertrophic scar in humans. J Invest Dermatol 1972; 59:323–331.

25. Majno G, Gabbiani G, Hirschel BJ, Ryan GB, Statkov PR. Contraction of granulation tissue in vitro: similarity to smooth muscle. Science 1971; 173:548–550.

26. Schurch W, Seemayer TA, Gabbiani G. Myofibroblast. In: Sternberg SS, ed. Histology for Pathologists. New York: Raven, 1992:109–144.

27. Gabbiani G, Ryan GB, Manjo G. Presence of modified fibroblasts in granulation tissue and their possible role in wound contraction. Experientia 1971; 27:549–550.

28. Lane BP. Alterations in the cytologic detail of intestinal smooth muscle cells in various stages of contraction. J Cell Biol 1965; 27:199–213.

29. Bloom S, Cancilla PA. Conformational changes in myocardial nuclei of rats. Circulation Res 1969; 24:189–196.

30. Majno G, Shea SM, Leventhal M. Endothelial contraction induced by histamine-type mediators: an electron microscope study. J Cell Biol 1969; 42:647–672.

31. Darby I, Skalli O, Gabbiani G. Alpha-smooth muscle actin is transiently expressed by myofibroblasts during experimental wound healing. Lab Invest 1990; 63:21–29.

32. Schmitt-Graff A, Desmouliere A, Gabbiani G. Heterogeneity of myofibroblast phenotypic features: an example of fibroblastic cell plasticity. Virchows Arch 1994; 425:3–24.

33. Hirschel BJ, Gabbiani G, Ryan GB, Manjo G. Fibroblasts of granulation tissue: immunofluorescent staining with antismooth muscle serum. Proc Soc Exp Biol Med 1971; 138:466–469.

34. Gabbiani G, Hirschel BJ, Ryan GB, Statkov PR, Manjo G. Granulation tissue as a contractile organ. J Exp Med 1972; 135:719–734.

35. Ryan GB, Cliffs J, Gabbiani G, Irle C, Montandon D, Statkov PR, Manjo G. Myofibroblasts in human granulation tissue. Hum Pathol 1974; 5:55–67.

36. Rungger-Brandle E, Gabbiani G. The role of cytoskeletal and cytocontractile elements in pathologic processes. Am J Pathol 1983; 110:361–392.

37. Singer II, Kawka D, Kazazis DM, Clark RAF. In vivo codistribution of fibronecrin and actin fibres in granulation tissue: immunofluorescence and electron microscope studies of the fibronexus at the myofibroblast surface. J Cell Biol 1984; 98:2091–2106.

38. Harris AK, Wild P, Stopak D. Silicone rubber substrata: a new wrinkle in the study of cell locomotion. Science 1980; 208:177–179.

39. Harris AK, Stopack D, Wild P. Fibroblast traction as a mechanism for collagen morphogenesis. Nature 1981; 290:249–251.

40. Izzard CS, Lochner LR. Cell-to-substrate contacts in living fibroblasts: an interference reflexion study with an evaluation of the technique. J Cell Sci 1976; 21:129–160.

41. Abercrombie M. The crawling movement of metazoan cells. Proc R Soc Lond [Biol] 1978; 207:129–147.

42. Herman IM, Crisona NJ, Pollard TD. Relation between cell activity and the distribution of cytoplasmic actin and myosin. J Cell Biol 1981; 90:84–91.

43. Geiger B. A 130 K protein from chicken gizzard. Its localization at the termini of microfilament bundles in cultured chicken cells. Cell 1979; 18:193–205.

44. Isenberg G, Rathke PC, Hulsmann N, Franke W, Wohlfarth-Botterman KE. Cytoplasmic actomyosin fibrils in tissue culture cells. Cell Tissue Res 1976; 166:427–443.

45. Kreis TE, Birchmeier W. Stress fiber sarcomeres of fibroblasts are contractile. Cell 1980; 22:555–561.

46. Ehrlich HP. Wound closure: evidence of cooperation between fibroblasts and collagen matrix. Eye 1988; 2:149–157.

47. Doillon CJ, Hembry RM, Ehrich HP, Burke JF. Actin filaments in normal dermis and during wound healing. Am J Pathol 1987; 126:164–170.

48. Desmoulière A, Gabbiani G. Smooth muscle cell and fibroblast biological and functional features: similarities and differences. In: Schwartz SM, Mecham RP, eds. The Vascular Smooth Muscle Cell: Molecular and Biological Responses to the Extracellular Matrix. San Diego: Academic, 1995:329–359.

49. Yokoyama Y, Ozawa S, Seyama Y, Namiki H, Hayashi Y, Kaji K, Shirama K, Shioda M, Kano K. Enhancement of apoptosis in developing chick neural retina cells by basic fibroblast growth factor. J Neurochem 1997; 68:2212–2215.

50. Muir DA, Compston DA. Growth factor stimulation triggers apoptotic cell death in mature oligodendrocytes. J Neurosci Res 1996; 44:1–11.

51. Imaizumi T, Jean-Louis LF, Dubertret ML, Bailly C, Cicurel L, Petchot BJ, Dubertret L. Effect of human basic fibroblast growth factor on fibroblast proliferation, cell volume, collagen lattice contraction: in comparison with acidic type. J Dermatol Sci 1996; 11:134–141.

52. Funato N, Moriyama K, Shimokawa H, Kuroda T. Basic fibroblast growth factor induces apoptosis in myofibroblastic cells isolated from rat palatal mucosa. Biochem Biophys Res Commun 1997; 240:21–26.

53. Rockwell WB, Cohen IK, Ehrlich HP. Keloids and hypertrophic scars: a comprehensive review. Plast Reconstr Surg 1989; 84:827–837.

54. Younai S, Venter G, Vu S, Nichter L, Nimni ME, Tuan TL. Role of growth factors in scar contraction: an in vitro analysis. Ann Plast Surg 1996; 36:495–501.

55. Squier CA. The stretching effect on formation of myofibroblasts in mouse skin. Cell Tissue Res 1981; 220:325–335.

56. Kischer CW, Bailey JF. The mast cell in hypertrophic scars. Tex Rep Biol Med 1972; 30:327–328.

57. Kischer CW, Bunce H, Shetlar MR. Mast cell analyses in hypertrophic scars, hypertrophic scars treated with pressure and mature scars. J Invest Dermatol 1978; 70:355–357.

58. Kischer CW, Shetlar MR, Chvapil M. Hyperthophic scars and keloids: a review and new concept concerning their origin. Scanning Electron Microsc 1982; 4:1699–1713.

59. Taipale J, Lohi J, Saarinen J, Kovanen PT, Keski-Oja J. Human mast cell chymase

and leukocyte elastase release latent transforming growth factor-β1 from the extracellular matrix of cultured human epithelial and endothelial cells. J Biol Chem 1995; 270:4689–4696.

60. Smith CJ, Smith JC, Finn MC. The possible role of mast cells (allergy) in the production of keloid and hypertrophic scarring. J Burn Care Rehabil 1987; 8:126–131.

61. Sandberg N. Accelerated collagen formation and histamine [letter]. Nature 1962; 194:183.

62. Hakanson R, Owman C, Sjoberg NO, Sporrong B. Direct histochemical demonstration of histamine in cutaneous mast cells: urticaria pigmentosa and keloids. Experientia 1969; 25:854–855.

63. Buffoni F, Faimondi L. A lysyl oxidase with histaminase activity in the pig aorta. Agents Actions 1981; 11:38–41.

64. Scott PG, Dodd CM, Tredget EE, Ghahary A, Rahemtulla F. Chemical characterization and quantification of proteoglycans in human post-burn hypertrophic and mature scars. Clin Sci 1996; 90:417–425.

65. Chung E, Rhodes RK, Miller EJ. Isolation of three collagenous components of probable basement membrane origin from several tissues. Biochem Biophys Res Commun 1976; 71:1167–1174.

66. Ehrlich HP, White BS. The identification of alphaA and alphaB collagen chains in hypertrophic scar. Exp Mol Pathol 1981; 34:1–8.

67. Madri JA, Furthmayr H. Isolation and tissue localization of type AB2 collagen from normal lung parenchyma. Am J Pathol 1979; 94:323–331.

68. Roll FJ, Madri JA, Albert J, Furthmayr H. Codistribution of collagen types IV and AB2 in basement membranes and mesangium of the kidney. An immunoferritin study of ultrathin frozen sections. Lab Invest 1980; 43:303–315.

69. Adachi E, Hayashi T. In vitro formation of hybrid fibrils of type V collagen and type I collagen. Limited growth of type I collagen into thick fibrils by type V collagen. Connect Tissue Res 1986; 14:257–266.

70. Birk DE, Fitch JM, Babiarz JP, Doane KJ, Linsenmayer TF. Collagen fibrillogenesis in vitro: interaction of types I and V collagen regulates fibril diameter. J Cell Sci 1990; 95:649–657.

71. Peltonen J, Hsiao LH, Jaakhola S, Sollberg S, Aumailley M, Timpl R, Chu M-L, Uitto J. Activation of collagen gene expression in keloids: colocalization of type I and VI collagen and transforming growth factor-β1 mRNA. J Invest Dermatol 1991; 97:240–248.

72. Furthmayr H, Wiedemann H, Timpl R, Odermatt E, Engel J. Electron-microscopical approach to a structural model of intima collagen. Biochem J 1983; 211:303–311.

73. Engel J, Furthmayr H, Odermatt E, von der Mark H, Aumailley M, Fleischmajer R, Timpl R. Structure and macromolecular organization of type VI collagen. Ann NY Acad Sci 1985; 460:25–37.

74. Kischer CW. Collagen and dermal patterns in the hypertrophic scar. Anat Rec 1974; 179:137–145.

75. Ehrlich HP, Desmouliere A, Diegelmann RF, Cohen IK, Compton CC, Garner WL, Kapanci Y, Gabbiani G. Morphological and immunochemical differences between keloid and hypertrophic scar. Am J Pathol 1994; 145:105–113.

76. Su CW, Alizadeh K, Boddie A, Lee R. The problem scar. Clin Plast Surg 1998; 25:451–65.
77. Shetlar MR, Shetlar CL, Kischer CW. Glycosaminoglycans in granulation tissue and hypertrophic scars. Burns 1981; 8:27–31.
78. Shetlar MR, Shetlar CL, Linares HA. The hypertrophic scar: location of glycosaminoglycans within scars. Burns 1977; 4:14–19.
79. Rajaraman R. In: Malhotra S, ed. Advances in Structural Biology. Greenwich, CT: JAI, 1991:117–174.
80. Fava RA, McClure DB. Fibronectin-associated transforming growth factor. J Cell Physiol 1987; 131:184–189.
81. Kischer CW, Hendrix MJC. Fibronectin (FN) in hypertrophic scars and keloids. Cell Tissue Res 1983; 231:29–37.
82. Tsuji T, Sawabe M. Elastic fibers in scar tissue: scanning and transmission electron microscopic studies. J Cutan Pathol 1987; 14:106–113.
83. DeVries HJC, Zeegelaar JE, Middelkoop E, Gijsbers G, VanMarle J, Wildevuur CHR, Weterhof W. Reduced wound contraction and scar formation in punch biopsy wounds. Native collagen dermal substitutes. A clinical study. Br J Dermatol 1995; 132:690–697.
84. DeVries HJC, Middelkoop E, Mekkes JR, et al. Dermal regeneration in native non-cross-linked collagen sponges with different extra-cellular matrix molecules. Wound Repair Regen 1994; 2:37–47.
85. Linares HA, Larson DL. Elastic tissue and hypertrophic scars. Burns 1976; 3:4–7.
86. Compton CC, Gill JM, Bradford DA, Regauer S, Gallico GG, O'Connor NE. Skin regenerated from cultured epithelial autografts on full-thickness burn wounds from 6 days to 5 years after grafting. A light electron microscopic and immunohistochemical study. Lab Invest 1989; 60:600–612.
87. McKay I. In: McKay I, Leigh I, eds. Growth Factors: A Practical Approach. Oxford: IRL, 1993:251.
88. Roberts AB, Sporn MB. Transforming growth factor-β. In: Clark RAF, ed. The Molecular and Cellular Biology of Wound Repair. New York: Plenum, 1996:275–298.
89. Postlethwaite AE, Keski-Oja J, Moses HL, Kang AH. Stimulation of the chemotactic migration of human fibroblasts by transforming growth factor-β. J Exp Med 1987; 165:251–256.
90. Wahl SM, Hunt DA, Wakefield LM, McCartney-Francis N, Wahl LM, Roberts AB, Sporn MB. Transforming growth factor-β (TGF-β) induces monocyte chemotaxis and growth factor production. Proc Natl Acad Sci USA 1987; 84:5788–5792.
91. Frank S, Madlener M, Werner S. Transforming growth factors 1, 2, and 3 and their receptors are differentially regulated during normal and impaired wound healing. J Biol Chem 1996; 271:10188–10193.
92. Zhou L, Ono I, Kaneko F. Role of transforming growth factor-β1 in fibroblasts derived from normal and hypertrophic scarred skin. Arch Dermatol Res 1997; 289: 646–652.
93. Ghahary A, Shen YJ, Nedelec B, et al. Collagenase production is lower in post-

burn hypertrophic scar fibroblasts than in normal fibroblasts and is reduced by insulin-like growth factor-1. J Invest Dermatol 1996; 106:476–481.

94. Ghahary A, Shen YJ, Scott PG, Gong Y, Tredget EE. Enhanced expression of mRNA for transforming growth factor-beta, type I and type III procollagen in human post-burn hypertrophic scar tissues. J Lab Clin Med 1993; 122:465–473.

95. Bloom BB, Humphries DE, Kuang PP, Fine A, Goldstein RH. Structure and expression of the promotor for the RI human type I transforming growth factor-β receptor: regulation by TGF-β. Biochim Biophys Acta 1996; 1312:243–248.

96. McWhirter A, Colosetti P, Rubin K, Miyazono K, Black C. Collagen type I is not under autocrine control by transforming growth factor-beta 1 in normal and scleroderma fibroblasts. Lab Invest 1994; 71:885–894.

97. Desmoulière A, Geinoz A, Gabbiani F, Gabbiani G. Transforming growth factor-β1 induces α-smooth muscle actin expression in granulation tissue myofibroblasts and in quiescent and growing cultured fibroblasts. J Cell Biol 1993; 122:103–111.

98. Tsuji T, Okada F, Yamaguchi K, Nakamura T. Molecular cloning of the large subunit of transforming growth factor type β masking protein and expression of the mRNA in various rat tissues. Proc Natl Acad Sci USA 1990; 87:8835–8839.

99. Purchio AF, Cooper JA, Brunner AM, Lioubin MN, Gentry LF, Kovacina KS, Roth RA, Marquardt H. Identification of mannose 6-phosphate in 2 asparagine-linked sugar chains of recombinant transforming growth factor-β-1 precursor. J Biol Chem 1988; 263:14211–14215.

100. Miyazono K, Olofsson A, Colosetti P, Heldin CH. A role of the latent TGF-β binding protein in the assembly and secretion of TGF-β. EMBO J 1991; 10:1091–1101.

101. Grainger DJ, Wakefield L, Bethell HW, Farndale RW, Metcalfe JC. Release and activation of platelet latent TGF-in blood clots during dissolution with plasmin. Nature Med. 1995; 1:932–937.

102. Okazaki R, Durham SK, Riggs BL, Conver CA. Transforming growth factor and forskolin increase all classes of insulin-like growth factor-1 transcripts in normal human osteoblast-like cells. Biochem Biophys Res Commun 1995; 207:963–970.

103. Dallas SL, Park-Snyder S, Miyazono K, Twardzik D, Mundy GR, Bonewald LF. Characterization and autoregulation of latent transforming growth factor beta (TGF-beta) complexes in osteoblast-like cell line: production of a latent complex lacking the latent TGF-β binding protein. J Biol Chem 1994; 269:6815–6821.

104. Wakefield LM, Smith DM, Masui T, Harris CC, Sporn MB. Distribution and modulation of the cellular receptor for transforming growth factor-β. J Cell Biol 1987; 105:965–975.

105. Wakefield LM, Winoker TS, Hollands RS, Christopherson K, Levinson AD, Sporn MB. Recombinant latent TGF-β1 has a longer half life in rats than active TGF-β1 and a different tissue distribution. J Clin Invest 1990; 86:1976–84.

106. Okubo H, Ishibashi H, Shibata J, Tsuda-Kawamura K, Yanase T. Distribution of alpha2-macroglobulin in normal, inflammatory, and tumor tissues in rats. Inflammation 1984; 8:171–179.

107. Feldman SR, Rosenberg MR, Ney KA, Michalopoulos G, Pizzo SV. Binding of alpha2-macroglobulin to hepatocytes: mechanism of in vivo clearance. Biochem Biophys Res Commun 1985; 128:795–802.

108. Dickson K, Philip A, Warshawsky H, O'Connor-McCourt M, Bergeron JJM. Spe-

cific binding of endocrine transforming growth factor-β1 to vascular endothelium. J Clin Invest 1995; 95:2539–2554.

109. Gamble JR, Vadas MA. Endothelial adhesiveness for blood neureophils is inhibited by transforming growth factor-beta 1. Science 1988; 242:97–99.

110. Lefer AM. Mechanisms of the protective effects of transforming growth factor-β in reperfusion injury. Biochem Pharmacol 1991; 42:1323–1327.

111. Lefer AM, Ma XL, Weyrich AS, Scalia R. Mechanism of the cardioprotective effect of TGF-β1 in feline myocardial ischemia and reperfusion. Proc Natl Acad Sci USA 1993; 90:1018–1022.

112. Gamble JR, Khew-Goodall Y, Vadas MA. Transforming growth factor β inhibits E-selectin expression on human endothelial cells. J Immunol 1993; 150:4494–4503.

113. Shull MM, Ormsby I, Kier AB, et al. Targeted disruption of the mouse transforming growth factor-β1 gene results in multifocal inflammatory disease. Nature 1992; 359:693–699.

114. Kulkarni AB, Huh CG, Becker D, et al. Transforming growth factor-β1 null mutation in mice causes excessive inflammatory response and early death. Proc Natl Acad Sci USA 1993; 90:770–774.

115. Wahl SM. Transforming growth factor β: the good, the bad, the ugly. J Exp Med 1994; 180:1587–1590.

116. Mustoe TA, Pierce GF, Thomason A, Gramates P, Sporn MB, Deuel TF. Accelerated healing of incisional wounds in rats induced by transforming growth factor β. Science 1987; 237:1333–1336.

117. Beck LS, DeGuzman L, Lee WP, Xu Y, Siegel MW, Amento EP. One systemic administration of transforming growth factor-β1 reverses age- or glucocorticoid-impaired wound healing. J Clin Invest 1993; 92:2841–2849.

118. Wahl SM, Wong JB, Allen JB, Ellingsworth LR. Antagonistic and agonistic effects of transforming growth factor β and IL-1 in rheumatoid arthritis. J Immunol 1990; 145:2514–2519.

119. Allen JB, Wong HL, Guyre PM, Simon GL, Wahl SM. Association of circulating FcγRIII-positive monocytes in AIDS patients with elevated levels of transforming growth factor-β. J Clin Invest 1991; 87:1773–1779.

120. Lowrance JH, O'Sullivan FX, Caver TE, Waegell W, Gresham HD. Spontaneous elaboration of transforming growth factor β suppresses host defense against bacterial infection in autoimmune MRL/1pr mice. J Exp Med 1994; 180:1693–1703.

121. Lyons RM, Oja JK, Moses HL. Proteolytic activation of latent transforming growth factor-β from fibroblast conditioned medium. J Cell Biol 1988; 106:1659–1665.

122. Lyons RM, Gentry LE, Purchio AF, Moses HL. Mechanism of activation of latent recombinant transforming growth factor-β1 by plasmin. J Cell Biol 1990; 110:1361–1367.

123. Sato Y, Rifkin DB. Inhibition of endothelial cell movement by pericytes and smooth muscle cells: activation of a latent transforming growth factor-1-like molecule by plasmin. J Cell Biol 1989; 109:309–315.

124. Sato Y, Tsuboi R, Lyons RM, Moses HL, Rifkin DB. Characterization of the activation of latent TGF-β by co-cultures of endothelial cells and pericytes or smooth muscle cells: a self-regulating system. J Cell Biol 1990; 111:757–763.

125. Tuan TL, Zhu JY, Sun B, Nichter LS, Nimni ME, Laug WE. Elevated levels of plasminogen activator inhibitor-1 may account for the altered fibrinolysis by keloid fibroblasts. J Invest Dermatol 1996; 106:1007–1011.

126. DeClerck YA, Laug WF. The role of extracellular matrix in tumor invasion and metastasis. In: Teicher RA, ed. Mechanism of Drug Resistance in Oncology. New York: Marcel Dekker, 1993:121–163.

127. Roberts AB, Sporn MB. The transforming growth factor betas. In: Sporn MB, Roberts AB, eds. Peptide Growth Factors and Their Receptors. Handbook of Experimental Pharmacology. New York: Springer-Verlag, 1990:419–472.

128. Schwartz LB, Austen KF. Structure and function of the chemical mediators of mast cells. Prog Allergy 1984; 34:271–321.

129. Salvesen G, Enghild JJ. An unusual specificity in the activation of neutrophil serine proteinase zymogens. Biochemistry 1990; 29:5304–5308.

130. Frommherz KJ, Faller B, Bieth JG. Heparin strongly decreases the rate of inhibition of neutrophil elastase by alpha 1-proteinase inhibitor. J Biol Chem 1991; 266:15356–15362.

131. Schechter NM, Sprows JL, Shoenberger OL, Lazarus GS, Cooperman BS, Rubin H. Reaction of human skin chymotrypsin-like proteinase chymase with plasma proteinase inhibitors. J Biol Chem 1989; 264:21308–21315.

132. Schechter NM, Irani AMA, Sprows JL, Abernethy J, Wintroub B, Schwartz LB. Identification of a cathepsin G-like proteinase in the MCTC type of human mast cell. J Immunol 1990; 8:2652–2661.

133. Dennis PA, Rifkin DB. Cellular activation of latent transforming growth factor-β requires binding to the cation-independent mannose 6-phosphate/insulin-like growth factor type II receptor. Proc Natl Acad Sci USA 1991; 88:580–584.

134. Ghahary A, Tredget EE, Shen Q. Insulin-like growth factor-II/mannose 6 phosphate receptors facilitate the matrix effects of latent transforming growth factor-β1 released from genetically modified keratinocytes in a fibroblast/keratinocyte co-culture system. J Cell Physiol 1999; 180:61–70.

135. Sato Y, Rifkin DB. Autocrine activities of basic fibroblast growth factor: regulation of endothelial cell movement, plasminogen activator synthesis, and DNA synthesis. J Cell Biol 1988; 107:1199–1205.

136. Kojima S and Rifkin DB. Mechanism of retinoid-induced activation of latent transforming growth factor-β in bovine endothelial cells. J Cell Physiol 1993; 155:323–332.

137. Bendixen E, Borth W, Harpel PC. Crosslinking of plasminogens to fibronectin by factor XIIIa and tissue transglutaminase. Blood 1991; 78(suppl):1–28.

138. Schultz-Cherry S, Ribeiro S, Gentry L, Murphy UJ. Thrombospondin binds and activates the small and large forms of latent transforming growth factor-β in a chemically defined system. J Biol Chem 1994; 269:26775–26782.

139. Caver TE, O'Sullivan FX, Gold LI, Gresham HD. Intracellular demonstration of active TGF-β1 in B cells and plasma cells of autoimmune mice. J Clin Invest 1996; 98:2496–2506.

140. Wrana JL, Attisano L, Wieser R, Ventura F, Massague J. Mechanism of activation of the TGF-β receptor. Nature 1994; 370:341–347.

141. Wieser R, Wrana JL, Massague J. GS domain mutations that constitutively activate

T beta R-I, the downstream signaling component in the TGF-beta receptor complex. EMBO J 1995; 14:2199–2208.

142. Attisano L, Wrana JL, Montalvo E, Massague J. Activation of signalling by the activin receptor complex. Mol Cell Biol 1996; 16:1066–1073.

143. Schmid P, Itin P, Cherry G, Bi C, Cox DA. Enhanced expression of transforming growth factor-β type I and type II receptors in wound granulation tissue and hypertrophic scar. Am J Pathol 1998; 152:485–493.

144. Kim SJ, Angel P, Lafyatis R, Hattori K, Kim KY, Sporn MB, Karin M, Roberts AB. Autoinduction of transforming growth factor-β1 is mediated by the AP-1 complex. Mol Cell Biol 1990; 10:1492–1497.

145. Wakefield LM, Letterio JJ, Chen T, Danielpour D, Allison RS, Pai LH, Denicoff AM, Noone MH, Cowan KH, O'Shaughnessy JA, Sporn MB. Transforming growth factor-β1 circulates in normal plasma and is unchanged in advanced metastatic breast cancer. Clin Cancer Res 1995; 1:129–136.

146. McCaffrey TA, Falcone DJ, Brayton CF, Agarwal LA, Welt FGP, Weksler BB. Transforming growth factor-β activity is potentiated by heparin via dissociation of the transforming growth factor-beta/alpha 2-macroglobulin inactive complex. J Cell Biol 1989; 109:441–448.

147. Kuby J. Hypersensitive reactions. In: Kuby J, ed. Immunology. (2nd ed). New York: WH Freeman, 1991:419–434.

148. Scott PG, Dodd CM, Ghahary A, Shen YJ, Tredget EE. Fibroblasts from post-burn hypertrophic scar tissue synthesize less decorin than normal dermal fibroblasts. Clin Sci 1998; 94:541–547.

149. Kahari V, Larjava H, Uitto J. Differential regulation of extracellular matrix proteoglycan (pg) gene expression. J Biol Chem 1991; 266:10608–10615.

150. Andres JL, Stanley K, Cheifetz S, Massague J. Membrane-anchored and soluble forms of betaglycan, a polymorphic proteoglycan that binds transforming growth factor-beta. J Cell Biol 1989; 109:3137–3145.

151. Saksela O, Moscatelli D, Sommer A, Rifkin DB. Endothelial cell-derived heparan sulphate binds basic fibroblast growth factor and protects it from proteolytic degradation. J Cell Biol 1988; 107:743–751.

152. Scott PG, Dodd CM, Tredget EE, Ghahary A, Rahemtulla F. Immunohistochemical localization of the proteoglycans decorin, biglycan and versican and transforming growth factor-β in human post-burn hypertrophic and mature scars. Histopathology 1995; 26:423–431.

153. Gartner MH, Benson JD, Caldwell MD. Insulin-like growth factors I and II expression in the healing wound. J Surg Res 1992; 52:389–394.

154. Makower AM, Wroblewski J, Pawlowski A. Effects of IGF-1, EGF, and FGF on proteoglycans synthesized by fractionated chondrocytes of rat rib growth plate. Exp Cell Res 1988; 179:498–506.

155. Ghahary A, Shen Y, Nedlec B, Scott PG, Tredget EE. Enhanced expression of mRNA for insulin-like growth factor-1 in post burn hypertrophic scar tissue and its fibrogenic role by dermal fibroblasts. Mol Cell Biochem 1995; 148:25–32.

156. D'Ercole AJ, Stiles AD, Underwood LE. Tissue concentrations of somatomedin C: further evidence for multiple sites of synthesis and paracrine or autocrine mechanisms of action. Proc Natl Acad Sci USA 1984; 81:935–939.

157. Murphy LJ, Murphy LC, Friesen HG. Estrogen induces insulin-like growth factor-1 expression in the rat uterus. Mol Endocrinol 1988; 1:445.

158. Martin L, Finn CA, Trinder G. Hypertrophy and hyperplasia in the mouse uterus after estrogen treatment: an autoradiographic study. J Endocrinol 1983; 56:133–144.

159. Murphy LJ, Ghahary A. Uterine insulin-like growth factor-1: regulation of expression and its role in estrogen-induced uterine proliferation. Endocr Rev 1990; 11:443–453.

160. Ghahary A, Murphy LJ. Uterine insulin-like growth factor-1 receptors: regulation by estrogen and variation throughout the estrous cycle. Endocrinology 1989; 125:597–604.

161. Burch WM, Correa J, Shively JE, Powell DR. The 25 kilodalton insulin-like growth factor (IGF)-binding protein inhibits both basal and IGF-1 mediated growth of chick embryo pelvic cartilage in vitro. J Clin Endocrinol Metab 1990; 70:173–180.

162. Murphy LJ, Friesen HG. Differential effects of estrogen and growth hormone on uterine and hepatic insulin-like growth factor-1 gene expression in the ovariectomized, hypophysectomized rat. Endocrinology 1988; 122:325–332.

163. Copeland KC, Johnson DM, Kuehl TJ, Castracane VD. Estrogen stimulates growth hormone and somatomedin-C in castrate and intact female baboons. J Clin Endocrinol Metab 1984; 58:698–703.

164. Rosenfield RL, Furlanetto R. Physiologic testosterone or estradiol induction of puberty increases plasma somatomedin-C. J Pediatr 1985; 107:415–417.

165. Ross JL, Cassorla FG, Skerda MC, Valk IM, Loriaux DL, Cutler GB. A preliminary study of the effect of estrogen dose on growth in Turner's syndrome. N Engl J Med 1983; 309:1104–1106.

166. Liu L, Merriam GR, Sherins RJ. Chronic sex steroid exposure increases in mean plasma growth hormone concentration and pulse amplitude in men with isolated hypogonadotropic hypogonadism. J Clin Endocrinol Metab 1987; 64:651–656.

167. Camacho-Hubner C, Busby WH, McCusker RH, Wright G, Clemmons DR. Identification of the forms of insulin-like growth factor-binding proteins produced by human fibroblasts and the mechanisms that regulate their secretion. J Biol Chem 1992; 267:11949–11956.

168. Jones JI, Gockerman A, Busby WH, Camacho-Hubner C, Clemmons DR. Extracellular matrix contains insulin-like growth factor binding protein-5: Potentiation of the effect of IGF-1. J Cell Biol 1993; 121:679–687.

169. Ghahary A, Shen YJ, Wang R, Scott PG, Tredget EE. Expression and localization of insulin-like growth factor-1 in normal and post-burn hypertrophic scar tissue in human. Mol Cell Biochem 1998; 183:1–9.

170. Barecca A, DeLuca M, Del Monte P, Bondanza S, Damonte G, Cariola G, DiMarco E, Giordano G, Canceda R, Minuto F. In vitro paracine regulation of human keratinocyte growth by fibroblast-derived insulin-like growth factors. J Cell Physiol 1992; 151:262–268.

171. Ghahary A, Shen YJ, Scott PG, Tredget EE. Expression of mRNA for transforming growth factor-β1 is reduced in hypertrophic scar and normal dermal fibroblasts following serial passage in vitro. J Invest Dermatol 1994; 103:684–686.

172. Sporn MB, Roberts AB, Wakefield LM, Crombrugghe B. Some recent advances

in the chemistry and biology of transforming growth factor-beta. J Cell Biol 1987; 105:1039–1045.

173. Nagoka I, Trapnell BC, Crystal RG. Regulation of insulin-like growth factor 1 gene expression in the human macrophage cell line U937. J Clin Invest 1990; 85:448–455.

174. Ghahary A, Shen Q, Shen YJ, Scott PG, Tredget EE. Induction of transforming growth factor-β1 by insulin-like growth factor-1 in dermal fibroblasts. J Cell Phys 1998; 174:301–309.

175. Kalvakolanu DV, Borden EC. An overview of the interferon system: signal transduction and mechanisms of action. Cancer Invest 1996; 14:25–53.

176. Berman B, Bieley HC. Keloids. J Am Acad Dermatol 1995; 33:117–123.

177. Berman B, Bieley HC. Adjunct therapies to surgical management of keloids. Dermatol Surg 1996; 22:126–130.

178. Nedelec B, Dodd CM, Scott PG, Ghahary A, Tredget EE. The effect of interferon-α2b on guinea pig wound closure and the expression of cytoskeletal proteins in vivo. Wound Repair Regen 1998; 6:202–212.

179. Nedelec B, Shen YJ, Ghahary A, Scott PG, Tredget EE. The effect of interferon-α2b on the expression of cytoskeletal proteins in an in vitro model of wound contraction. J Lab Clin Med 1995; 126:474–484.

180. Fu XY, Kessler DS, Veals SA, Levy DA, Darnell JE. ISGF3, the transcriptional activator induced by interferon-α, consists of multiple interacting polypeptide chains. Proc Natl Acad Sci USA 1990; 87:8555–8559.

181. Kessler DS, Veals SA, Fu XY, Levy DE. Interferon-α regulates nuclear translocation and DNA-binding affinity of ISGF3, a multimeric transcriptional activator. Genes Dev 1990; 4:1753–1765.

182. Williams BRG. Transcriptional regulation of interferon-stimulated genes. Eur J Biochem 1991; 200:1–11.

183. Sahara K, Kuckukcelebi A, Ko F, Phillips L, Robson M. Suppression of in vitro proliferative scar fibroblast contraction by interferon α-2b. Wound Repair Regen 1993; 1:22–27.

184. Hansson GK, Hellstrand M, Rymo L, Rubbia L, Gabbiani G. Interferon-γ inhibits the proliferation and expression of differentiation-specific α-smooth muscle actin in arterial smooth muscle cells. J Exp Med 1989; 170:1595–1608.

185. Tomasek JJ, Hay ED. Analysis of the role of microfilaments and microtubules in acquisition of bipolarity and elongation of fibroblasts in hydrated collagen gels. J Cell Biol 1984; 99:536–549.

186. Morgan CJ, Pledger WJ. Fibroblast proliferation. In: Wound Healing. Philadelphia: Saunders, 1992:63–73.

187. Telasky C, Tredget EE, Shen Q, Khorramizadeh MR, Iwashina T, Scott PG, Ghahary A. IFN-α2b suppresses the fibrogenic effects of insulin-like growth factor-1 in dermal fibroblasts. J Interferon Cytokine Res 1998; 18:571–577.

188. Ghahary A, Shen YJ, Nedelec B, Scott PG, Tredget EE. Interferons gamma and alpha-2b differentially regulate the expression of collagenase and tissue inhibitor of metalloproteinase-1 messenger RNA and in human hypertrophic and normal dermis. Wound Repair Regen 1995; 3:176–184.

189. Moncada S, Palmer RMJ, Higgs EA. Nitric oxide: physiology, pathophysiology, and pharmacology. Pharmacol Rev 1991; 43:109–142.

190. Stadler J, Stefanovic-Racic M, Billiar TR, Curran RD, McIntyre LA, Georgescu HI, Simmons RL, Evans CH. Articular chondrocytes synthesize nitric oxide in response to cytokines and lipopolysaccharides. J Immunol 1991; 147:3915–3920.

191. Palmer RM, Hickery MS, Charles IG, Moncada S, Bayliss MT. Induction of nitric oxide synthase in human chondrocytes. Biochem Biophys Res Commun 1993; 193: 398–405.

192. Bani D, Bigazzi M, Masini E, Bani G, Sacchi T. Relaxin depresses platelet aggregation: in vitro studies on isolated human and rabbit platelets. Lab Invest 1995; 73: 709–716.

193. Salvemini D, Masini E, Pistelli A, Mannaioni PF, Vane JR. Nitric oxide: a regulatory mediator of mast cell reactivity. J Cardiovasc Pharmacol 1991; 17:258–264.

194. Murrell GAC, Jang D, Williams RJ. Nitric oxide activates metalloproteases enzymes in articular cartilage. Biochem Biophys Res Commun 1995; 206:15–21.

195. Wang R, Ghahary A, Shen YJ, Scott PG, Tredget EE. Nitric oxide synthase expression and nitric oxide production are reduced in hypertrophic scar tissue and fibroblasts. J Invest Dermatol 1997; 108:438–444.

196. Wang R, Ghahary A, Shen YJ, Scott PG, Tredget EE. Human dermal fibroblasts produce nitric oxide and express both constitutive and inducible nitric oxide synthase isoforms. J Invest Dermatol 1996; 106:419–427.

197. Berman B, Flores F. Recurrence rates of excised keloids treated with postoperative triamcinolone acetonide injections or interferon alpha-2b injections. J Am Dermatol 1997; 37:755–757.

198. McCauley RL, Chopra V, Li Y-Y, Herndon DN, Robson MC. Altered cytokine production in black patients with keloids. J Clin Immunol 1992; 12:300–308.

199. Granstein RD, Murphy GF, Margolis RJ, Byrne MH, Amento EP. Gamma-interferon inhibits collagen synthesis in vivo in the mouse. J Clin Invest 1987; 79:1254–1258.

200. Harrop AR, Ghahary A, Scott PG, Forsyth N, Uji-Friedland A, Tredget EE. Regulation of collagen synthesis and mRNA expression in normal and hypertrophic scar fibroblasts in vitro by interferon-γ. J Surg Res 1995; 58:471–477.

201. Tredget EE, Wang R, Shen Q, Scott PG, Ghahary A. Transforming growth factor-beta mRNA and protein in hypertrophic scar tissues and fibroblasts: antagonism by interferon-alpha and -gamma in vitro and in vivo. J Interferon Cytok Res. In press.

202. Tredget EE, Shankowsky HA, Pannu R, Nedelec B, Iwashina T, Ghahary A, Taerum T, Scott PG. Transforming growth factor-β in thermally injured patients with hypertrophic scars: effects of interferon α-2b. Plast Reconstr Surg 1998; 102: 1317–1328.

203. Vitale M, Fields-Blache C, Luterman A. Servere itching in the patient with burns. J Burn Care Rehabil 1991; 12:330–333.

204. Blundell TL, Humbel RE. Hormone families: pancreatic hormones and homologous growth factors. Nature 1980; 287:781–787.

205. Vasilenko P, Mead JP. Growth-promoting effects of relaxin and related compositional changes in the uterus, cervix, and vagina of the rat. Endocrinology 1987; 120:1370–1376.

206. Whitby DJ, Ferguson MWJ. The extracellular matrix of lip wounds in fetal, neonatal and adult mice. Development 1991; 112:651–668.
207. Whitby DJ, Ferguson MWJ. Immunohistochemical localisation of growth factors in fetal wound healing. Dev Biol 1991; 147:207–215.
208. Krummel TM, Michna BA, Thomas BL, Sporn MB, Nelson JM, Salzberg AM, Cohen IK, Diegelmann RF. Transforming growth factor beta (TGF-β) induces fibrosis in a fetal wound model. J Pediatr Surg 1988; 23:647–652.
209. Shah M, Foreman DM, Ferguson WJ. Control of scarring in adult wounds by neutralizing antibody to transforming growth factor β. Lancet 1992; 339:213–214.
210. Shah M, Foreman DM, Ferguson WJ. Neutralising antibody to TGF-β1,2 reduces cutaneous scarring in adult rodents. J Cell Sci 1994; 107:1137–1157.
211. Kovacina KS, Steele-Perkins G, Purchio AF, Lioubin M, Miyazono K, Heldin CH, Roth RA. Interactions of recombinant and platelet transforming growth factor-β1 precursor with the insulin-like growth factor II/mannose 6-phosphate. Biochem Biophys Res Commun 1989; 160:393–403.
212. Bowen-Pope DF, Malpass TW, Foster DM, Ross R. Platelet-derived growth factor in vivo: levels, activity, and rate of clearance. Blood 1984; 64:458–469.
213. Eming SA, Morgan JR, Berger A. Gene therapy for tissue repair: approaches and prospects. Br J Plast Surg 1997; 50:491–500.
214. Heath TD, Fraley RT, Papahdjopoulos D. Antibody targeting of liposomes: cell specificity obtained by conjugation of F(ab′)2 to vesicle surface. Science 1980; 210:539–541.
215. Heath TD, Bragman KS, Matthay KK, et al. Antibody-directed liposomes: the development of a cell-specific cytotoxic agent. Biochem Soc Trans 1984; 12:340–342.
216. Du Plessis J, Egbaria K, Weiner N. Influence of formulation factors on the deposition of liposomal components into the different strata of the skin. J Soc Cosmet Chem 1992; 43:93–100.
217. Lieb LM, Ramachandran C, Egbaria K, Weiner N. Topical delivery enhancement with multilamellar liposomes into pilosebaceous units: I. In vitro evaluation using fluorescent techniques with the hamster ear model. J Invest Dermatol 1992; 99:108–113.
218. Li L, Hoffman RM. Model of selective gene therapy of hair growth: liposome targeting of the active lac-z gene to hair follicles of histoculture skin. In Vitro Cell Dev Biol 1995; 31A:11–13.
219. Wilson T, Papahadjopoulos D, Taber R. The introduction of poliovirus RNA into cells via lipid versicles (liposomes). Cell 1979; 17:77–84.
220. Frahley R, Subramani S, Berg P, Papahadjopoulos D. Introduction of liposome-encapsulated SV40 DNA into cells. J Biol Chem 1980; 255:10431–10435.
221. Frahley R, Straubinger RM, Rule G, Springer EL, Papahadjopoulos D. Liposome-mediated delivery of deoxyribonucleic acid to cells: enhanced efficiency of delivery related to lipid composition and incubation conditions. Biochemistry 1981; 20:6978–6987.
222. Felgner PL, Gedek TR, Holm M, Roman R, Chan HW, Wenz M, Northrop JP, Ringold GM, Danielsen M. Lipofection: a novel highly efficient lipid mediated DNA transfection procedure. Proc Natl Acad Sci USA 1987; 84:7413–7417.

223. Malone R, Felgner PL, Verma I. Lipofection mediated RNA transfection. Proc Natl Acad Sci USA 1989; 86:6077–6081.

224. Duzgunes N, Goldstein JA, Friend DS, Felgner PL. Fusion of liposomes containing a novel cationic lipid, N-[2,3-(dioleyloxy)propyl]-N,N,N-trimethylammonium: induction by multivalent anions and asymmetric fusion with acidic phospholipid vesicles. Biochemistry 1989; 28:9179–9184.

225. Zhou X, Huang L. DNA transfection mediated by cationic liposomes containing lipopolylysine: characterization and mechanism of action. Biochim Biophys Acta 1994; 1189:195–203.

226. Felgner JH, Kumar R, Sridhar CN, Wheeler CJ, Tsai YJ, Border R, Ramsey P, Martin M, Felgner PL. Enhanced gene delivery and mechanism studies with a novel series of cationic lipid formulations. J Biol Chem 1994; 269:2550–2561.

227. Behr J, Demeneix B, Loeffler J, Perez-Mutul J. Efficient gene transfer into mammalian primary endocrine cells with lipopolyamine-coated DNA. Proc Natl Acad Sci USA 1989; 86:6982–6986.

228. Gao XA, Huang L. A novel cationic liposome reagent for efficient transfection of mammalian cells. Biochem Biophys Res Commun 1991; 179:280–285.

229. Rose JK, Buonocore L, Witt MA. A new cationic liposome reagent mediating nearly quantitative transfection of animal cells. Biotechniques 1991; 10:520–525.

230. Zhou X, Klibanov AL, Huang L. Lipophilic polylysines mediate efficient DNA transfection in mammalian cells. Biochim Biophys Acta 1991; 1965:8–14.

231. Debs R, Pian M, Gaensler K, Clements J, Friend DS, Dobbs L. Prolonged transgene expression in rodent lung cells. Am J Resp Cell Mol Biol 1992; 7:406–413.

232. Ruysschaert JM, EI Ouahbi A, Willeaume V, et al. A novel cationic ampiphile for transfection of mammalian cells. Biochem Biophys Res Commun 1994; 203:1622–1628.

233. Caplen NJ, Kinrade E, Sorgi F, Gao X, Gruenert D, Geddes D, Coutelle C, Huang L, Alton EW, Williamson R. In vitro liposome-mediated DNA transfection of epithelial cell lines using the cationic liposome DC-Chol/DOPE. Gene Ther 1995; 2:603–613.

234. Fasbender AJ, Zabner J, Welsh MJ. Optimization of cationic lipid-mediated gene transfer to airway epithelia. Am J Physiol 1995; 269:L45–L51.

235. Lu D, Benjamin R, Kim M, Conry RM, Curiel DT. Optimization of methods to achieve mRNA-mediated transfection of tumor cells in vitro and in vivo employing cationic liposome vectors. Cancer Gene Ther 1994; 1:245–252.

236. Debs RJ, Freedman LP, Edmunds S, Gaensler KL, Duzgunes N, Yamamoto KR. Regulation of gene expression in vivo by liposome-mediated delivery of a purified transcription factor. J Biol Chem 1990; 265:10189–10192.

237. Farhood H, Gao X, Barsoum J, Huang L. Codelivery to mammalian cells of a transcriptional factor with *cis*-acting element using cationic liposomes. Anal Biochem 1995; 225:889–893.

238. Scheule RK, Cheng SH. Unpublished data.

239. Yang NS. Gene transfer into mammalian somatic cells in vivo. Crit Rev Biotechnol 1992; 12:211–25.

240. Miller AD. Human gene therapy comes of age. Nature 1992; 375:455–460.

241. Morgan RA, Anderson WF. Human gene therapy. Annu Rev Biochem 1993; 62: 191–217.

242. Miller AD. Retrovirus packaging cells. Hum Gene Ther 1990; 1:5–14.

243. Mulligan RC. The basic science of gene therapy. Annu Rev Biochem 1993; 62: 191–217.

244. Coffin JM. Structure and classification of retroviruses. In: Levy JA, ed. The Retroviridae. New York: Plenum, 1992:19.

245. Roe T, Reynolds TC, Yu G, Brown PO. Integration of murine leukaemia virus DNA depends on mitosis. EMBO J 1993; 12:2099–2108.

246. Lewis PF, Emerman M. Passage through mitosis is required for oncoretroviruses but not for the human immunodeficiency virus. J Virol 1994; 68:510–516.

247. Naldini L, Blomer U, Gallay P, Ory D, Mulligan R, Gage FH, Verma IM, Trono D. In vivo delivery and stable transduction of nondividing cells by a lentiviral vector. Science 1996; 272:263–7.

248. Günzburg WH, Salmons B. Retroviral vectors. In: Lemoine NR, Cooper DN, eds. Gene Therapy. Oxford: BIOS Scientific, 1996:33–60.

249. Bett AJ, Prevec L, Graham FL. Packaging capacity and stability of human adenovirus type 5 vectors. J Virol 1993; 67:5911–5921.

250. Cotton M, Wagner E, Zatloukai K, Phillips S, Curiel DT, Birnsteil ML. High-efficiency receptor-mediated delivery of small and large (48 kb) gene constructs using the endosome disruption activity of defective or chemically inactivated adenovirus particles. Proc Natl Acad Sci USA 1992; 89:6094–6098.

251. Yu CL, Prochownik EV, Imperiale M, Jove R. Attenuation of serum inducibility of immediate early genes by oncoproteins in tyrosine kinase signaling pathways. Mol Cell Biol 1993; 13:2011–2019.

252. Dai Y, Schwarz EM, Gu D, Zhang WW, Sarvetnick N, Berma IM. Cellular and humoral immune responses to adenoviral vectors containing factor IX and vector antigens allows for long term expression. Proc Natl Acad Sci USA 1995; 92:1401–1405.

253. Prince GA, Porter DD, Jenson AB, et al. Pathogenesis of adenovirus type 5 pneumonia in cotton rats. J Virol 1993; 67:101–111.

254. Ginsberg HS, Prince GA. The molecular basis of adenovirus pathogenesis. Infect Agents Dis 1994; 3:1–8.

255. Yamaguchi Y, Mann DM, Ruoslahti E. Negative regulation of transforming growth factor-beta by the proteoglycan decorin. Nature 1990; 346:281–284.

256. Isaka Y, Brees DK, Ikegaya K, et al. Gene therapy by skeletal muscle expression of decorin prevents fibrotic disease in rat kidney. Nature Med 1996; 2:418–423.

257. Noble NA, Harper JR, Border WA. In vivo interactions of TGF-β and extracellular matrix. Prog Growth Factor Res 1992; 4:369–382.

258. Border WA and Noble NA. Targeting TGF-β1 for treatment of disease. Nature Med 1995; 1:1000–1001.

259. Tsutsumi Y, Kakumu S, Yoshioka K, Arao M, Inoue M, Wakita T. The effects of various cytokines on collagen synthesis by rat hepatocytes in primary cultures and fibroblasts. Digestion 1989; 44:191–199.

260. Tredget EE, Shen YJ, Liu G, Forsyth N, Smith C, Harrop RA, Scott PG, Ghahary A. Regulation of collagen synthesis and mRNA levels in normal and

hypertrophic scar fibroblasts in vitro by interferon-α2b. Wound Repair Regen 1993; 1:156–165.

261. Rosenbloom J, Feldman G, Freundlich B, Jimenez SA. Transcriptional control of human diploid fibroblast collagen synthesis by gamma-interferon. Biochem Biophys Res Commun 1984; 123:365–372.

262. Ghahary A, Tredget EE, Scott PG, Shen Q. Liposome associated interferon-alpha-2b functions as an antifibrogenic factor in dermal wounds in the guinea pig. J Invest Dermat. Under review.

263. Ahmed T, Lutton JD, Feldman E, Tani K, Asano S, Abraham NG. Gene transfer of alpha-interferon into hematopoietic stem cells. Leuk Res 1998; 22:119–124.

264. Broxmeyer HE, Lu E, Platzer E, Feit C, Juliano L, Rubin BY. Comparative analysis of the influences of human gamma, alpha and beta interferons on human multipotential (CFU-GEMM), erythroid (BFU-E) and granulocyte macrophage (CFU-GM) progenitor cells. J Immunol 1983; 131:1300–1305.

265. Geissler D, Gastl G, Aulitzky W, Tilg H, Gaggl S, Konwalinka G, Huber C. Recombinant interferon-alpha-2C in chronic myelogenous leukemia: relationship of sensitivity of committed haematopoietic precursor cells in vitro (BFU-E, CFU-GM, CFU-Meg) and clinical response. Leuk Res 1990; 14:629–636.

10

The Role of Transforming Growth Factors–Beta in Cutaneous Scarring

Mamta Shah, Patricia Rorison, and Mark W. J. Ferguson
University of Manchester, Manchester, England

I. INTRODUCTION

Recent advances in the molecular and cellular biology of fetal wound healing and the fetal phenotype of scarless healing have opened up new avenues in our understanding of the mechanisms for preventing/controlling scarring following postnatal injury. Fetal wounds heal rapidly, without formation of a scab, with reduced inflammatory and angiogenic responses, with different extracellular matrix composition, with enhanced regeneration of epithelial and mesenchymal tissues, and with a different growth factor profile compared with adult wounds (1–3). Over the last decade, the role of growth factors in wound healing has been studied extensively. Whitby and Ferguson (2) used immunolocalization techniques to compare the differences among the growth factor profiles of healing upper lip wounds in fetal, neonatal, and adult mice. While platelet-derived growth factor (PDGF) was detected in fetal, neonatal, and adult wounds, transforming growth factor-β1,2 (TGF-β1,2) was only detected in neonatal and adult wounds, which heal with scar formation, and not in the fetal wounds, which heal without scar formation (2). Using in situ hybridization and immunolocalization techniques, Martin et al. (4) reported a rapid but transient expression of TGF-β1 in fetal wounds compared with adult wounds in which the expression of TGF-β1 appeared much slower and was sustained for a longer period of time. Moreover, Krummel et al. (5), Adolph et al. (6), Houghton et al. (7), and Haynes et al. (8) have demonstrated that fetal wounds can be made to heal with scar formation by exogenous addition of TGF-β or PDGF. This suggests that growth factors not only play a crucial role in wound healing, but also appear to influence the quality of healing.

II. TRANSFORMING GROWTH FACTOR-BETA

Of the various growth factors that are implicated in the process of wound healing, TGF-β appears to play a central role (9). Transforming growth factor-β is released from degranulating platelets and secreted by most cells involved in the process of wound healing: neutrophils, lymphocytes, macrophages, fibroblasts, epithelial cells, smooth muscle cells, and endothelial cells. Transforming growth factor-β itself influences the migration, proliferation, and differentiation of these cells and the expression of other growth factors and their receptors involved in wound healing, thereby orchestrating the healing of wounds.

Transforming growth factor-β represents a highly homologous family of peptides that are differentially expressed. Three isoforms of TGF-β are expressed by mammalian cells: TGF-β1, TGF-β2, and TGF-β3. Transforming growth factor-β1 was the first isoform to be isolated from several cell lines and from platelets (10,11). Transforming growth factor-β2 was isolated from bovine bone and later from porcine platelets (12), while TGF-β3 was identified by complementary deoxyribonucleic acid (cDNA) characterization and human umbilical cord analysis (13,14). The three isoforms of TGF-β display 70 to 80% sequence homology and have similar biological effects in most experimental systems (15).

Transforming growth factor-β is expressed by virtually every cell, and almost all cells are responsive to TGF-β. Hence, it is not surprising that there exist several mechanisms to control the expression and effects of TGF-β. The regulatory mechanisms can be summarized as

1. Production of TGF-β in the latent form and subsequent activation
2. Sequestration of activated TGF-β by extracellular matrix and circulating proteins
3. Regulation of TGF-β gene transcription
4. Expression of antagonists of TGF-β signaling (e.g., SMADs 6,7)

Natural TGF-β is secreted as a biologically latent form consisting of either a 2- or 3-component complex known as the small or large latent complex, respectively. The active TGF-β is noncovalently associated with the processed precursor (75-kDa dimer) called the latency-associated peptide (LAP) and forms the small latent complex. In the large latent complex, the LAP is disulphide bonded to an unrelated modulator protein called the latent TGF-β–binding protein (LTBP) (16,17). Miyazono and Heldin (18) have postulated that the carbohydrates of LAP may be important in maintaining the latency of TGF-β, as enzymatic removal of these carbohydrates by sialidases activates TGF-β. The exact role of LTBP in the activation of TGF-β is not known, though it has been shown to be important for the proper assembly and secretion of TGF-β (19) and may promote binding of TGF-β to the matrix and facilitate its activation, analogous to fibrillin to which it shows homology (20).

The bioavailability of active TGF-β isoforms in vivo depends on the balance of secretion of latent complexes by cells, activation of these complexes, as well as inactivation and clearance of the active TGF-βs. Latent TGF-β can be activated by transient acidification, proteolysis, and chaotropic agents (21). Removal of the carbohydrate residues from LAP by glycosidases or sialase can activate TGF-β. The removal of the phosphates from the mannose 6-phosphate (M6P) residues of the LAP by phosphatases has also been shown to activate latent TGF-β (19). However, the exact mechanism of activation of TGF-β in vivo is still not well understood. Most cells secrete inactive TGF-β but activated macrophages and neutrophils can secrete active TGF-β1 (22,23). Treatment of cells with retinoic acid, 1,25-dihydroxy vitamin D_3, tamoxifen, or gestodene also results in activation of TGF-β (24–26).

More recent studies have shown that activation of latent TGF-β by the coculture system of endothelial cells and smooth muscle cells requires binding of the latent TGF-β to the cation-independent mannose 6-phosphate/insulin-like growth factor-2 (IGF-2) receptor in the presence of plasmin/urokinase (27). Activation could be blocked by mannose 6-phosphate or by antibodies to the mannose 6-phosphate receptor. Furthermore, this group has also reported the requirement of LTBP for activation of latent TGF-β in this coculture system (20). Using an antibody to native platelet LTBP, they observed inhibition of activation of latent TGF-β. When they added transglutaminase inhibitors or a neutralizing antibody to transglutaminase to these coculture systems, they found inhibition of activation of latent TGF-β, suggesting a role for transglutaminase in the activation of latent TGF-β in this system (28). From these observations, they have proposed the following hypothesis: LTBP targets latent TGF-β to a molecular assembly on the cell surface where the LAP region binds to the mannose 6-phosphate receptors. Transglutaminase may concentrate the latent TGF-β on the cell surface by cross-linking to the membrane proteins and also mediate the cross-linking of plasminogen to the cell surface, where plasmin cleavage may take place and release active TGF-β.

Another form of latent TGF-β is that associated with α_2-macroglobulin (α_2-M) (29). It is believed that the α_2-macroglobulin may be acting as a scavenger of active TGF-β or as a carrier for delivering TGF-β to the liver. The bioavailability of TGF-β is also regulated by the extracellular matrix. Fibronectin (30) and thrombospondin (31) associated TGF-β can exhibit biological activity. By contrast, decorin, biglycan, α-fetoprotein, and soluble betaglycan also bind TGF-β but neutralize the biological activity of TGF-β (32,33). Binding of TGF-β1 to collagen IV has also been reported (34).

Transforming growth factors-β themselves regulate the expression of their messenger ribonucleic acid (mRNA) and protein. While TGF-β1 up-regulates the expression of TGF-β1 mRNA and TGF-β1 protein synthesis (35), the regulation of the TGF-β isoforms by each other is complex and cell dependent (36–38). The autoinduction of TGF-β1 appears to be mediated by the AP-1 sites in its promoter region (39); by contrast, TGF-β2 and 3 promoter regions each contain a TATA box with cyclic AMP–responsive element/activating transcription factor site just 5′ of the TATA box (38,40).

Transforming growth factors-β initiate their cellular action by binding to receptors with intrinsic serine/threonine kinase activity (41,42). This receptor family consists of two subfamilies, type I and type II receptors. Both receptors have an extracellular domain, a transmembrane domain, and a cytoplasmic kinase domain and belong to the serine/threonine kinase family of receptors. Transforming growth factor-β first binds to the type II receptor (TβRII), which occurs in the cell membrane with activated kinase. Then, the type I receptor (TβRI), which cannot bind TGF-β in the absence of type II receptor, is recruited into the complex; TβRII phosphorylates TβRI in the GS domain to activate it. The assembly of the receptor complex is triggered by ligand binding, but the complex is also stabilized by the direct interaction of the cytoplasmic parts of the receptors. Transforming growth factor-β2 binds with low affinity to TβRII and requires the cooperation of betaglycan for high affinity binding.

Betaglycan, or type III receptor, is heterogeneous in nature and also exists in the soluble form, which is found in serum and in the extracellular matrices (43). The role of betaglycan is not yet known; due to its structural features, relative abundance, and secretory nature, betaglycan could function as a reservoir or clearance system for bioactive TGF-β as well as facilitate binding of TGF-β to its signaling receptors as described above (44). Endoglin is another cell surface protein that binds TGF-β with high affinity though it lacks a kinase domain (41).

The signaling pathway for TGF-β from the cell surface to the nucleus has recently been unraveled. The key components in these signal transduction pathways are identified as SMADs. After phosphorylation and activation by receptor kinases, hetero-oligomeric SMAD complexes migrate into the nucleus and, either directly or in complex with other proteins, affect transcription of specific genes. SMAD6 and SMAD7 serve as inhibitors in the signal transduction by preventing the interaction between the serine/threonine kinase receptors and the pathway-restricted SMADs. As the expression of the inhibitory SMADs is induced by ligand stimulation, they may have a negative-feedback role in signal transduction (44), thus forming another regulatory pathway for TGF-β activity.

III. BIOLOGICAL EFFECTS OF TRANSFORMING GROWTH FACTOR-BETA IN WOUND HEALING

Relatively large amounts of TGF-β are present in platelets, and these are released by degranulation of the α-granules after injury. TGF-β is a potent chemoattractant of macrophages, neutrophils, and fibroblasts, and these cells in turn secrete TGF-β when activated. Transforming growth factor-β induces activation and autocrine release of other growth factors by macrophages, fibroblasts, and endothelial cells, and by its direct and indirect effects induces proliferation of cells and angiogenesis. Transforming growth factor-β stimulates extracellular matrix synthesis and prevents its degradation by up-regulating the expression of tissue inhibitors of metalloproteinases (TIMPs) and down-regulating the expression of proteases (9).

Cromack et al. (45) implanted wound chambers subcutaneously in rats and measured the levels of TGF-β in the wound fluid at various times after implantation. This and other reports (46,47) demonstrate the presence of TGF-β and suggest an intrinsic role during wound healing. Transforming growth factor-β itself, can initiate the cascade of events resulting in wound healing as demonstrated by several studies. Subcutaneous injection of TGF-β into the necks of newborn mice (48) induced the formation of granulation tissue; injection of TGF-β into wound chambers accelerated the accumulation of total protein, collagen, and DNA content of the chambers (49–51).

IV. TRANSFORMING GROWTH FACTOR-BETA AND FIBROSIS

While TGF-β appears to play a key role in tissue repair, excessive or abnormal production of TGF-β can be detrimental. Excessive production of TGF-β1 has been implicated in the pathogenesis of mesangial proliferative glomerulonephritis (52). Border et al. (53,54) showed that neutralizing antibody to TGF-β or decorin could prevent the increase in extracellular matrix deposition seen in experimental glomerulonephritis, thereby suppressing the disease. Transforming growth factor-β has also been implicated in bleomycin-induced pulmonary fibrosis (55), idiopathic pulmonary fibrosis (56), fibrosis in the eye (57), fibrosis in the central nervous system following trauma (58), cirrhosis of the liver (59), hepatic fibrosis (60), human vascular restenosis lesions (61), systemic sclerosis (62), and diffuse fasciitis and eosinophilia myalgia syndrome (63). In all these fibrotic disease processes, TGF-β appears to be responsible for excess extracellular matrix deposition. Anscher et al. (64) measured plasma TGF-β levels in advanced breast cancer patients prior to high-dose chemotherapy and bone marrow transplantation and found significantly high levels of TGF-β in patients who developed hepatic veno-occlusive disease or idiopathic interstitial pneumonitis posttreatment. Thus, plasma TGF-β can be used as a predictor of lung and liver fibrosis in these patients prior to treatment. Transforming growth factor-β has also been implicated in synovial inflammation (65). Wahl et al. (65) have demonstrated reversal of acute and chronic synovial inflammation by administration of neutralizing antibody to TGF-β in an experimental model of chronic erosive polyarthritis. Logan and Berry (66) administered neutralizing antibody to TGF-β after experimental injury to the central nervous system and found a reduction in fibrosis. TGF-β1 has been co-localized with collagens I and VI in hypertrophic scars and keloids (67,68). It is clear from the above examples that while TGF-β is required for the repair process, uncontrolled expression can have pathological consequences.

V. REDUCTION OF CUTANEOUS SCARRING BY MODULATION OF TRANSFORMING GROWTH FACTOR-BETA PROFILE OF ADULT WOUNDS

Local intradermal infiltration of a polyclonal neutralizing antibody to TGF-β1,2 into the wound margins of full-thickness cutaneous wounds in adult rodents just prior to wounding or within 24 hr of wounding and repeated daily for two days postwounding, resulted in reduced inflammatory response, reduced angiogenic response, less extracellular matrix deposition without reduction in the tensile strength of the wounds, with an improved architecture of the neodermis resembling normal dermis, and, most importantly, with markedly reduced cutaneous scarring (69,70). By contrast, the untreated wounds and wounds treated similarly but with an irrelevant antibody (sham control) healed with obvious cutaneous scarring. When these wounds were immunostained for the TGF-β1 protein, wounds treated with the neutralizing antibody to TGF-β demonstrated a marked reduction in the immunoreactivity for TGF-β1 on day 7 postwounding compared with the control group of wounds. This suggests that early neutralization of TGF-β1 prevents the autocatalytic induction of TGF-β1, thereby possibly reducing the effects of TGF-β1 on the inflammatory and angiogenic responses and induction of extracellular matrix deposition in the wounds. The reduced levels of TGF-β may, in turn, reduce the levels of plasminogen activator inhibitor-1 (PAI-1) resulting in a relative increase in the levels of plasminogen and plasmin, leading to increased fibrinolysis, making the provisional scaffold less compact for the migrating fibroblasts to organize the neodermis in a more reticular pattern (70).

A second approach to reduce autoinduction of TGF-β1 early in the process of wound healing utilized antisense technology. Antisense oligonucleotides to TGF-β1 injected intradermally prior to wounding adult rodent skin also resulted in reduced immunoreactivity to TGF-β1 protein at day 7 postwounding and some improvement in cutaneous scarring at day 70 postwounding compared with scrambled or sense oligonucleotide control treated wounds (Chamberlain, Ph.D. thesis, University of Manchester, 1993). More recently, Choi et al. (71) have also reported reduction in cutaneous scarring following administration of antisense TGF-β1 oligodeoxynucleotides to adult wounds.

The active form of TGF-β needs to be released from its latent complex before TGF-β can bind to its receptors and exhibit any biological effects. As described above, the activation process involves the binding of mannose 6-phosphate (M6P) residues on the LAP of the latent TGF-β complex to the M6P/IGF-2 receptor (27). Excess M6P can compete with the LAP and inhibit the activation of TGF-β. Thus, when full-thickness incisional wounds in adult rodents were injected intradermally with mannose 6-phosphate, the inflammatory response was reduced, collagen deposition was accelerated, the architecture of the neodermis was found to be more akin to that of normal dermis, and there was a marked reduction in cutaneous scarring. By contrast, sham control wounds treated with either mannose 1-phosphate (which binds to the mannose receptor but not the M6P receptor) or glucose 6-phosphate and untreated control wounds healed with obvious cutaneous scarring (72,73). The early modulation of collagen synthesis seen in wounds treated with either M6P or M1P may have been a direct effect of the mannose sugars binding to the mannose receptors, while the antiscarring effect seen exclusively with M6P may well be due to competitive binding to the M6P receptor and thereby preventing the activation of the latent TGF-β at the wound sites.

Kojima et al. (28) demonstrated the role of tissue transglutaminase in the activation of latent TGF-β in the endothelial cell–smooth muscle cell coculture system. They proposed that tissue transglutaminase binds latent TGF-β complex to the cell surface through LTBP or LAP as well as cross-links plasminogen to the cell surface where it is converted to plasmin, thereby increasing the local concentration of plasmin in the vicinity of latent TGF-β and thus facilitating plasmin-mediated activation of TGF-β. Nunes et al. (74) have also shown that activation of latent TGF-β by lipopolysaccharide-stimulated peritoneal macrophages requires tissue transglutaminase.

Full-thickness incisional wounds on the dorsum of adult rodents were treated with tissue transglutaminase inhibitors, monodansylcadaverine and cystamine, at the time of wounding and once daily for four days postwounding. Compared with the untreated control wounds, tissue transglutaminase inhibitor–treated wounds had a lower inflammatory response, decreased extracellular matrix deposition, improved architecture of the neodermis, and reduced cutaneous scarring. Moreover, the tissue levels of active TGF-β were significantly reduced in tissue transglutaminase inhibitor–treated wounds compared with control wounds on day 5 postwounding. By contrast, the levels of latent TGF-β were markedly higher in the treated wounds compared with control wounds. These data suggest that inhibiting tissue transglutaminase at the wound site prevents the activation of latent TGF-β and thereby reduces cutaneous scarring (Yang, Ph.D. thesis, University of Manchester, 1998).

There are three isoforms of TGF-β expressed by mammalian cells. In order to investigate which of the three isoforms are implicated in cutaneous scarring, Shah et al. (75) treated adult rodent wounds with isoform-specific neutralizing antibodies either alone or in combination. Exogenous addition of neutralizing antibody to TGF-β1 alone resulted in some reduction in the inflammatory and angiogenic responses as well as reduction of extracellular matrix deposition in the early stages with a marginal reduction in cutaneous scarring. By contrast, neutralizing antibody to TGF-β2 alone had little effect on the inflammatory or angiogenic responses and no effect on the resultant scar. However, when neutralizing antibody to TGF-β1 and neutralizing antibody to TGF-β2 were administered together, there was a marked reduction in the inflammatory response, neovascularization and extracellular matrix deposition in the early stages of healing; the architecture of the neodermis resembled that of normal dermis and the wounds healed with markedly reduced scarring. This demonstrates the synergistic effects of both TGF-β1 and TGF-β2 on cutaneous scarring. When wounds were treated with an antibody that neutralized all three isoforms of TGF-β, there was no effect on the resultant scar.

In most in vitro experiments, the three isoforms of TGF-β appear to have similar biological activities albeit with different potencies. Surprisingly, exogenous addition of TGF-β3 to cutaneous wounds in adult rodents reduced the inflammatory response and extracellular matrix deposition in the early stages of healing, altered the architecture of the neodermis to resemble that of the normal dermis, and markedly reduced cutaneous scarring. By contrast, treatment of wounds with either TGF-β1 or TGF-β2 increased the extracellular matrix deposition in the early stages of healing but had no effect on the architecture of the neodermis at later stages or on the resultant cutaneous scar (75). Wounds treated with TGF-β3 showed a marked reduction in the immunoreactivity for TGF-β1 and TGF-β2 on days 5 and 7 postwounding compared with untreated control wounds. Moreover, the antiscarring effects of TGF-β3 can be abrogated by the addition of TGF-β1, suggesting a down-regulation of TGF-β1 by TGF-β3 (Shah et al., submitted).

More recently, Shah et al. (76) found that cutaneous wounds in transgenic mice that have high circulating levels of plasma active TGF-β1 (77) heal with reduced cutaneous scarring compared to wounds in the wild type control mice, which heal with obvious scars. The exact mechanism of this apparently paradoxical effect of high systemic levels of TGF-β1 is currently not known. However, compared with wounds from control mice, wounds from the transgenic mice, harvested seven days postinjury, were more immunoreactive for TGF-β3 and less immunoreactive for TGF-β1. These data further corroborate the previously observed findings that the relative ratio of the three TGF-β isoforms is more important for control of cutaneous scarring than the absolute levels of individual TGF-β isoforms. TGF-β1 and TGF-β2 appear to be implicated in cutaneous scarring, while TGF-β3 reduces scarring.

By interfering with the transcription/translation of TGF-β, activation of latent TGF-β, neutralization of active TGF-β by neutralizing antibodies or binding proteins, such as decorin (66), or by local addition of TGF-β3, and alteration of the ratios of the three TGF-β isoforms, adult cutaneous wounds can be manipulated to heal with reduced scarring. Another strategy to alter the TGF-β levels would be to use cytokines that antagonize the effects of TGF-β directly and/or indirectly. Transforming growth factor-β is chemotactic to macrophages and monocytes, and induces the expression of other cytokines, such as PDGF, which is also a potent chemoattractant of inflammatory cells and a mitogen for fibroblasts. Shah et al. (78) injected neutralizing antibody to PDGF intradermally into the margins of cutaneous wounds of adult rodents and reported some reduction in cutaneous scarring. Interestingly, Tredget et al. (79) reported a reduction of the high systemic levels of TGF-β1 found in thermally injured patients with hypertrophic scars when treated systemically with interferon-α2b which improved the scars. The mechanism by which systemic interferon-α2b reduces systemic levels of TGF-β1 was not determined by the authors. Interferon-α has previously been shown to up-regulate collagenase production and down-regulate production of TIMP-1 by dermal fibroblasts (67) and this may have contributed to the improvement in the scars.

REFERENCES

1. Whitby DJ, Ferguson MWJ. The extracellular matrix of lip wounds in fetal, neonatal and adult mice. Development 1991; 112:651–668.
2. Whitby DJ, Ferguson MWJ. Immunohistochemical localization of growth factors in fetal wound healing. Dev Biol 1991; 147:207–215.
3. Longaker MT, Whitby DJ, Adzick NS, Crombleholme TM, Langer JC, Duncan BW, Bradley SM, Stern R, Ferguson MWJ, Harrison MR. Studies in fetal wound healing: VI. Second and early third trimester fetal wounds demonstrate rapid collagen deposition without scar formation. J Pediatr Surg 1990; 25:63–69.
4. Martin P, Dickson MC, Millan FA, Ackhurst R. Rapid induction and clearance of TGF beta 1 is an early response to wounding in the mouse embryo. Dev Genet 1993; 14:225–238.
5. Krummel TM, Michna BA, Thomas BL, Sporn MB, Nelson JM, Salzberg AM, Cohen IK, Diegelmann RF. Transforming growth factor β (TGF-β) induces fibrosis in a fetal wound model. J Pediatr Surg 1988; 23:647–652.
6. Adolph VR, DiSanto SK, Bleacher JC, Dillon PW, Krummel, TM. The potential role of the lymphocyte in fetal wound healing. J Pediatr Surg 1993; 28:1316–1320.

7. Houghton PE, Keefer KA, Krummel TM. The role of transforming growth factor beta (TGFβ) in the conversion from scarless healing to healing with scar formation. Wound Repair Regen 1995; 3:229–236.

8. Haynes JH, Johnson DE, Flood LC, Mast BA, Habacker TA, Diegelmann RF, Cohen IK, Krummel TM. Platelet-derived growth factor induces fibrosis at a fetal wound site. Surg Forum 1990; 41:641–643.

9. Roberts AB, Sporn MB. Transforming Growth Factor-β. In: Clark RF, ed. The Molecular and Cellular Biology of Wound Repair. 2d ed. New York: Plenum, 1996: 275–308.

10. Moses HL, Branum EL, Proper JA, Robinson RA. Transforming growth factor production by chemically transformed cells. Cancer Res 1981; 41:2842–2848.

11. Roberts AB, Anzano MA, Lamb LC, Smith JM, Sporn MB. New class of transforming growth factors potentiated by epidermal growth factor. Proc Natl Acad Sci USA 1981; 78:5339–5343.

12. Cheifetz S, Weatherbee JA, Tsang MLS, Anderson JK, Mole JE, Lucas R, Massague J. The transforming growth factor β system, a complex pattern of cross reactive ligands and receptors. Cell 1987; 48:409–415.

13. Derynck R, Lindquist PB, Lee A, Wen D, Tamm J, Graycar JL, Rhee L, Mason AJ, Miller DA, Coffey RJ, Moses HL, Chen EY. A new type of transforming growth factor-β, TGF-β3. EMBO J 1988; 7:3737–3743.

14. ten Dijke P, Hansen P, Iwata KK, Pieler C, Foulkes GJ. Identification of another member of the transforming growth factor type β gene family. Proc Natl Acad Sci USA 1988; 85:4715–4719.

15. Roberts AB, Sporn MB. Physiological actions and clinical applications of transforming growth factor-beta (TGF-beta). Growth Factors 1993; 8:1–9.

16. Wakefield LM, Smith DM, Flanders KC, Sporn MB. Latent transforming growth factor-β from human platelets. J Biol Chem 1988; 263:7646–7654.

17. Miyazono K, Hellman U, Wernstedt C, Heldin C-H. Latent high molecular weight complex of transforming growth factor β1. J Biol Chem 1988; 263:6407–6415.

18. Miyazono, K, Heldin, C-H. Interaction between TGF-β1 and carbohydrate structures in its precursor renders TGF-β1 latent. Nature 1989; 338:158–160.

19. Miyazono K, Olofsson A, Colosetti P, Heldin C-H. A role of the latent TGFβ1 binding protein in the assembly and secretion of TGFβ1. EMBO J 1991; 10:1091–1101.

20. Flaumenhaft R, Abe M, Sato Y, Miyazono K, Harpel J, Heldin C-H, Rifkin DB. Role of the latent TGF-β binding protein in the activation of latent TGF-β by co-cultures of endothelial and smooth muscle cells. J Cell Biol 1993; 120:995–1002.

21. Brown PD, Wakefield LM, Levinson AD, Sporn MB. Physicochemical activation of recombinant latent transforming growth factor beta's 1, 2, and 3. Growth Factors 1990; 3:35–43.

22. Assoian RK, Fleurdelys BE, Stevenson HC, Miller PJ, Madtes DK, Raines EW, Ross R, Sporn MB. Expression and secretion of type beta transforming growth factor by activated human macrophages. Proc Natl Acad Sci USA 1987; 84:6020–6024.

23. Grotendorst GR, Smale G, Pencev D. Production of transforming growth factor beta

by human peripheral blood monocytes and neutrophils. J Cell Physiol 1989; 140: 396–402.

24. Glick AB, Flanders KC, Danielpour D, Yuspa SH, Sporn MB. Retinoic acid induces transforming growth factor-β2 in cultured keratinocytes and mouse epidermis. Cell Reg 1989; 1:87–97.

25. Colletta AA, Wakefield LM, Howell FV, Roozendaal KEPV, Danielpour D, Ebbs SR, Sporn MB, Baum M. Anti-oestrogens induce the secretion of active transforming growth factor beta from human fetal fibroblasts. Br J Cancer 1990; 62:405–409.

26. Kojima S, Rifkin DB. Mechanism of retinoid-induced activation of latent transforming growth factor β in bovine endothelial cells. J Cell Physiol 1993; 155:323–332.

27. Dennis PA, Rifkin DB. Cellular activation of latent transforming growth factor-β requires binding to the cation-independent mannose 6 phosphate/insulin-like growth factor type II receptor. Proc Natl Acad Sci USA 1991; 88:580–584.

28. Kojima S, Nara K, Rifkin DB. Requirement for transglutaminase in the activation of latent transforming growth factor β in bovine endothelial cells. J Cell Biol 1993; 121:439–448.

29. O'Connor-McCourt MD, Wakefield LM. Latent transforming growth factor β in serum. J Biol Chem 1987; 262:14090–14099.

30. Fava RA, McClure DB. Fibronectin-associated transforming growth factor. J Cell Physiol 1987; 131:184–189.

31. Murphy-Ullrich JE, Schultz-Cherry S, Hook M. Transforming growth factor-β complexes with thrombospondin. Mol Biol Cell 1992; 3:181–188.

32. Yamaguchi Y, Mann DM, Ruoslahti E. Negative regulation of transforming growth factor β by the proteoglycan decorin. Nature 1990; 346:281–284.

33. Miyazono K, Ichijo H, Heldin C-H. Transforming growth factor-beta: latent forms, binding proteins and receptors. Growth Factors 1993; 8:11–22.

34. Paralkar VM, Vukicevic S, Reddi AH. Transforming growth factor β type 1 binds to collagen IV of basement membrane matrix: implications for development. Dev Biol 1991; 143:303–308.

35. Van-Obberghen-Schilling E, Roche NS, Flanders KC, Sporn MB, Roberts AB. Transforming growth factor β1 positively regulates its own expression in normal and transformed cells. J Biol Chem 1988; 263:7741–7746.

36. Bascom CC, Wolfshohl JR, Coffey RJ, Madisen L, Webb NR, Purchio AR, Derynck R, Moses HL. Complex regulation of transforming growth factor β1, β2 and β3 mRNA expression in mouse fibroblasts and keratinocytes by transforming growth factors β1 and β2. Mol Cell Biol 1989; 9:5308–5515.

37. Roberts AB, Kim SJ, Takafumi N, Glick AB, Lafyatis R, Lechleider R, Jakowlew SB, Geiser AO, O'Reilly MA, Danielpour D, Sporn MB. Multiple forms of TGFβ: distinct promoters and differential expression. In: Clinical Applications of TGFβ. CIBA Foundation Symposium. Chichester: Wiley, 1991:7–28.

38. O'Reilly MA, Danielpour D, Roberts AB, Sporn MB. Regulation of expression of transforming growth factor-β2 by transforming growth factor-β isoforms is dependent upon cell type. Growth Factors 1992; 6:193–201.

39. Kim SJ, Jeang KT, Glick AB, Sporn MB, Roberts AB. Promoter sequences of the

human transforming growth factor-beta 1 gene responsive to transforming growth factor-beta 1 autoinduction. J Biol Chem 1989; 264:7041–7045.

40. Lafyatis R, Lechleider R, Kim SJ, Jakowlew S, Roberts AB, Sporn MB. Structural and functional characterisation of the transforming growth factor beta 3 promoter. A cAMP-responsive element regulates basal and induced transcription. J Biol Chem 1990; 265:19128–19136.

41. Lin HY, Moustakas A. TGFβ receptors: structure and function. Cell Mol Biol 1994; 40:337–349.

42. Massague J, Attisano L, Wrana JL. The TGFβ family and its composite receptors. Trends Cell Biol 1994; 4:172–178.

43. Andres JL, Stanley K, Cheifetz S, Massague J. Membrane-anchored and soluble forms of betaglycan, a polymorphic proteoglycan that binds transforming growth factor-β. J Cell Biol 1989; 109:3137–3145.

44. Heldin C-H, Miyazono K, ten Dijke P. TGF-β signalling from cell membrane to nucleus through SMAD proteins. Nature 1997; 390:465–471.

45. Cromack DT, Sporn MB, Roberts AB, Merino MJ, Dart LL, Norton JA. Transforming growth factor β levels in rat wound chambers. J Surg Res 1987; 42:622–628.

46. Grotendorst GR, Grotendorst CA, Gilman T. Production of growth factors (PDGF and TGFβ) at the site of tissue repair. In: Barbul A, Pines, Caldwell, Hunt T, eds. Growth Factors and Other Aspects of Wound Healing. Biological and Clinical Implications. New York: Liss, 1988:47–54.

47. Quaglino D, Nanney LB, Ditesheim JA, Davidson JM. Transforming growth factor-β stimulates wound healing and modulates extracellular matrix gene expression in pig skin: incisional wound model. J Invest Dermatol 1991; 97:34–42.

48. Roberts AB, Sporn MB, Assoian RK, Smith JM, Roche NS, Wakefield LM, Heine UI, Liotta LA, Falanga V, Kehrl JH, Fauci AS. Transforming growth factor type β: rapid induction of fibrosis and angiogenesis in vivo and stimulation of collagen formation in vitro. Proc Natl Acad Sci USA 1986; 83:4167–4171.

49. Sporn MB, Roberts AB, Shull JH, Smith JM, Ward JM, Sodek J. Polypeptide transforming growth factors isolated from bovine sources and used for wound healing in vivo. Science 1983; 219:1329–1331.

50. Lawrence WT, Sporn MB, Gorschboth C, Norton JA, Grotendorst GR. The reversal of an adriamycin induced healing impairment with chemoattractants and growth factors. Ann Surg 1986; 203:142–147.

51. Sprugel KH, McPherson JM, Clowes AW, Ross R. Effects of growth factors in vivo—cell ingrowth into porous subcutaneous chambers. Am J Pathol 1987; 129:601–613.

52. Okuda SL, Ranguino R, Ruoslahti E, Border WA. Elevated expression of transforming growth factor-β and proteoglycan production in experimental glomerulonephritis. Possible role in expansion of the mesangial extracellular matrix. J Clin Invest 1990; 86:453–462.

53. Border WA, Noble NA, Yamamoto T, Harper JR, Yamaguchi Y, Pierschbacher MD, Ruoslahti E. Natural inhibitor of transforming growth factor β protects against scarring in experimental kidney disease. Nature 1992; 360:361–364.

54. Border WA, Okuda S, Languino LR, Sporn MB, Ruoslahti E. Suppression of experi-

mental glomerulonephritis by antiserum against transforming growth factors β1. Nature 1990; 346:371–374.

55. Raghow R. Role of transforming growth factor β in repair and fibrosis. Chest 1991; 99:61S–65S.

56. Broekelmann TJ, Limper AH, Colby TV, McDonald JA. Transforming growth factor β1 is present at sites of extracellular matrix gene expression in human pulmonary fibrosis. Proc Natl Acad Sci USA. 1991; 88:6642–6646.

57. Connor TB, Roberts AB, Sporn MB, Danielpour D, Dart LL, Michels RG, de Bustros S, Enger C, Kato H, Lansing M, Hayashi H, Glaser BM. Correlation of fibrosis and transforming growth factor β type 2 levels in the eye. J Clin Invest 1989; 83:1661–1666.

58. Logan A, Frautschy SA, Gonzalez AM, Sporn MB, Baird A. Enhanced expression by transforming growth factor β1 in the rat brain after a localized cerebral injury. Brain Res 1992; 587:216–225.

59. Castilla A, Prieto J, Fausto N. Transforming growth factors β and α in chronic liver disease. N Engl J Med 1991; 324:933–940.

60. Czaja MJ, Weiner FR, Flanders KC, Giabrone MA, Wind R, Blempica L, Zern MA. In vitro and in vivo association of transforming growth factor-β with hepatic fibrosis. J Cell Biol 1989; 108:2477–2482.

61. Nikol S, Isner JM, Pickering JG, Kearney M, Leclerc G, Weir L. Expression of transforming growth factor-β1 is increased in human vascular restenosis lesions. J Clin Invest 1992; 90:1582–1592.

62. Smith EA, Leroy EC. A possible role for transforming growth factor β in systemic sclerosis. J Invest Dermatol 1990; 95:1255–1275.

63. Peltonen J, Varga J, Sollberg S, Uitto J, Jimenez SA. Elevated expression of the genes for transforming growth factor-β1 and type VI collagen in diffuse fasciitis associated with the eosinophilia-myalgia syndrome. J Invest Dermatol 1991; 96:20–25.

64. Anscher MS, Peters WP, Reisenbichler H, Petros WP, Jirtle RL. Transforming growth factor β as a predictor of liver and lung fibrosis after autologous bone marrow transplantation for advanced breast cancer. N Engl J Med 1993; 328:1592–1598.

65. Wahl SM, Allen JB, Costa GL, Wong HL, Dasch JR. Reversal of acute and chronic synovial inflammation by anti-transforming growth factor β. J Exp Med 1993; 177:225–230.

66. Logan A, Berry M. Transforming growth factor-beta1 and basic fibroblast growth factor in the injured CNS. Trends Pharmacol Sci 1993; 14:337–342.

67. Tredget EE, Nedelec B, Scott PG, Ghahary A. Hypertrophic scars, keloids and contractures: the cellular and molecular basis for therapy. Surg Clin North Am 1997; 77:701.

68. Peltonen J, Hsiao LL, Jaakkola S, Sollberg S, Aumailley M, Timpl R, Chu M-L, Uitto J. Activation of collagen gene expression in keloids: co-localization of type I and VI collagen and transforming growth factor-β1mRNA. J Invest Dermatol 1991; 97:240–248.

69. Shah M, Foreman DM, Ferguson MWJ. Control of scarring in adult wounds by neutralising antibody to transforming growth factor β. Lancet 1992; 339:213–214.

70. Shah M, Foreman DM, Ferguson MWJ. Neutralising antibody to TGFβ1,2 reduces cutaneous scarring in adult rodents. J Cell Sci 1994; 107:1137–1157.

71. Choi BM, Kwak HJ, Jun CD, et al. Control of scarring in adult wounds using anti-sense transforming growth factor-beta 1 oligodeoxynucleotides. Immunol Cell Biol 1996; 74(2):144–150.

72. Foreman DM, Shah M, Ferguson MWJ. Reduction of scar tissue formation in adult rodent wound healing by mannose-6-phosphate. 2d Annual Meeting of European Tissue Repair Society Malmo, Sweden, 1992. (ISBN 095 2620901)

73. McCallion R, Ferguson MWJ. Fetal wound healing. In: Clark RF, ed. The Molecular and Cellular Biology of Wound Repair. 2d ed. New York: Plenum, 1996:570–595.

74. Nunes I, Shapiro RL, Rifkin DB. Characterization of latent TGF-β activation by murine peritoneal macrophages. J Immunol 1995; 155:1450–1459.

75. Shah M, Foreman DM, Ferguson MWJ. Neutralisation of TGF-β_1 and TGF-β_2 or exogenous addition of TGF-β_3 to cutaneous rat wounds reduces scarring. J Cell Science 1995; 108:985–1002.

76. Shah M, Revis D Jr, Herrick S, Baillie R, Thorgeirsson S, Ferguson MWJ, Roberts AB. The role of elevated levels of active TGFβ1 in the plasma on wound healing. Am J Pathol 1999; 154:1115–1124.

77. Sanderson N, Factor V, Nagy P et al. Hepatic expression of mature transforming growth factor beta 1 in transgenic mice results in multiple tissue lesions. Proc Natl Acad Sci USA 1995; 92:2572.

78. Shah M, Foreman DM, Ferguson MWJ. Reduction of scar tissue formation in adult rodent wound healing by manipulation of the growth factor profile. J Cell Biochem 1991; 15F(suppl):198.

79. Tredget EE, Shankowsky RN, Pannu R, Nedelec B, Iwashina T, Ghahary A, Taerum TV, Scott PG. Transforming growth factor-β in thermally injured patients with hypertrophic scars: effects of interferon α-2b. Plast Reconstr Surg 1998; 102:1317–1328.

11
Recent Advances in Embryonic Wound Healing

Alison M. Shaw

St. Andrew's Centre for Plastic Surgery and Burns, Broomfield Hospital, Chelmsford, Essex, England

I. INTRODUCTION

The observation that mammalian embryos can heal wounds perfectly, without apparent scar formation was first made more than 20 years ago (1,2). This exciting finding has subsequently fueled much experimental work to determine the mechanisms whereby this phenomenon might occur, as well as to try and elucidate the differences between the processes occurring in the healing of adult and embryonic wounds.

Clearly, the implications of producing wounds that heal without forming scars are immense (3). For example, it is hoped that light may be shed on the pathogenesis of debilitating fibrotic diseases that are known to occur in man, such as idiopathic pulmonary fibrosis. Also exciting is the possibility that studies of embryonic wound healing may help reveal the mechanisms that underlie the numerous morphogenetic processes that occur naturally during embryonic development. Indeed, wound healing models may be used to observe cellular processes that are involved in morphogenesis, and may ultimately lead to the identification of factors that regulate these morphogenetic events (4).

II. STRUCTURE OF THE DERMAL–EPIDERMAL JUNCTION

In an early mammalian embryo, the epidermis consists of a single layer of cuboidal epithelial cells with a thin layer of squamouslike periderm cells overlying it

"

(5). Below this bilayered epidermis is a homogeneous mesenchyme that subsequently develops into the dermis. Later on, the epidermis differentiates to form four well-defined layers of cells (stratum basale, stratum spinosum, stratum granulosum, and stratum corneum). The cells in these layers are connected to one another by tight junctions, adherent junctions, and desmosomes. In the basal surface of the cells of the stratum basale are special adherent junctions called hemidesmosomes, which are recognized from 9 weeks of gestation onward in the human embryo (6,7) and increase fourfold in number from 9 to 15 weeks of gestation (8). These hemidesmosomes provide an attachment from the basal cells to the basal lamina, which overlies the mesenchyme.

Beneath the epithelial layer, the basal lamina itself consists of a complex arrangement of molecules, which, when viewed by transmission electron microscopy, appear to be composed of two layers, the lamina lucida and the lamina densa (9). Various laminins form a network in a sheetlike manner in the lamina lucida (10). Collagen IV appears to do the same in the lamina densa. Both laminin and collagen IV are detected as early as 6 weeks of gestation in humans (11,12).

Beneath the basal lamina, the ''primitive'' dermis consists principally of mesenchyme cells along with fibrils of collagen, particularly of types I and III (13). Additionally, fibronectin is particularly found around developing hair follicles. By 16 weeks of gestation, the human dermis is recognizable as the complex bilayered arrangement seen in the adult dermis and contains epidermal appendages, such as hair follicles (14).

III. EMBRYONIC WOUND HEALING

Classically, adult wound closure is described as being composed of two main components; one being reepithelialization, whereby front row keratinocytes crawl forward by means of lamellipodia; and the other being a contractile process occurring in the granulation tissue of the newly repairing mesenchyme. In contrast, it has been demonstrated that, although embryonic wound healing involves both epithelial and mesenchymal elements, which take place in the primitive tissue layers already described, the nature of these movements is markedly different from those occurring in an adult wound. Additionally, the extent of the acute inflammatory reaction provoked by wounding is significantly reduced, or even absent, in embryonic wounds in comparison with adult wounds.

A. The Embryonic Epithelial Wound Is Closed by an Actin Purse-String

In 1977, England and Cowper (15) described how incisional wounds to the endoderm of chick embryos close by a process whereby the endoderm sweeps over the underlying mesoderm without apparent formation of lamellipodia. Stanisstreet et al. (16) demonstrated a similar mechanism occurring at the wound edge in neurula-stage frog embryos. Clearly, the lamellipodial crawling that drives reepithelialization of adult wounds (17) is not essential for embryonic repair.

Martin and Lewis (18), observing excisional wounds in 4-day-old chick embryos, also found no evidence of lamellipodial crawling by wound edge epithelial cells. In addition, unlike adult cells with lamellipodia, these embryonic cells remained adherent to the underlying basement membrane. In fact, the wounds created in the chick wing buds were seen to rapidly form a smooth edge, and by 24 hr, the majority of these wounds were closed. By marking the boundary mesenchyme with a lipophillic dye, DiI, it was seen that the epidermal cells moved independently of and over the underlying mesenchyme. Fluorescently labeled phalloidin, which binds filamentous actin, revealed the rapid assembly of a cable of actin in the basal epithelial cells of the leading wound edge. This cable appeared continuous from one cell to the next and apparently acted as a purse-string to draw the epithelial wound margins closed.

A similar actin purse-string was seen in tissue culture by Bement et al. (19) after wounding a confluent monolayer of the gut epithelial cell line Caco-2BBe. Additionally, it seems that various morphogenic processes, most clearly dorsal closure in the fruitfly *Drosophila*, which occurs about 12 hr after egglaying, might also be driven by contraction of a similar actin purse-string (20,21).

Further work by McCluskey and Martin (22) has shown that an actin cable is also rapidly assembled in excisional wounds in mouse embryos (Fig. 1). Importantly, addition of cytochalasin D, which prevents new polymerization of actin, results in complete failure of reepithelialization of the wound, providing good evidence that the actin cable is required for reepithelialization of embryo wounds.

B. Characterization of the Actin Purse-String

In order to clarify further the role of actin filaments in the healing of embryonic wounds, Brock et al. (23) have studied incisional wounds in the dorsum of chick embryo wing buds. Since these wounds are quick to create, they allowed the early timecourse of actin cable assembly to be studied in more detail. In fresh wounds fixed within 30 sec of wounding, no visible specialization of actin was seen, but by 2 min postwounding, actin began to concentrate and form a linear cable passing from cell to cell along an axis parallel to the wound margin. By 5 min, the actin cable appeared 3 times brighter than the cortical actin at the margin of an unwounded cell, reaching a maximum of 4 times brighter than cortical actin by 30 min (Fig. 2a). This rapidity of actin cable assembly indicates that it is probably formed by reorganization of preexisting filamentous actin and/ or polymerization of actin monomer, since the timecourse is too rapid for the up-regulation of actin at the transcriptional or translational level. The stimulus

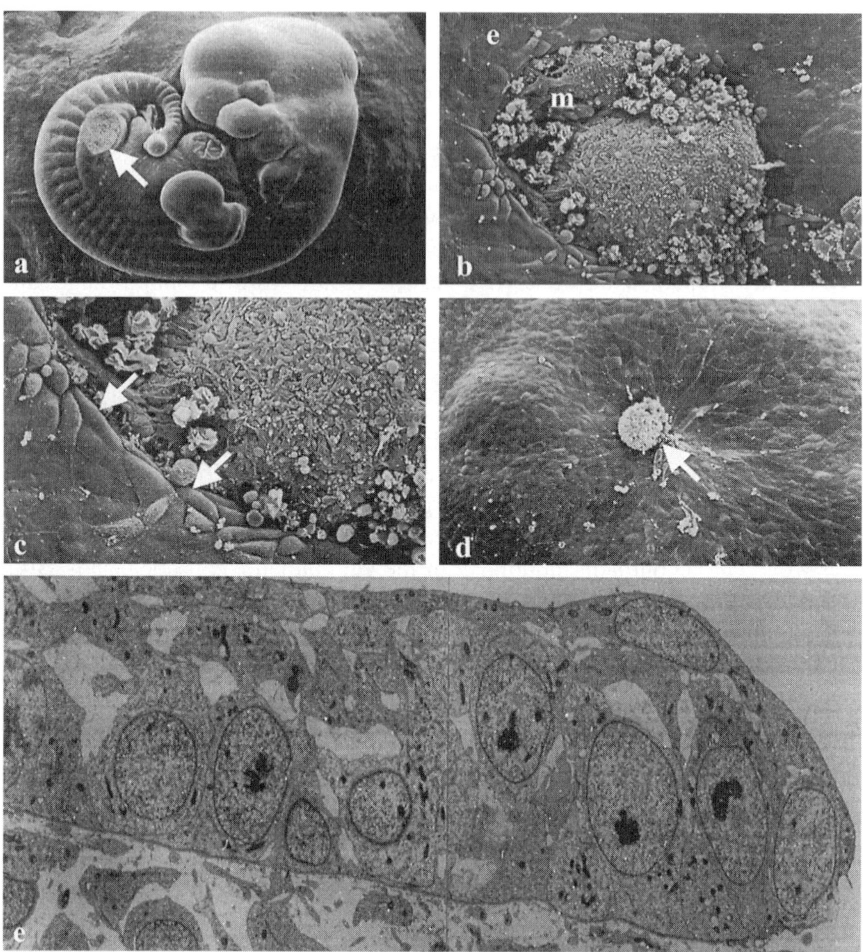

Figure 1 (a) Scanning electron micrograph (SEM) of whole mouse embryo at embryonic day 11.5. Arrow marks wound formed by amputation of hindlimb bud. (b) SEM of wound 12 hours postamputation; e = epithelium, m = mesenchyme. (c) High-power magnification of b showing elongation of wound margin cells (arrows). (d) By 24 h, the wound is closed leaving only a central clumping of debris marking the original wound site (arrow). (e) Transmission electron micrograph (TEM) of epidermal wound margin showing the blunt face of the leading edge cell and no evidence of lamellipodial extension. (From Ref. 4. Copyright Springer-Verlag GmbH & Co.)

for wound-induced actin cable assembly is very likely the rapid changes in epithelial cell tensions at the time of wounding, since wound edge cells are clearly seen to be stretched as the wound gapes open. Evidence in support of such mechanical cues being responsible for cable assembly at the wound edge comes from Kolega (24), who demonstrated that if tension is applied to fish keratinocytes in culture, the arrangement of the actin filaments changes and the filaments become organized into bundles running parallel to the line of tension.

Immunocytochemistry using anti-cadherin antibodies on the above described embryonic chick wounds (23) demonstrated that, in addition to an increase in actin concentration, there was a concomitant increase in the concentration of e-cadherin molecules in the leading edge of the basal epithelial cells. This increase was localized to the site of insertion of intracellular segments of the actin cable into adherent junctions. This arrangement results in continuity of the actin cable, from one cell to the next, along the length of the wound edge.

Normally, contractility of actin filaments is dependent upon their association with members of the myosin family. The work of Bement et al. (19) with gut epithelial cell lines demonstrated an association of myosin II to actin cables in tissue culture. Furthermore, *Drosophila* zipper mutant embryos, which lack a functional copy of the zygotic myosin gene, fail in dorsal closure (21). In the chick embryo wounds of Brock et al. (23), immunocytochemistry revealed nonmuscle myosin II localizing to the actin cable within approximately 10 min of wounding, a time when reepithelialization begins.

Most recently, efforts have been made in order to understand the molecular switches within epithelial cells that transduce primary wound signals, such as stretch, and which might lead to the rapid cytoskeletal reorganizations of the sort described above. Obvious candidates are the Rho family of small GTPases, since work by Ridley and Hall (25) has shown that Rho will mediate actin stress fiber assembly in serum-starved fibroblasts in culture, when the cells are exposed to serum factors. Indeed, when Rho is blocked by loading of the inhibitor C3-transferase into healing embryo wound edge cells, cable assembly fails and reepithelialization is prevented (23).

C. The Inflammatory Response

All adult tissue repair is accompanied by a rapid and sustained inflammatory response; initially neutrophils invade the wound site and subsequently macrophages become the major inflammatory cell type. Growth factors initially released by degranulating platelets and subsequently by the inflammatory macrophages provide some of the chemotactic signals that draw neutrophils and macrophages into the wound (26).

In the embryo, tissue repair occurs in the absence of an inflammatory response (27,28). The reason for this is not clear, although it is known that megakar-

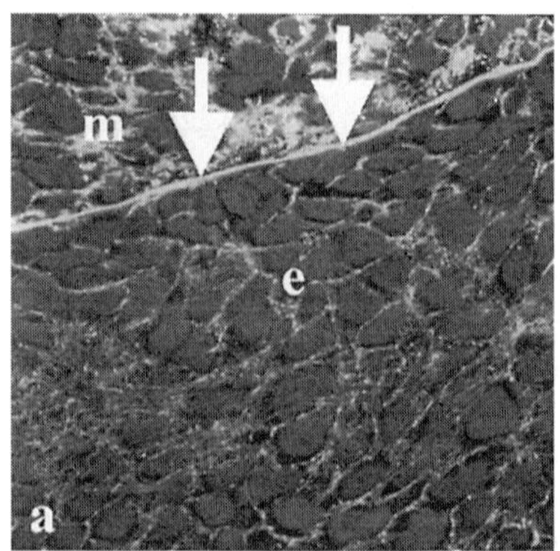
m
e
a

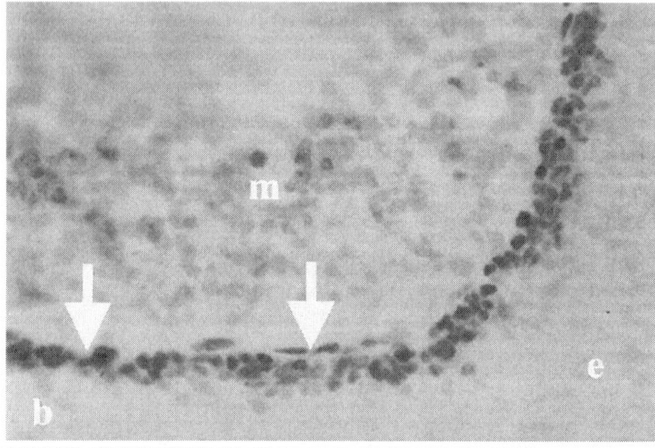
m
e
b

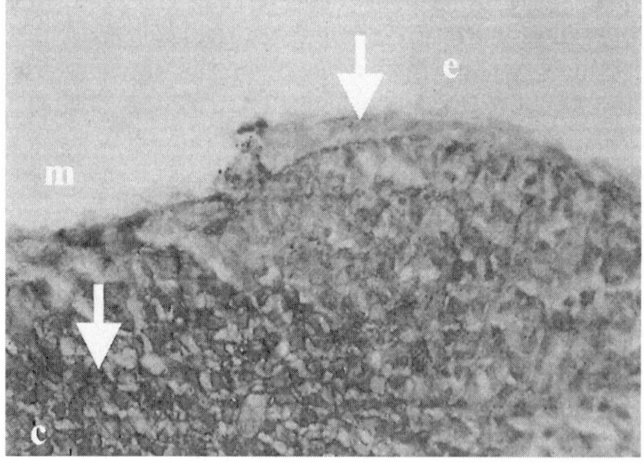
e
m
c

yocytes, the precursors of platelets, do not begin to differentiate until embryonic gestational day (E) 13.5 (29), and while macrophages are present within the embryo from around E10 (30), they are not recruited to the wound site until after the wound has closed (31). In fact, the earliest stage at which macrophages start to appear at embryonic wound sites is around E14.5. Since platelets are some of the key cells that initiate a cytokine response to wounding, it may be that the presence of macrophages at an early wound is dependent on the platelet-activated inflammatory response. Not surprisingly, it is at this same stage of development that embryonic wounds are first seen to heal with scar formation.

D.   The Role of the Mesenchyme

The granulation tissue characteristic of a healing adult wound, the formation of which is stimulated by the cytokines and growth factors of the acute inflammatory response, is not seen in embryonic wounds (28,32). In particular, no sign of fibroblast conversion into contractile myofibroblasts is seen at any stage of embryonic repair (22). Myofibroblasts in adult wounds ressemble smooth muscle cells, and with their expression of α–smooth muscle actin are able to provide a strong contractile force (33). Nevertheless, in the absence of such cells, mesenchymal contraction is known to occur in embryonic wounds and can be demonstrated by tagging the mesenchymal boundary with the lipophillic dye, DiI (22). Such studies reveal that mesenchymal contraction of up to 50% of initial wound area can occur during the 24 hr it takes for an embryo hindlimb bud amputation wound to heal.

In an attempt to identify what might be the kick-start signals that drive this mesenchymal contractile process in the absence of myofibroblasts, Martin and Nobes (34) looked specifically at levels of the c-fos protein in rat embryos after wounding. They demonstrated a rapid and transient induction of c-fos in epider-

---

Figure 2   (a) Confocal laser scanning micrograph of a wound in an E4 chick embryo. Fluorescein isothiocyanate (FITC) phalloidin stains for filamentous actin; e = epithelium (basal cells), m = mesenchyme in wound base. Arrows mark the actin cable within cells of the epidermal wound margin. (b) Immunostaining for the immediate early gene c-fos demonstrates its upregulation by epithelial cells of the wound margin; e = epithelium, m = mesenchyme, arrows mark wound margin. (c) Immunostaining for TGF-β1 demonstrates its presence within the mesenchyme of the wound base; e = epithelium, m = mesenchyme, arrows mark the expressing epidermis and the mesenchymal tissue into which this growth factor is released. (From Ref. 4. Copyright Springer-Verlag GmbH & Co.)

mal cells of the wound margin, as early as 15 min after wounding, with cells staining positive up to four rows back from the margin of the wound (Fig. 2b).

Downstream of immediate early genes, such as c-fos, is presumably a battery of effector genes that directly regulate the various tissue movements required to repair the wound. Work by Whitby and Ferguson (35) compared growth factor profiles in lip wounds of E16-fetal, neonatal, and adult mice and found that platelet-derived growth factor (PDGF) was present in all wounds, whereas both transforming growth factor-β (TGF-β) and fibroblast growth factor-2 (FGF-2) were not seen in wounds in the E16 fetuses. However, in situ hybridization and immunocytochemistry by Martin et al. (36) revealed an induction of TGF-β1 in the embryonic wound epithelium of E11.5 mice and positive staining for protein in the wound mesenchyme within hours of wounding (Fig. 2c). Since exogenous TGF-β1 is known to stimulate cultured fibroblasts to contract a collagen gel (37), it is likely that it may also directly signal mesenchymal contraction at the embryo wound site in vivo. Interestingly, TGF-β is one of the growth factor signals that is believed to stimulate conversion of fibroblasts to the myofibroblast phenotype in an adult wound (38).

In contrast to the profile of growth factors at an adult wound site, where levels are high throughout, the TGF-β1 signal at an embryonic wound is only transient, and the levels drop away, so that by the time wound closure is achieved, at around 18 to 24 hr after wounding, only low levels persist. This reduced expression of TGF-β1 may explain why embryonic wounds are able to contract closed, but do not overcontract, resulting in a scar.

A recent exciting finding in support of this theory has been the finding that addition of neutralizing antibody to TGF-β1 and -β2 to adult rat wounds results in reduced scarring (39).

IV. LESSONS FOR SCARLESS HEALING OF ADULT SKIN

The stage at which transition from scarless embryonic healing to adultlike healing with scar formation occurs is at around E14 to 16 in mouse embryos (in the third trimester in primates) (31,40,41). As already described, this is also approximately the stage at which platelets are first seen in the embryo. The presence of platelets, which may initiate an, albeit primitive, acute inflammatory response, is one of the factors in the transition from scarless healing to healing with scar.

An acute inflammatory response involving neutrophil and macrophage invasion leads to a sustained release of many of the growth factors and cytokines that are key signals in activating the various cell and tissue movements that lead to wound closure. However, at least one of these growth factors, TGF-β1, is now known to be released in excess at the wound site, since reduction of its activity results in more perfect healing with less scar formation (39). It may be that modulation of the levels of other growth factors, for example PDGF, at the wound site, so that they more closely ressemble the levels at embryonic wounds, will also prove beneficial to healing. An alternative strategy to blocking specific growth factors would be to consider local modulation of the inflammatory response at the wound site. Clearly, comparing how embryonic and adult tissues heal will supply us with excellent clues as to possible therapeutic strategies for preventing excessive fibrosis and scarring in clinical medicine.

ACKNOWLEDGMENTS

Dr. Paul Martin—for his valuable time, patience, and advice in the preparation and proofreading of this chapter.

REFERENCES

1. Burrington JD. Wound healing in the fetal lamb. J Pediatr Surg 1971; 6:523–528.
2. Goss AN. Intra-uterine healing of fetal rat oral mucosal, skin and cartilage wounds. J Oral Pathol 1977; 6:35–43.
3. Hedrick MH, Longaker MT, Harrison MR. A fetal surgery primer for plastic surgeons. Plast Reconstr Surg 1998; 101:1709–1729.
4. Nodder S, Martin P. Wound healing in embryos: a review. Anat Embryol 1997; 195: 215–228.
5. Sengel P. Morphogenesis of Skin. Cambridge University Press, Cambridge, England, 1976.
6. Smith LT, Sakai LY, Burgeson RE, Holbrook KA. Ontogeny of structural components at the dermal-epidermal junction in human embryonic and fetal skin: the appearance of anchoring fibrils and type VII collagen. J Invest Dermatol 1985; 90: 480–485.
7. Eady RAJ, McGrath JA, McMillan JR. Ultrastructural clues to genetic disorders of skin: the dermal-epidermal junction. J Invest Dermatol 1994; 103:13S–18S.
8. MacMillan JR and Eady RAJ. Hemidesmosome ontogeny in digit skin of the human fetus. Arch Dermatol Res 1996; 288:91–97.
9. Yurchenco PD and O'Rear JJ. Basal lamina assembly. Curr Opin Cell Biol 1994; 6:674–681.
10. Aumailley M and Krieg T. Laminins: a family of diverse multifunctional molecules of basement membranes. J Invest Dermatol 1996; 106:209–214.
11. Fine JD, Smith LT, Holbrook KA, Katz SI. The appearance of four basement membrane zone antigens in developing human fetal skin. J Invest Dermatol 1984; 83: 66–69.
12. Hertle MD, Adams JC, Watt FM. Integrin expression during human epidermal development in vivo and in vitro. Development 1991; 112:193–206.

13. Smith LT, Holbrook KA, Madri JA. Collagen types I, III, and V in human embryonic and fetal skin. Am J Anat 1986; 175:507–521.

14. Smith LT, Holbrook KA. Development of dermal connective tissue in human embryonic and fetal skin. Scan Electron Microsc 1982; 4:1745–1751.

15. England MA, Cowper SV. Wound healing in the early chick embryo studied by scanning electron microscopy. Anat Embryol 1977; 152:1–14.

16. Stanisstreet M, Wakely J, England MA. Scanning electron microscopy of wound healing in Xenopus and chicken embryos. J Embryol Exp Morphol 1980; 59:341–353.

17. Grinnell F. Wound repair, keratinocyte activation and integrin modulation. J Cell Science 1992; 101:1–5.

18. Martin P, Lewis J. Actin cables and epidermal movement in embryonic wound healing. Nature 1992; 360:179–182.

19. Bement WM, Forscher P, Mooseker MS. A novel cytoskeletal structure involved in purse-string wound closure and cell polarity maintenance. J Cell Biol 1993; 121:565–578.

20. Young PE, Pesacreta TC, Kiehart DP. Dynamic changes in the distribution of cytoplasmic myosin during *Drosophila* embryogenesis. Development 1991; 111:1–14.

21. Young PE, Richman AM, Ketchum AS, Kiehart DP. Morphogenesis in *Drosophila* requires nonmuscle myosin heavy chain function. Genes Dev 1993; 7:29–41.

22. McCluskey J, Martin P. Analysis of the tissue movements of embryonic wound healing—DiI studies in the limb bud stage mouse embryo. Dev Biol 1995; 170:102–114.

23. Brock J, Midwinter K, Lewis J, Martin P. Healing of incisional wounds in the embryonic chick wing bud: characterization of the actin purse-string and demonstration of a requirement for Rho activation. J Cell Biol 1996; 135:1097–1107.

24. Kolega J. Effects of mechanical tension on protrusive activity and microfilament and intermediate filament organization in an epidermal epithelium moving in culture. J Cell Biol 1986; 102:1400–1411.

25. Ridley AJ, Hall A. The small GTP-binding protein rho regulates the assembly of focal adhesions and actin stress fibers in response to growth factors. Cell 1992; 70:389–399.

26. Martin P. Wound healing—aiming for perfect skin regeneration. Science 1997; 276:75–81.

27. Somasundaram K, Prathap K. Intra-uterine healing of skin wounds in rabbit foetuses. J Pathol 1970; 100:81–86.

28. Robinson BW, Goss AN. Intra-uterine healing of fetal rat cheek wounds. Cleft Palate J 1981; 18:251–255.

29. Rugh R. The mouse: its reproduction and development. Oxford University Press, Oxford, England, 1990.

30. Morris L, Graham CF, Gordon S. Macrophages in haemopoietic and other tissues of the developing mouse detected by the monoclonal antibody F4/80. Development 1991; 112:517–526.

31. Hopkinson-Woolley J, Hughes D, Gordon S, Martin P. Macrophage recruitment during limb development and wound healing in the embryonic and fetal mouse. J Cell Sci 1994; 107:1159–1167.

32. Hallock GH. In utero cleft lip repair in A/J mice. Plast Reconstr Surg 1985; 75: 785–788.
33. Skalli O, Gabbiani G. The biology of the myofibroblast. Relationship to wound contraction and fibrocontractive diseases. In: Clark RAF, Henson PM, eds. The Molecular and Cellular Biology of Wound Repair. New York: Plenum, 1988.
34. Martin P, Nobes CD. An early molecular component of the wound healing response in rat embryos—induction of c-fos protein in cells at the epidermal wound margin. Mech Dev 1992; 38:209–216.
35. Whitby DJ, Ferguson MWJ. Immunohistochemical localization of growth factors in fetal wound healing. Dev Biol 1991; 147:207–215.
36. Martin P, Dickson MC, Millan FA, Akhurst RJ. Rapid induction and clearance of TGFβ1 in response to wounding in the mouse embryo. Dev Genet 1993; 14:225–238.
37. Montesano R, Orci L. Transforming growth factor β stimulates collagen-matrix contraction by fibroblasts: implications for wound healing. Proc Natl Acad Sci USA 1988; 85:4894–4897.
38. Desmouliere A, Geinoz A, Gabbiani F, Gabbiani G. Transforming growth factor-beta 1 induces alpha-smooth muscle actin expression in granulation tissue myofibroblasts and in quiescent and growing cultured fibroblasts. J Cell Biol 1993; 122: 103–111.
39. Shah M, Foreman DM, Ferguson MWJ. Neutralizing antibody to TGF-β1,2 reduces cutaneous scarring in adult rodents. J Cell Sci 1994; 107:1137–1157.
40. Whitby DJ, Ferguson MWJ. The extracellular matrix of lip wounds in fetal, neonatal and adult mice. Development 1991; 112:651–668.
41. Lorenz HP, Whitby DJ, Longaker MT, Adzick NS. Fetal wound healing. The ontogeny of scar formation in the non-human primate. Ann Surg 1993; 217:319–398.

12
Characteristics of Fetal Wound Repair

Gyu S. Chin, Eric J. Stelnicki, George K. Gittes, and Michael T. Longaker
New York University School of Medicine, New York, New York

I. INTRODUCTION

Intensive research is being focused on unraveling the mechanisms that underlie scarless fetal skin wound repair. Recent advances in prenatal diagnosis initiated these endeavors. The ability to diagnose and repair congenital anomalies in utero, such as cleft lip, with scarless healing would revolutionize the field of reconstructive plastic surgery. Furthermore, if the biologic characteristics of scarless fetal skin healing are determined, these properties might be replicated in the adult environment with tremendous clinical benefits.

In 1979, Rowlatt (1) first observed that the human fetus appears to heal without scarring. That report documented that the midgestation fetus healed by mesenchymal proliferation, without the formation of adultlike scar. Over the past two decades, advances in fetal surgery for highly selected life-threatening conditions have confirmed the scarless nature of fetal skin healing. Subsequently, numerous animal models, including chick, guinea pig, opossum, rabbit, sheep, monkey, mouse, and rat, have been used to study fetal repair (2). However, differences in wounding techniques and inherent variations among the different species make comparison with human repair difficult. Despite this variability, a broad understanding of fetal healing biology is slowly emerging. This chapter summarizes the current knowledge of the defining characteristics that may determine fetal wound healing.

II. THE FETAL ENVIRONMENT: EXTRINSIC AND INTRINSIC DIFFERENCES

Initial research in fetal wound healing has centered around the concept that the in utero environment is uniquely conducive to scarless wound repair. This concept arose from the fact that fetal wounds are continuously bathed in a sterile amniotic fluid that may contain all the necessary components to achieve scarless healing. Since amniotic fluid provides a warm, moist environment rich with growth factors and extracellular matrix components, such as fibronectin and hyaluronic acid (HA), the intrauterine environment was thought to be critical in the scarless healing process (3–5). Although appealing in concept, this idea has now been proven invalid by several researchers.

One of the first experiments to address this concept of amniotic fluid as a mediator of scarless healing made use of a marsupial model in which a fetus develops partially outside the uterus in the maternal pouch (6). Armstrong and Ferguson (7) demonstrated that scarless healing proceeded outside of the uterus, in the American opossum (*Monodelphis domestica*). At birth, the opossum is functionally a fetus, yet it thrives in a nonsterile pouch environment free of amni-

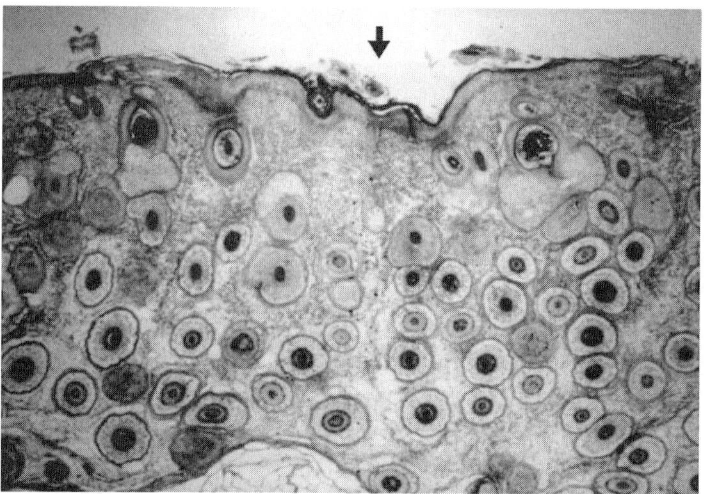

Figure 1 Photomicrograph of 19-week gestational age human fetal skin subcutaneous graft wound, harvested 14 days after wounding and stained with Mallory's trichrome. India ink marks the wound location (arrow) in which no scar is present. India ink is present in the dermis between and around hair follicles in the wound. No scar formation is evident. The reticular collagen staining pattern is unchanged from the surrounding unwounded dermis, demonstrating scarless tissue repair can occur in human fetal skin. (From Ref. 9.)

otic fluid. Even fetuses of day-2 pouch gestation healed without scar formation when wounded (7). Rat in vitro studies also have shown that fetal skin explants can heal without scar formation after removal from the fetal environment (8). Further evidence was gained from experiments in which human fetal skin at 15 to 22 weeks of gestation was transplanted cutaneously and subcutaneously into nude mice (9). The grafts were wounded 1 week after transplantation. Tissue analysis revealed that the subcutaneously grafted human fetal skin healed with donor-specific fetal fibroblasts without a scar, despite occurring in an environment free of amniotic fluid (Figs. 1 and 2). Thus, the fetal fibroblast healed fetal skin wounds without a scar, despite being perfused by adult serum in an adult environment. Longaker et al. (10) pursued this finding in the sheep model by placing adult tissue into a fetal environment. Adult sheep skin was grafted onto 60-day-gestation fetal sheep (term = 145 days). The graft was incorporated without rejection, and was perfused by fetal serum and bathed in amniotic fluid. Incisional wounds were created in the adult skin grafts at 100 days of gestation, a time in gestation when fetal sheep incisional wounds heal without scar formation (Fig. 3). Histological analysis of the wounded adult skin grafts revealed that they healed with scar formation, suggesting that the fetal environment may not be a critical determinant of scarless repair (Fig. 4). Taken together, these experimental studies support the hypothesis that it is the intrinsic properties of the fetal skin that determine scarless repair, rather than the unique fetal environment.

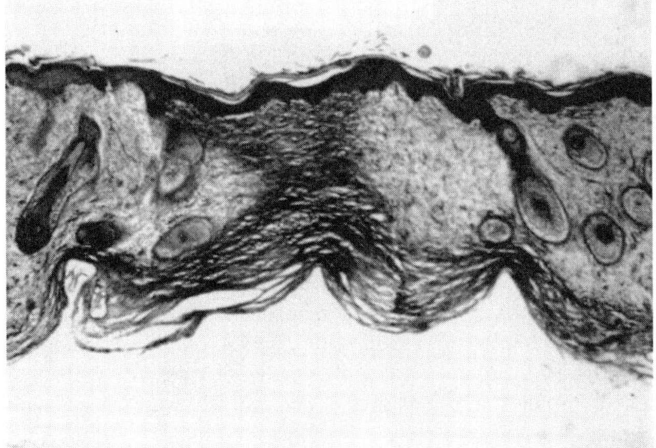

Figure 2 Photomicrograph of 19-week human fetal skin cutaneous graft wound, harvested 14 days after wounding and stained with Mallory's trichrome. In contrast to subcutaneous graft, the cutaneous wound healed with an obvious scar, which was also present along the bases of the grafts. (From Ref. 9.)

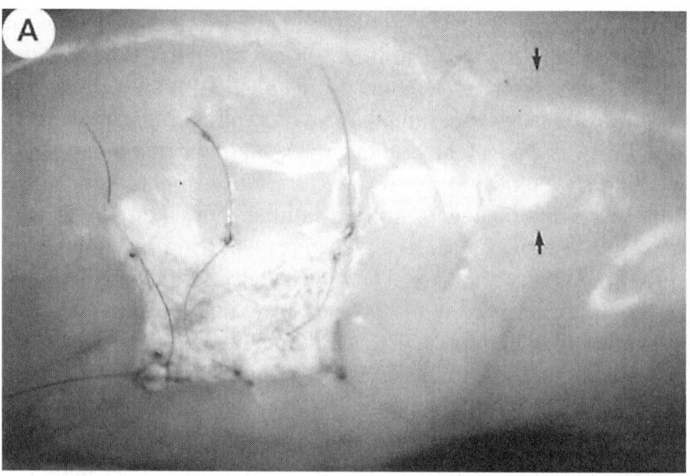

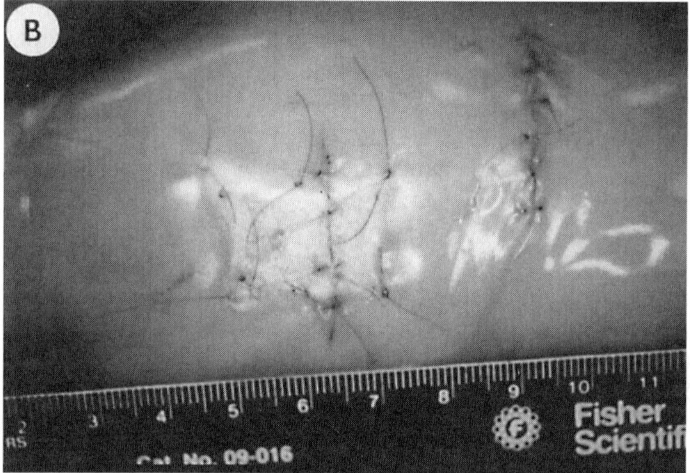

Figure 3 Photographic description of surgery to transplant adult (maternal) skin into the fetal environment. (A) At 40 days posttransplantation (100 days of gestation), the adult skin (left) had maintained its phenotype and is easily distinguished from surrounding fetal skin. The fetal autograph (right) is almost indistinguishable, marked only by the four sutures used to secure the graft (arrows). No scar is evident at the graft edges. (B) Incisional wounds were created across both adult and fetal grafts. The wounds were closed with interrupted sutures. (From Ref. 10.)

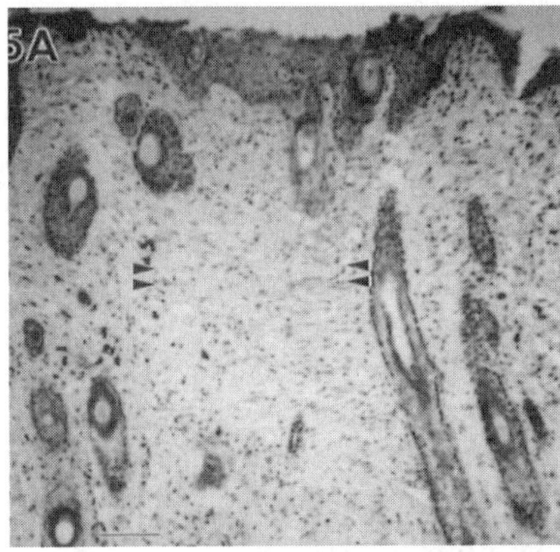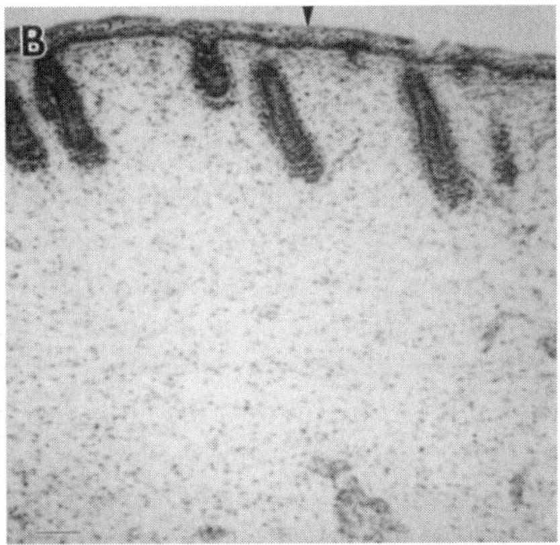

Figure 4 Adult and fetal wounds at 14 days. (A) Adult wound stained by hematoxylin and eosin. The wound site, marked by the arrows, has healed. The epidermis is thickened, and a band of scar tissue (between double arrows) is present. The parallel packed collagen fibers and fibroblasts in this area are oriented perpendicularly to the original wound surface. Note the lack of hair follicles within the scar. (B) Fetal wound stained by hematoxylin and eosin. The wound site (arrowhead) has healed and is indistinguishable from the surrounding skin. (From Ref. 10.)

III. CHARACTERIZING THE INTRINSIC FACTORS

There are a number of intrinsic factors that may be important in determining whether a wound heals with or without scar. Some of these differentiating factors in scarless wound healing may be related to gestational age, species, or tissue type. Other critical factors may include the interaction of extracellular matrix (ECM) components released after wounding, the cytokines released, and the size of the wound created for evaluation. An example of an intrinsic environmental difference is tissue oxygenation. Human fetal tissue appears to be markedly hypoxemic, with an arterial partial pressure of oxygen (pO_2) of 20 mm Hg (11). Using a miniaturized oximeter probe, it has been determined that the tissue pO_2 in the midgestation fetal sheep is 16 mm Hg, whereas the tissue pO_2 of the adult is between 45 and 60 mm Hg (12). Although this relative hypoxia is partially compensated by the greater affinity of fetal hemoglobin for oxygen, it is nevertheless intriguing that fetal wounds heal so rapidly, given the importance of tissue oxygenation and perfusion in postnatal wound healing and resistance to infection (12).

It is logical to assume that if the intrinsic properties of skin determine how wounds heal, then these properties must change with gestational age. In fact, a gradual transition from scarless healing in the early-gestation embryo to scar-forming repair in the late-gestation fetus has been documented in sheep (Figs. 5 and 6) (13), opossum (7), monkey (14), and rat (8). In the monkey model (14), wounds made at 75 days of gestation (term = 165 days) revealed fully restored tissue architecture. However, the ability to form hair follicles and sebaceous glands at the site of repair was lost at 85 to 100 days of gestation (the ''transition wound''). At 107 days of gestation, wounds healed with a thin scar.

In short, the transition from scarless to scarring phenotypes of repair in fetal skin has been correlated with three factors: 1) gestational-age-related changes in the cytokine response to wounding, 2) the complexity of dermal and subdermal tissue architecture, and 3) the ability of the fetus to generate an acute inflammatory response. In addition, the role of the fibroblast, the specific organ wounded, and the particular species of animals used are important factors that may determine whether fetal skin wounds heal with or without a scar.

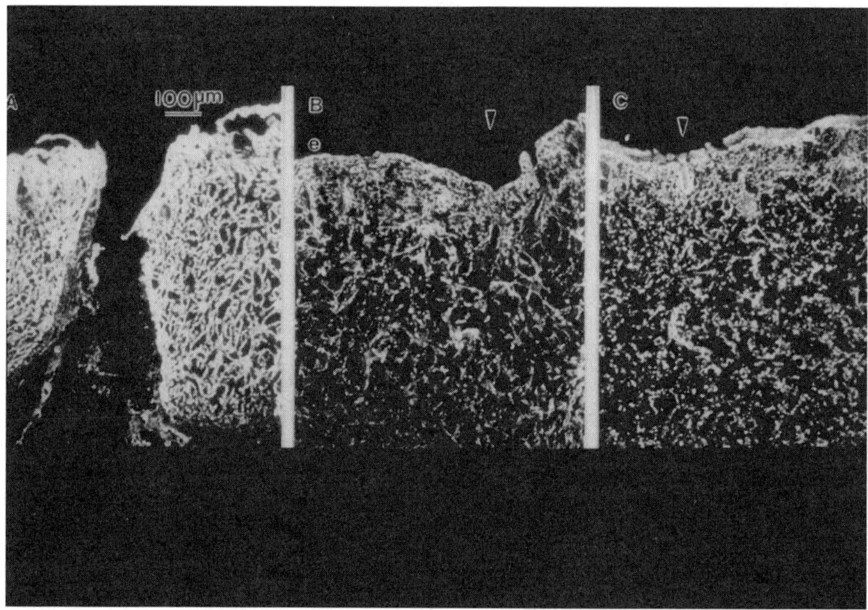

Figure 5 Fetal lamb incisional wounding model at 75 days of gestation. (A) 75-Day fetus 24 hr postwounding. Collagen type VI staining throughout the dermis. No collagen deposition is seen in the wound. (B) 75-Day fetus 15 days postwounding. Collagen type VI staining shows the wound well healed and a normal collagen pattern without scar formation. (C) 75-Day fetus 15 days postwounding. Collagen type I staining was similar to type VI. Again note the lack of scar formation. Bar = 100 μm, arrow marks wound sites. (From Ref. 13.)

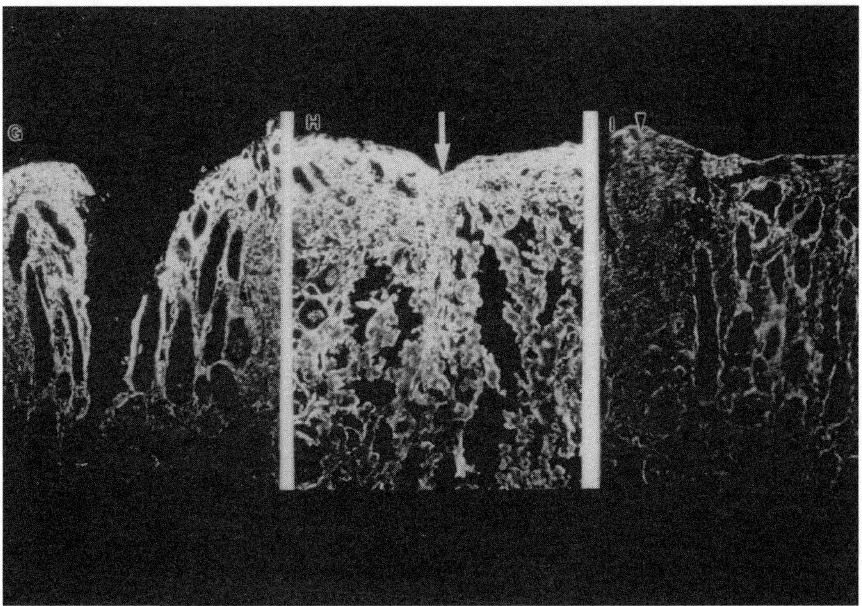

Figure 6 Fetal lamb incisional wounding model at 120 days of gestation. (G) 120-Day fetus 24 hr postwounding. Collagen type VI staining throughout the dermis without collagen deposition in the wound. (H) 120-Day fetus 7 days postwounding. Collagen type VI staining showed the wound epithelialized and collagen deposited in the wound as bands parallel to the original wound (arrow). (I) 120-Day fetus 14 days postwounding. Collagen type VI staining showed a narrow band of scar tissue at the wound site (arrow). Normal tissue is shown on the right for comparison. (From Ref. 13.)

A. Species Differences

Although there are distinct differences between the fetal and adult tissue response to wound healing, additionally, there are differences in the fetal response to injury among different animal models (2,6–8,13–17). This fetal variability might be related to differences in placentation, amniotic fluid content, or intrinsic wound healing characteristics of different animal species (18). This lack of uniformity is most apparent in excisional wound healing models. For example, fetal rabbit wounds do not contract in the presence of amniotic fluid, but do contract when excluded from amniotic fluid (19,20). This difference is due to a characteristic of rabbit amniotic fluid that appears to inhibit fibroblast contraction. This inhibition has been confirmed in vitro using a fibroblast-populated collagen lattice model (12). Rabbit amniotic fluid is known to contain large numbers of high-molecular-weight proteins, such as immunoglobulins, that may be responsible for inhibiting fibroblast contraction. In contrast, amniotic fluid in sheep stimulates contraction of sheep fibroblasts in collagen lattices in vitro in a dose-dependent manner (21). This stimulation may be due to a 40-kDa protein that has been isolated from sheep amniotic fluid and is thought to stimulate fibroblast contraction.

It is important to realize that, when applying animal models toward human wound healing, differences in breeding technique may affect individual variability in healing. Most laboratory animals used in wound healing research are inbred, to eliminate genetic variability (18). However, even laboratory sheep, pigs, and monkeys that are outbred, still show less individual variation than humans (22). For example, the fetal opossum *Monodelphis domestica* (7), an outbred animal, shows significant individual variability in the transition time from scarless to scar-forming healing, as well as in the extent of scarring. Nevertheless, one consistent aspect of all animal models of fetal wound healing is that fetal incisional skin wounds, made early in gestation, heal without scar and more rapidly than adult incisional wounds.

B. Organ Specificity

It is clear that the regenerative capacity of fetal skin is different from that of the adult. However, it was unclear whether different fetal organs possess different regenerative patterns. Thus, researchers have attempted to evaluate the ability of the fetus to heal defects in other organs. In the fetal sheep, at 100 days of gestation, incisional diaphragmatic wounds made in utero healed with scar formation, whereas incisional skin wounds healed flawlessly (23). This finding suggested that there are differences in the timing or mechanism of repair in wounds from different types of fetal tissues. In contrast to other tissues of mesodermal origin, midgestation fetal sheep long bones heal with minimal callus, and demonstrate both intramembranous and endochondral ossification. Furthermore, fetal sheep long bones can heal defects that are 3 times the bony width (what would be a critical size defect in adult animals), including periosteum (24). In addition, gastric or intestinal wounds made in early-gestation fetal lambs also have been shown to heal with scar formation (25,26). These studies confirm our observation that the fetal healing response is an organ-specific response and is not uniformly scarless in early gestation.

C. Fetal Fibroblasts

It is becoming clear that fetal fibroblasts may be crucial for scarless repair. A number of studies have begun to define functional intrinsic differences between fetal and adult fibroblasts. One major difference is the regulation of collagen production. Early-gestation fetal fibroblasts synthesize greater total collagen than their adult counterparts, and have a greater prolyl hydroxylase enzyme activity, a known rate-limiting step in collagen synthesis (27,28). Moreover, fetal fibroblasts migrate faster through collagen matrices than adult fibroblasts, probably due to greater levels of hyaluronic acid in the fetal environment (29).

Hyaluronic acid is a major component of the extracellular matrix of fetal skin and stimulates the migration of fibroblasts. While adult fibroblasts decrease HA synthesis as cell density increases, fetal cells do not. In fact, subconfluent fetal fibroblasts continue to produce approximately the same amount of HA as confluent cells. This finding led some authors to suggest that the increased migratory ability of fetal fibroblasts may be related to increased HA synthesis (29). In addition, fetal fibroblasts have fourfold greater density of HA receptors than adult cells by Western blotting analysis. This finding was corroborated by fluorescence-activated cell sorting for the HA receptor, which determined that fetal cells had 2.5 times the HA receptor levels of adult cells (30). The increased number of HA receptors, increased amount of HA, and increased migratory ability of fetal fibroblasts may all play important roles in the increased rate and efficiency of fetal healing (31,32).

Another important role for fetal fibroblasts was discovered in the fetal lamb model. Fibroblast gene expression studies demonstrated that the onset of expression of α-smooth muscle actin (α-SMA) coincided with the onset of scar formation. In adult wound healing, the myofibroblast is thought to play a role in wound contraction and scar formation and is characterized by α-SMA production. Excisional wounds in 75-day-gestation fetal lambs showed an absence of both scar and contraction in the absence of α-SMA expression. At 100 days of gestation, when α-SMA first appeared, scars began to form (33). Thus, the correlation between the presence of myofibroblasts and scar formation suggests that the contractile forces generated by myofibroblasts may alter the orientation of collagen fibrils and may contribute to scarring. This suggestion was initially made by Longaker et al. (34) with the observation that fetal lamb wounds contract in utero and the documentation of wound myofibroblasts.

Understanding the genetic regulation of fetal tissues is important. Once a defect is created, the fibroblasts surrounding the defect must recognize that there is an injury that needs to be corrected in a specific way. Ultimately, this regulation of repair and regeneration must be at the genetic level. Some animals (newts, for example) retain their ability to heal massive defects throughout adult life. How this occurs is not completely understood, but what is clear is that this type of tissue regeneration is characterized by the induction of patterning genes, such as homeobox (HOX) gene expression, in the advancing newt limb blastema (35). It is likely that fetal mammals have the same ability to heal large skin defects made early in gestation because transcription factor patterning genes, such as homeobox genes, are also more active in the fetal environment. As a result, researchers have hypothesized that transcription factors, like homeobox genes, may be the "first domino" in the fetal cutaneous wound repair regulatory cascade (36).

D. Homeobox Genes

In order to identify transcription factors that may control skin development and possibly mediate scarless fetal tissue regeneration, Stelnicki et al. screened human skin samples at a variety of developmental stages by reverse transcriptase polymerase chain reaction (RT-PCR) for *HOX* and non-*HOX* patterning gene expression (35,37). The goal of the initial experiments was to find patterning genes expressed in developing skin, categorize them, and then identify genes whose expression patterns correlated temporally with the process of scarless wound repair. Using this method, they were able to identify four *HOX*– and four non-*HOX*–containing patterning genes as potential candidates (35,37).

The *HOX* genes identified were all expressed in the fetal dermis only during the time of scarless wound repair, i.e., the first and second trimesters of human fetal skin development. In situ hybridization of second trimester human fetal skin detected the transcripts of these genes throughout the dermis and epidermis. *HOX* expression was down-regulated in the basal and stratum spinosum layers of the newborn and adult skin, where expression appeared to be localized only in the upper granular layers of the epidermis. Therefore, *HOX* expression in the developing dermis was restricted only to the period of dermal generation or formation, whereas expression in the epidermis, which has the ability to renew itself throughout life, extended beyond the period of fetal development.

The non-*HOX* homeobox gene transcripts most frequently detected during fetal skin development were *MSX-1*, *MSX-2*, *MOX-1*, and *PRX-2*. The *MSX-1*, *MSX-2*, and *PRX-2* signals in both fetal and adult epidermis may represent self-renewing stem cells. However, dermal expression of these three genes was limited to the first and second trimesters of development. In the early and mid-second trimester of gestation, *MSX-1* and *MSX-2* were both clearly expressed in the cells of the dermal stroma. At this stage, both the reticular and papillary dermis are developing and the dermal signals for both *MSX-1* and *MSX-2* appeared to be localized to fibroblasts. Both *MSX-1* and *MSX-2* were also detected in the hair follicles that were beginning to grow downward from the overlying epithelium. Within each follicle, the expression of both genes appeared to be in the dermal papilla, the collar epithelium that lines the inner root sheath, and in the papillary ectoderm.

Interestingly, *MOX-1* expression was also only detected in the first and early second trimesters of development. During these developmental periods, *MOX-1* was expressed in the dermal fibroblasts, the epithelial and mesenchymal cells of the developing hair follicles, and in the overlying epithelium, including the periderm. However, in late-second-trimester human fetal skin, *MOX-1* expression was dramatically down-regulated and was detected only in a few specific epithelial cells located at the innermost layer of the outer root sheath. In adult skin, its expression was conspicuously absent by both ribonuclease (RNase) protection and RT-PCR analysis. Thus, just as in *HOX* gene expression, dermal expression of *MOX* and *MSX* was limited to the time of scarless fetal wound repair.

PRX-2 expression, however, was barely detected in normal fetal skin as a weak signal concentrated over the papilla of the developing hair shaft, with no signal detected in the epidermis, and little signal above background in the dermal fibroblasts. However, *PRX-2* expression was detected in cultured fibroblasts, suggesting that a portion of the *PRX-2* signal is also mesodermal. In the adult, no dermal *PRX-2* signal was detected, but in situ hybridization showed a strong localization of *PRX-2* expression throughout all layers of the epidermis.

Stelnicki et al. (38) then characterized homeobox gene expression in wounded fetal versus adult skin. Probing wounded fetal and adult skin, they noted that the homeobox genes *HOX-B13* and *PRX-2* were the most differentially expressed, out of the candidate genes previously mentioned. Both genes were expressed in the fetal fibroblast and in the fetal, rather than the adult, dermis. In wounded human fetal skin, *PRX-2* expression was strongly up-regulated compared with unwounded fetal and wounded adult skin. In situ hybridization showed a marked increase in *PRX-2* transcription throughout the fetal dermis 12 hr after wounding. This result implies that *PRX-2* activation is an important stimulant to dermal generation. Conversely, *HOX-B13*, which was strongly expressed in normal second trimester fetal skin, was markedly down-regulated in response to wounding. Thus, *HOX-B13* may be an inhibitor of dermal proliferation, and its constant expression may be involved in maintaining a static dermal architecture rather than promoting dermal growth.

How these homeobox genes may coordinate scarless fetal wound repair is currently the focus of intense investigation. Several possible targets have been identified including the promoter regions of members of the transforming growth factor-β (TGF-β) superfamily, various cellular adhesion molecules, and cell surface proteins such as integrins. Several cell adhesion molecule (CAM) regulatory regions are activated in vitro by HOX proteins, including N-CAM by Hoxb8, Hoxb9 and Hoxc6, and L-CAM by Hoxd9 (39–42). The promoter region of the α_2-integrin gene contains both activator and repressor regions with putative homeodomain binding sites (39). Analysis of both in vitro transgenic cell lines and in vivo knockout animal models may provide important clues as to how these proteins interrelate.

IV. EXTRACELLULAR MATRIX COMPONENTS

The ECM is a cross-linked network of structural proteins, polysaccharides, and adhesion molecules. These include collagen, tenascin, fibronectin, and HA. Although the fetal wound synthesizes many of the same extracellular matrix components seen in adult wounds, the timing and relative concentration of these various molecules in fetal wounds are distinct. In short, understanding the mechanisms of deposition, synthesis, and degradation of ECM components may bring us closer to understanding the mechanisms supporting fetal skin repair.

A. Collagen

Collagen is the most abundant protein in adult extracellular matrix, and its lack of organization at the site of repair dictates scar formation. It is of particular interest in fetal healing, since the relative quantity and pattern of collagen deposition are different from that of the adult. Fetal wounds demonstrate a more orderly and rapid collagen deposition than adult wounds, with a reticular pattern indistinguishable from surrounding intact skin (43). In contrast, postnatal and adult wounds demonstrate excessive, disorganized collagen bundles aligned perpendicularly to the plane of injury. Furthermore, the relative expression of different subtypes of collagen may have an important role in the ability of the fetus to perform scarless repair.

Immunohistochemistry using antibodies to collagen types I, III, IV, and VI showed rapid deposition in fetal lamb incisional wounds at 75, 100, and 120 days of gestation (13). Two weeks postwounding, there was a pattern of collagen deposition in the 75- and 100-day groups that was indistinguishable from normal fetal skin (see Figure 5). In contrast, wounds created on 120-day fetuses showed a transition to adult pattern healing with formation of a collagen scar (see Figure 6) (13). Other studies have revealed that the relative ratio of collagen III to collagen I is higher in early fetal wounds (44). This finding is significant due to the fact that the most abundant subtype of collagen in the mature adult wounds is collagen I.

In vitro, first-passage fetal fibroblasts have been found to produce higher levels of collagen III and collagen V than adult fibroblasts (45). Furthermore, collagen I gene expression in fetal cells is up-regulated compared with adult cells. Hydroxy-L-proline, a marker of collagen synthesis, is detected earlier in fetal rabbit than in similar adult rabbit fibroblasts in vitro (28). In summary, in vitro studies of fetal dermal fibroblasts show a greater capacity for collagen synthesis than their adult counterparts. The ability of the fetus to modulate and organize collagen synthesis and deposition is important to supporting a scarless repair.

B. Adhesion Molecules

The ECM provides the three-dimensional lattice for cell attachment and migration. Adhesion glycoproteins found in the ECM, such as tenascin and fibronectin, are thought to be necessary for migration and cell anchoring, respectively. During development, the presence of tenascin along migratory pathways facilitates cell movement, whereas fibronectin facilitates cell anchoring and is seen in association with fibrin clot formation and platelet granules. Fibronectin is normally present in adult wounds, but is deposited in larger amounts in fetal than in neonatal or adult wounds. Topical application of fibronectin to adult rat wounds has been observed to accelerate healing (12). In one wounding model, Whitby and Ferguson (43) created incisional lip wounds on fetal, neonatal, and adult mice. They always observed the deposition of fibronectin within 1 hr after wounding, in all groups. However, tenascin appeared 1 hr after wounding in the fetus, after 12 hr in the neonate, and after 24 hr in the adult. Thus, they concluded that the timecourse of tenascin's first appearance paralleled the rate of wound healing, which was fastest in the fetus and slowest in the adult. This observation was supported by other experiments in which trunk wounds of fetal and adult sheep showed a similar distribution of fibronectin in both wounds, but a more rapid deposition of tenascin in the fetal wounds (46). In summary, the large amounts of fibronectin in fetal wounds may stimulate immediate cell attachment, whereas the rapid deposition of tenascin may allow cells to migrate and fully epithelialize the fetal wound more rapidly than in the adult wound.

C. Proteoglycans and Glycosaminoglycans

Proteoglycans are macromolecules consisting of a protein core to which sulfated glycosaminoglycans (GAGs) are covalently bound. They are thought to be important factors in wound healing that modulate cell migration and proliferation, collagen synthesis, collagen and fibril organization, and the rate of collagen degradation. In fact, fetal wound matrix is rich in GAGs. Fetal rabbit wounds, for example, demonstrate 3 times the level of GAGs seen in adult wounds and 10 times the level of GAGs in unwounded fetal skin (47).

Hyaluronic acid is the most abundant glycosaminoglycan in the fetal extracellular matrix (31,32,47). Composed of alternating units of N-acetylglucosamine and glucuronic acid residues, HA is thought to provide stability and elasticity to the extracellular matrix and regulate the hydration and movement of substances within the extracellular matrix. By the nature of its hygroscopic properties, HA can occupy 1000 to 10,000 times its own volume. Thus, HA allows proliferating cells to avoid inhibitory contacts (48). Hyaluronic acid synthesis precedes mitosis and dissociates the dividing cell from its substratum, permitting cell movement. Most HA is linked to collagen; however, HA levels are elevated immediately after wounding. The CD44 receptor, a glycoprotein present on the surface of fibroblasts, is a member of the immunoglobulin superfamily and one of the two major HA receptors. It acts via a protein kinase and binds HA (49). As previously mentioned, the density measurements of CD44 receptors by Western blotting has shown that fetal rabbit fibroblasts have 4 times the number of CD44 receptors that adult fibroblasts have (30). It has been hypothesized that increased CD44 receptor expression may facilitate scarless repair by increasing fetal cell motility during wound repair.

The extended presence of HA in fetal wounds may provide the matrix signal needed for scarless repair (32,50). Polyvinyl alcohol (PVA) sponges placed in fetal rabbit wounds contained 3 times the HA levels of adult rabbit wounds (47). Hyaluronic acid was determined to be the predominant glycosaminoglycan in these sponges. Degradation of HA by the addition of hyaluronidase to PVA sponges in fetal wounds led to increased fibroblast infiltration, collagen deposition, and capillary formation (51). Likewise, the addition of HA degradation products to PVA sponges in fetal wounds also increased fibrosis and neovascularization (51). Furthermore, HA increased rapidly within 24 hr in fetal sheep wound fluid and remained elevated for 3 weeks, whereas HA in adult wound fluid peaked at 3 days after wounding and decreased to zero by 7 days (Fig. 7) (32). To further test the effects of HA on adult wound repair, King et al. (48) applied exogenous HA to adult hamster cheek pouch wounds. They determined that microcirculatory perfusion was improved at the site of tissue repair with accelerated wound closure. Taken together, these data support the hypothesis that the prolonged pres-

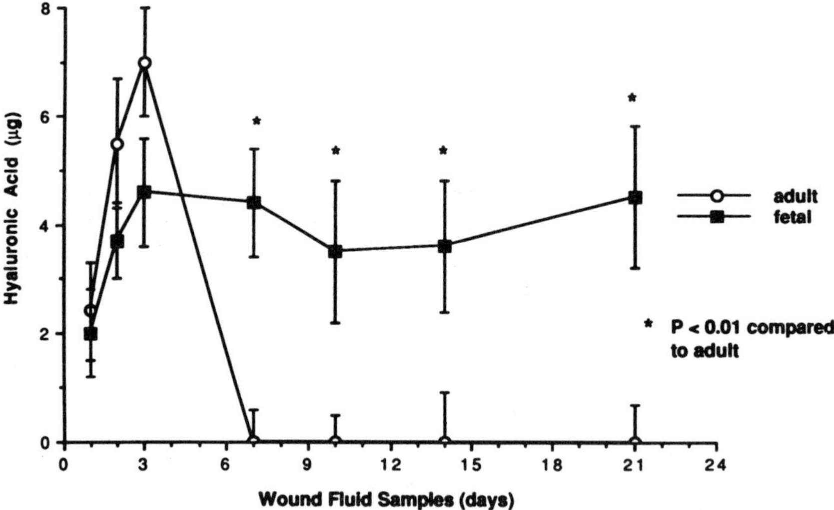

Figure 7 Hyaluronic acid levels in adult and fetal wound fluid. One hundred µL of wound fluid at each time point was assayed using HA-binding protein assay. Error bars represent the standard deviation of each value in triplicate. Student's *t* test was used for statistical analysis. Hyaluronic acid was not detectable in the adult after day 7. (From Ref. 33.)

ence of an HA-rich fetal wound ECM may create a permissive environment in which fibroblast movement is facilitated, and may promote scarless fetal repair.

V. THE IMMUNE RESPONSE

The fetal immune response to injury differs markedly from that of the adult. It is characterized by a lack of self–nonself immunological identity (at least until midgestation) and fetal skin repair proceeds with minimal acute inflammation, minimal fibroblast proliferation, and without excessive collagen deposition. Although the sequence of events in adult wound healing is well defined, and thought to be controlled in part by potent polypeptide cytokines, relatively little information exists regarding scarless fetal repair. Fetal wounds are relatively neutropenic, and fetal neutrophils may not possess the chemotactic ability of adult neutrophils. In addition, minimal scarring in some fetal skin wounds has also been associated with a markedly reduced mononuclear infiltrate and absence of endogenous immunoglobulin expression (27). Several investigators have shown that the level of inflammation in wounds correlates directly with gestational age (12,13,52,53). In the fetal rabbit and monkey, there is an increasing inflammatory response to foreign stimuli with advancing gestational age (54–57). This increase is accompanied by a different inflammatory cell composition in the fetal wound matrix in contrast to the adult (58–62). Furthermore, others have shown that neutrophils are less abundant in fetal sheep wounds, and fetal neutrophils show a limited ability to phagocytose opsonized *Staphylococcus aureus* until the third trimester (63). At the same time that neutrophil phagocytic ability is compromised, fetal serum is unable to opsonize bacteria effectively (63). In fetal opossum, virtually no inflammation was observed in wounds made in pouch-day-0, -1, and -2 animals (7). Cellular infiltrates of the early-pouch-day fetuses contained proportionately more mononuclear inflammatory cells than neutrophils (7). The altered acute inflammatory response and increased presence of macrophages in fetal wounds may provide a unique fetal wound microenvironment with modified cytokine profiles regulating a highly organized collagen deposition promoting scarless healing.

VI. CYTOKINES

Cytokines are polypeptides with multiple regulatory roles in cell growth and differentiation, and in developmental processes. Differences in cytokine expression may be responsible for the reduced acute inflammation seen in fetal wounds. Numerous investigators have sought to examine the role of cytokines in fetal wound repair. In fact, several cytokines have been studied, including transforming growth factor-β, transforming growth factor-α (TGF-α), epidermal growth factor (EGF), fibroblast growth factor (FGF), and platelet-derived growth factor (PDGF) (12,64–69).

Transforming growth factor-β is the most studied of all the growth factors in wound healing. It is produced by a variety of cell types and its activities are variable, depending on the local environment and target cell. The effects of the various types of TGF-β on scarless wound healing remain unclear. Three highly homologous TGF-β genes in mammals, designated TGF-β1, -β2, and -β3, have been identified. Transforming growth factor-β1 biological activity promotes ECM accumulation, fibrosis, and scarring (70,71). In one study, TGF-β placed into PVA sponges in rabbits at 24 days of gestation, a time when cutaneous fetal rabbit wounds heal without scarring, produced inflammation and fibrosis (72). Likewise, when TGF-β was added to human fetal skin wounds in vivo as a slow-release disk, scar formed (73). It has been shown that TGF-β up-regulates collagen expression in cultured fetal dermal fibroblasts, signifying that the response of fetal fibroblasts to TGF-β is similar to the adult. Fetal fibroblasts respond to exogenous TGF-β by increased collagen synthesis and cell proliferation (74). Furthermore, researchers discovered that TGF-β production by fetal fibroblasts may be blunted in hypoxemic conditions (75). This observation led to the theory that the decreased oxygen tension in the fetal environment may inhibit TGF-β production and, thus, decrease scar formation.

Initially, immunohistochemical studies supported the hypothesis that TGF-β was decreased in fetal wounds (45,76). Researchers discovered that there was a deficiency of TGF-β in the fetal mouse and rabbit wounds, as well as human skin transplanted onto nude mice, relative to adult wounds (45,73,77). However, recent studies have contradicted these earlier data. Now, it appears that TGF-β is not only present in fetal wounds, but also may be present in a greater quantity (64,78). Immunohistochemical localization for TGF-β isoforms in unwounded fetal mouse lips at day 16 of gestation (term = 19 days) demonstrated strong positive staining for all three isoforms of TGF-β (64). In contrast, little staining was found in unwounded adult skin. Upon wounding, fetal skin showed minimally increased staining at the wound margins. By 48 hours postwounding, a normal (i.e., unwounded) fetal TGF-β staining pattern was observed. However, the adult wounds remained strongly positive for all three isoforms of TGF-β through day 7 after wounding. This study suggested that changes in the expression of TGF-β isoforms, rather than the mere presence of TGF-β, may be important in explaining histological differences in fetal and adult repair (64).

Wound fluid analysis in fetal sheep wounds also demonstrated greater amounts of TGF-β when compared with adult wounds (78). Transforming growth factor-β was found in significantly greater concentration in 100-day and 120-day fetal sheep wound fluids than in adult wound fluids (78). Using a sandwich enzyme-linked immunosorbent assay technique, wound fluid was analyzed for specific TGF-β1 and -β2 isoform concentrations. The highest concentration of total TGF-β1 and TGF-β2 was found in 100-day fetal wound fluid, followed by 120-day fetal wounds, with the least amount detected in adult wounds. These data further suggested that the relative concentration of TGF-β isoforms in wound fluid may determine the biological activity and scarring. In summary, as new data continually emerge, we are gaining a greater understanding of the complex role of TGF-β isoforms in fetal wound repair.

Bone morphogenetic protein-2 (BMP-2), a member of the TGF-β super-family, is believed to have an important role in normal skin development and fetal wound healing. Stelnicki et al. (79) used ribonucleic acid in situ hybridization to demonstrate that BMP-2 was expressed at low levels in the developing hair follicles and in the epidermis of normal human fetal skin. In addition, they showed by histological analysis that exogenously added BMP-2 induced increased scarring and cellular proliferation in fetal lamb skin wounds. Specifically, the changes in skin histology in responses to BMP-2 were characterized by marked epidermal thickening, increased keratinization, a dramatic increase in the number of hair follicles, and more than 50% thickening of the dermis. Furthermore, wounds treated with both BMP-2 and TGF-β healed with an adultlike repair, indicating that there was not an additive effect of combining BMP-2 and TGF-β. Thus, they concluded that BMP-2 is a pleomorphic growth factor that induces cellular growth, maturation, and fibroplasia in both the dermis and epidermis. Further analysis of this growth factor in both fetal and adult wound healing may lead to important discoveries regarding the control of scar formation and fibrosis.

Epidermal growth factor has been shown to induce rapid epithelialization in adult wounds. When applied to fetal rabbit excisional wounds, EGF has been shown to accelerate the reepithelialization rate (65). This observation has led some to conclude that EGF can accelerate fetal wound healing. In contrast to EGF, TGF-α, a factor structurally similar to EGF, has been shown to induce mesenchymal cell infiltrates without reepithelialization in fetal excisional wounds (80). Thus, the mechanism of action of these growth factors needs to be examined in greater detail.

In addition to its mitogenic action on fibroblasts, PDGF stimulates important cellular metabolic activities, including protein, lipid, and prostaglandin synthesis (81–84). Platelet-derived growth factor is thought to be an important factor in early embryonic development and in vivo appears to modulate tissue regeneration and remodeling during wound healing and osteogenesis (83). Thus, investigators have sought to examine the effect of PDGF, a putative adult wound healing regulator, on the cellular and extracellular matrix events at a fetal wound site. Haynes et al. (66) subcutaneously implanted Silastic sponges containing PDGF into 24-day-gestation fetal rabbits (term = 31 days). They found that when compared with controls implanted with Silastic sponges alone, the PDGF-treated implants had a marked increase in acute inflammation, fibroblast recruitment, and collagen and hyaluronic acid deposition. These differences appeared to be largely time- and PDGF dose-dependent. Thus, they concluded that the fetal system is responsive to an adult wound healing mediator, and that scarless fetal repair may require the absence of PDGF.

In summary, cytokine profiles in fetal wounds have been shown to differ from adult wounds. However, the definitive role of cytokines in fetal wound healing has been obscured by the complexity of the cytokine milieu. It is important to realize that there is probably no one factor solely responsible for scarless repair. Rather, it is likely the balance of numerous known and, as yet, unknown cytokines that may provide the answer.

VII. WOUND SIZE

Recently, the effect of varying excisional wound size on the fetal healing response has been studied in the fetal sheep (85). Cass et al. (85) produced circular excisional wounds of 2-, 4-, 6-, and 10-mm diameter on the backs of fetal sheep at 60, 70, and 90 days of gestation (term = 145 days). After 14 days, the wounds were harvested and analyzed histologically for scar formation. In addition, the *wound-size threshold*, defined as the diameter of excised skin at which 50% of the wounds healed scarlessly at a given gestational age, was determined. The wound-size threshold was between 6 and 10 mm in 60- and 70-day-gestation animals and between 4 and 6 mm in 80- and 90-day-gestation animals. The data support the concept that the 60- and 70-day-gestation fetal lambs have a greater capacity for scarless repair than the 80- and 90-day-gestation animals.

How wound size actually affects the repair response is unknown. However, it is not unreasonable to assume that larger wounds may extend the time of the healing response, thus exposing wound tissues to a different extracellular matrix and growth factor profile. In addition, the larger excisional fetal wounds may stimulate the formation of myofibroblasts in the wound, resulting in scar formation.

VIII. SUMMARY

The expansion of our knowledge of scarless wound repair in fetal skin will have wide-reaching applications in therapeutic interventions. Understanding how the fetus is able to heal early-gestation cutaneous injury without scar formation may hold the key to scarless repair in children and adults. Several important unique characteristics central to the fetal wound healing response have been discussed. The scarless repair capabilities of the fetus appear to be influenced by the intrinsic properties of the fetal tissues, not by extrinsic factors. The fetal fibroblast may modulate the wound healing response through the organization of collagen and extracellular matrix deposition. The fetal immune response is characterized by a primarily mononuclear cell infiltrate, lacking the influence of polymorphonuclear leukocytes. Furthermore, we are beginning to understand the complex cytokine milieu during the wound healing cascade, and recognize that the cytokine profile of the fetal wound may differ markedly from that of the adult wound. Lastly, recent experiments involving patterning genes have improved our knowledge of the scarless phenomenon. Patterning genes involved in skin organogenesis may prove integral to fetal healing, and are emerging as an active area of research.

Many clinicians hope that an understanding of these remarkable reparative capabilities of the fetus may lead to the development of new wound healing therapies that reduce or prevent scar formation and fibrosis in the management of children. Equally intriguing is the possibility for future application toward improving adult wound healing and preventing scar formation after surgery or trauma.

REFERENCES

1. Rowlatt U. Intrauterine wound healing in a 20 week human fetus. Virchows Arch [A] 1979; 381:353–361.
2. Adzick NS, Longaker MT. Animal models for the study of fetal tissue repair. J Surg Res 1991; 51:216–222.
3. Dahl L, Hopwood JJ, Laurent UB, Lilja K, Tengblad A. The concentration of hyaluronate in amniotic fluid. Biochem Med 1983; 30:280–283.
4. Harris MC, Mennuti MT, Kline JA, Polin RA. Amniotic fluid fibronectin concentrations with advancing gestational age. Obstet Gynecol 1988; 72:593–595.
5. Mulvihill SJ, Stone MM, Fonkalsrud EW, Debas HT. Trophic effect of amniotic fluid on fetal gastrointestinal development. J Surg Res 1986; 40:291–296.
6. Block M. Wound healing in the newborn opossum (*Didelphis virginianam*). Nature 1960; 187:340.
7. Armstrong JR, Ferguson MW. Ontogeny of the skin and the transition from scar-free to scarring phenotype during wound healing in the pouch young of a marsupial, *Monodelphis domestica*. Dev Biol 1995; 169:242–260.
8. Ihara S, Motobayashi Y, Nagao E, Kistler A. Ontogenetic transition of wound healing pattern in rat skin occurring at the fetal stage. Development 1990; 110:671–680.
9. Lorenz HP, Longaker MT, Perkocha LA, Jennings RW, Harrison MR, Adzick NS. Scarless wound repair: a human fetal skin model. Development 1992; 114:253–259.
10. Longaker MT, Whitby DJ, Ferguson MW, Lorenz HP, Harrison, MR, Adzick, NS. Adult skin wounds in the fetal environment heal with scar formation. Ann Surg 1994; 219:65–72.
11. Nelson NM. Respiration and circulation before birth. In: Smith CA, Nelson NM, eds. The physiology of the newborn infant. Springfield: Thomas, 1976.

12. Longaker MT, Adzick NS. The biology of fetal wound healing: a review. Plast Reconstr Surg 1991; 87:788–798.

13. Longaker MT, Whitby DJ, Adzick NS, Crombleholme TM, Langer JC, Duncan BW, Bradley SM, Stern R, Ferguson MW, Harrison MR. Studies in fetal wound healing. VI. Second and early third trimester fetal wounds demonstrate rapid collagen deposition without scar formation. J Pediatr Surg 1990; 25:63–68; discussion 68–69.

14. Lorenz HP, Whitby DJ, Longaker MT, Adzick NS. Fetal wound healing. The ontogeny of scar formation in the non-human primate. Ann Surg 1993; 217:391–396.

15. Krummel TM, Nelson JM, Diegelman RF, Lindblad WJ, Salzberg AM, Greenfield LJ, Cohen LK. Fetal response to injury in the rabbit. J Pediatr Surg 1987; 22:640–644.

16. Hess A. Reactions of mammalian fetal tissues to injury. II. Skin. Anat Res 1958; 119:435.

17. Hallock GG. In utero cleft lip repair in A/J mice. Plast Reconstr Surg 1985; 75:785.

18. Ferguson MW, Whitby DJ, Shah M, Armstrong J, Siebert JW, Longaker MT. Scar formation: the spectral nature of fetal and adult wound repair. Plast Reconstr Surg 1996; 97:854–860.

19. Somasundaram K, Prathap K. Intra-uterine healing of skin wounds in rabbit foetuses. J Pathol 1970; 100:81.

20. Somasundaram K, Prathap K. The effect of exclusion of amniotic fluid on intra-uterine healing of skin wounds in rabbit foetuses. J Pathol 1972; 107:127.

21. Rittenberg T, Longaker MT, Adzick NS, Ehrlich HP. Sheep amniotic fluid has a protein factor which stimulates human fibroblast populated collagen lattice contraction. J Cell Physiol 1991; 149:444–450.

22. Adzick NS. Fetal animal and wound implant models. In: Adzick NS, Longaker MT, eds. Fetal Wound Healing. New York: Elsevier, 1991:71–82.

23. Longaker MT, Whitby DJ, Jennings RW, Duncan BW, Ferguson MW, Harrison MR, Adzick NS. Fetal diaphragmatic wounds heal with scar formation. J Surg Res 1991; 50:375–385.

24. Longaker MT, Moelleken BR, Cheng JC, Jennings RW, Adzick NS, Montorovich J, Levinsohn DG, Gordon L, Harrison MR, Simmons DJ. Fetal fracture healing in a lamb model. Plast Reconstr Surg 1992; 90:161–171; discussion 172–173.

25. Meuli M, Lorenz HP, Hedrick MH, Sullivan KM, Harrison MR, Adzick NS. Scar formation in the fetal alimentary tract. J Pediatr Surg 1995; 30:392–395.

26. Mast BA, Albanese CT, Kapadia S. Tissue repair in the fetal intestinal tract occurs with adhesions, fibrosis, and neovascularization. Ann Plast Surg 1998; 41:140–147.

27. Adzick NS, Lorenz HP. Cells, matrix, growth factors, and the surgeon. The biology of scarless fetal wound repair. Ann Surg 1994; 220:10–18.

28. Thomas BL, Krummel TM, Melany M, Cawthorn JW, Nelson JM, Cohen IK, Diegelman RF. Collagen synthesis and type expression by fetal fibroblasts in vitro. Surg Forum 1998; 39:642–644.

29. Chen WY, Grant ME, Schor AM, Schor SL. Differences between adult and foetal fibroblasts in the regulation hyaluronate synthesis: correlation with migratory activity. J Cell Sci 1989; 94:577.

30. Alaish SM, Yager D, Diegelman RF, Cohen IK. Biology of fetal wound healing: hyaluronate receptor expression in fetal fibroblasts. J Pediatr Surg 1994; 29:1040–1043.

31. Longaker MT, Chiu ES, Harrison MR, Crombleholme TM, Langer JC, Duncan BW, Adzick NS, Verrier ED, Stern R. Studies in fetal wound healing. IV. Hyaluronic acid-stimulating activity distinguishes fetal wound fluid from adult wound fluid. Ann Surg 1989; 210:667–672.

32. Longaker MT, Chiu ES, Adzick NS, Stern M, Harrison MR, Stern R. Studies in fetal wound healing. V. A prolonged presence of hyaluronic acid characterizes fetal wound fluid. Ann Surg 1991; 213:292–296.

33. Estes JM, Vande Berg JS, Adzick NS, MacGillivray TE, Desmouliere A, Gobbiani G. Phenotypic and functional features of myofibroblasts in sheep fetal wounds. Differentiation 1994; 56:173–181.

34. Longaker MT, Burd DA, Gown AM, Yen TS, Jennings RW, Duncan BW, Harrison MR, Adzick NS. Midgestational excisional fetal lamb wounds contract in utero. J Pediatr Surg 1991; 26:942–947; discussion 947–948.

35. Stelnicki EJ, Komuves LG, Kwong AO, Holmes D, Klein P, Rozenfeld S, Lawrence HJ, Adzick NS, Harrison M, Largman C. HOX homeobox genes exhibit spatial and temporal changes in expression during human skin development. J Invest Dermatol 1998; 110:110–115.

36. Weeks PM, Nath RK. Fetal wound repair: a new direction. Plast Reconstr Surg 1993; 91:922–924.

37. Stelnicki EJ, Komuves LG, Holmes D. The human homeobox genes MSX-1, MSX-2, and MOX-1 are differentially expressed in the dermis and epidermis in fetal and adult skin. Differentiation 1997; 62:33–41.

38. Stelnicki EJ, Arbeit J, Cass DL, Saner C, Harrison M, Largman C. Changes in expression of human homeobox genes PRX-2 and HOX B-13 are associated with scarless fetal wound healing. J Invest Dermatol 1998; 111:57–63.

39. Zutter MM, Santoro SA. The human α_2 integrin gene promoter. Identification of positive and negative regulatory elements important for cell type and developmentally restricted gene expression. J Biol Chem 1994; 269:463–469.

40. Goomer RS, Holst BD, Wood IC, Jones FS, Edelman GM. Regulation in vitro of an L-CAM enhancer by homeobox genes HoxD9 and HNF-1. Proc Natl Acad Sci USA 1994; 91:7985–7989.

41. Jones FS, Prediger EA, Bittner DA, De Robertis EM, Edelman GM. Cell adhesion molecules as targets for Hox genes: neural cell adhesion molecule promoter activity is modulated by cotransfection with Hox-2.5 and -2.4. Proc Natl Acad Sci USA 1992; 89:2086–2090.

42. Jones FS, Holst BD, Minowa O, De Robertis EM, Edelman GM. Binding and transcriptional activation of the promoter for the neural cell adhesion molecule by HoxC6 (Hox-3.3). Proc Natl Acad Sci USA 1993; 90:6557–6561.

43. Whitby DJ, Ferguson MW. The extracellular matrix of lip wounds in fetal, neonatal and adult mice. Development 1991; 112:651.

44. Merkel JR, DiPaolo BR, Hallock GG, Rice DC. Type I and type III collagen content of healing wounds in fetal and adult rats. Proc Soc Exp Biol Med 1988; 187:493.

45. Olutoye OO, Cohen IK. Fetal wound healing: an overview. Wound Repair Regen 1996; 4:66.

46. Whitby DJ, Longaker MT, Harrison MR, Adzick NS, Ferguson MW. Rapid epithelialisation of fetal wounds is associated with the early deposition of tenascin. J Cell Sci 1991; 99:583–586.

47. DePalma RL, Krummel TM, Durham LA, Michna BA, Thomas BL, Nelson BL, Diegelman RF. Characterization and quantitation of wound matrix in the fetal rabbit. Matrix 1989; 9(3):224–231.

48. King SR, Hickerson WL, Proctor KG. Beneficial actions of exogenous hyaluronic acid on wound healing. Surgery 1991; 109:76.

49. Shepard S, Becker H, Hartman JX. Using hyaluronic acid to create a fetal-like environment in vitro. Ann Plast Surg 1996; 36:65.

50. Mast BA, Flood LC, Haynes JH, DePalma RL, Cohen IK, Diegelman, RF, Krummel TM. Hyaluronic acid is a major component of the matrix of fetal rabbit skin and wounds: implications for healing by regeneration. Matrix 1991; 11:63–68.

51. Mast BA, Haynes JH, Krummel TM, Diegelman RF, Cohen IK. In vivo degradation of fetal wound hyaluronic acid results in increased fibroplasia, collagen deposition, and neovascularization. Plast Reconstr Surg 1992; 89:503–509.

52. Miller ME. Chemotactic function in the human neonate: humoral and cellular aspects. Pediatr Res 1971; 5:487.

53. Flake AW, Harrison MR, Adzick NS, Zanjani ED. Transplantation of fetal hematopoietic stem cells in utero: the creation of hematopoietic chimeras. Science 1986; 233:776–778.

54. Bracaglia R, Montemari G, Rotoli M, Petrosino R. Variation in acute phlogistic reactions in the skin of rabbit fetuses. Ann Plast Surg 1982; 9:175–179.

55. Schwartz LW, Osburn BI. An ontogenic study of the acute inflammatory reaction in the fetal Rhesus monkey. I. Cellular response to bacterial and nonbacterial irritants. Lab Invest 1974; 31:441–453.

56. Schwartz LW, Osburn BI, Frick OL. An ontogenic study of histamine and mast cells in the fetal Rhesus monkey. J Allergy Clin Immunol 1975; 56:381–386.

57. Schwartz LW, Osburn BI. An ontogenic study of the acute inflammatory response in the fetal Rhesus monkey. II. The mediation of increased vascular permeability by histamine, compound 48/80 and bradykinin. Vet Pathol 1978; 15:358–366.

58. Leibovich SJ, Ross R. The role of the macrophage in wound repair. A study with hydrocortisone and antimacrophage serum. Am J Pathol 1975; 78:71–100.

59. Knighton DR, Fiegel VD. The macrophages: effector cell wound repair. Prog Clin Biol Res 1989; 299:217–226.

60. Diegelman RF, Cohen IK, Kaplan AM. The role of macrophages in wound repair: a review. Plast Reconstr Surg 1981; 68:107.

61. Borchelt BD, Krummel TM, Cawthorn JW, Thomas BL, Diegelman RF, Cohen IK. Transposition of an early adult wound to a fetal rabbit wound site does not result in recruitment of fibroblasts. Surg Forum 1989; 40:555.

62. Simpson DM, Ross R. The neutrophilic leukocyte in wound repair, a study with antineutrophil serum. J Clin Invest 1972; 51:2009.

63. Jennings RW, Adzick NS, Longaker MT, Duncan BW, Scheuenstuhl H, Hunt TK.

Ontogeny of fetal sheep polymorphonuclear leukocyte phagocytosis. J Pediatr Surg 1991; 26:853–855.

64. Whitby DJ, McMullen HF, Sung JJ, Gold LI, Siebert JW, Longaker MT. Localization of TGF-beta isoforms in adult and fetal mouse lip wounds. Surg Forum 1994; 45:651.

65. Delozier J, Nanney LB, Hagan K, Reese RS. Epidermal growth factor enhances fetal epithelization. Surg Forum 1987; 38:623.

66. Haynes JH, Johnson DE, Mast BA, Diegelman RF, Salzberg DA, Cohen IK, Krummel TM. Platelet-derived growth factor induces fetal wound fibrosis. J Pediatr Surg 1994; 29:1405.

67. Shah M, Foreman DM, Ferguson MW. Control of scarring in adult wounds by neutralizing antibody to transforming growth factor beta. Lancet 1992; 339:213.

68. Shah M, Foreman DM, Ferguson MW. Neutralising antibody to TGF-beta 1,2 reduces cutaneous scarring in adult rodents. J Cell Sci 1994; 107:1137–1157.

69. Shah M, Foreman DM, Ferguson MW. Neutralisation of TGF-beta 1 and TGF-beta 2 or exogenous addition of TGF-beta 3 to cutaneous rat wounds reduces scarring. J Cell Sci 1995; 108:985–1002.

70. Border WA, Noble NA. Fibrosis linked to TGF-beta in yet another disease [editorial; comment]. J Clin Invest 1995; 96:655–656.

71. Roberts AB, Anzano MA, Wakefield LM, Roche NS, Stern DF, Sporn MB. Type beta transforming growth factor: a bifunctional regulator of cellular growth. Proc Natl Acad Sci USA 1985; 82:119–123.

72. Krummel TM, Michna BA, Thomas BL, Sporn MB, Nelson JM, Salzberg AM, Cohen IK, Diegelman RF. Transforming growth factor beta (TGF-beta) induces fibrosis in a fetal wound model. J Pediatr Surg 1988; 23:647–652.

73. Lin RY, Sullivan KM, Argenta PA, Meuli M, Lorenz HP, Adzick NS. Exogenous transforming growth factor-beta amplifies its own expression and induces scar formation in a model of human fetal skin repair. Ann Surg 1995; 222:146–154.

74. Lorenz HP, Chang J, Longaker MT, Banda MJ. Transforming growth factors beta-1 and beta-2 synergistically increase gene expression of collagen types I and III in fetal but not adult fibroblasts. Surg Forum 1993; 44:723–725.

75. Chang J, Longaker MT, Lorenz HP, Anita RB, Harrison MR, Adzick S, Banda MJ. Fetal and adult sheep fibroblast TGF-beta 1 gene expression in vitro: effects of hypoxia and gestational age. Surg Forum 1995; 46:720–722.

76. Whitby DJ, Ferguson MW. Immunohistochemical localization of growth factors in fetal wound healing. Dev Biol 1991; 147:207–215.

77. Sullivan KM, Lorenz HP, Meuli M, Lin RY, Adzick NS. A model of scarless human fetal wound repair is deficient in transforming growth factor beta. J Pediatr Surg 1995; 30:198–202; discussion 202–203.

78. Longaker MT, Bouhana KS, Harrison MR. Wound healing in the fetus. Possible role for macrophages and transforming growth factor-beta isoforms. Wound Repair Reg 1994; 2:104–112.

79. Stelnicki EJ, Longaker MT, Holmes D, Vanderwall K, Harrison MR, Largman C, Hoffman WY. Bone morphogenetic protein-2 induces scar formation and skin maturation in the second trimester fetus. Plast Reconstr Surg 1998; 101:12–19.

80. Dietsheim JA, Delozier JB, Rees RS. Fetal Excisional Wounds Can Respond to

Intrauterine Injury. Annual Meeting of the American Society of Plastic and Reconstructive Surgeons. San Francisco, CA: Oct 29–Nov 3, 1989.

81. Antoniades HN. PDGF: a multifunctional growth factor. Baillieres Clin Endocrinol Metab 1991; 5:595–613.

82. Bennett NT, Schultz GS. Growth factors and wound healing: biochemical properties of growth factors and their receptors. Am J Surg 1993; 165:728–737.

83. Moulin V. Growth factors in skin wound healing. Eur J Cell Biol 1995; 68:1–7.

84. Steenfos HH. Growth factors and wound healing. Scand J Plast Reconstr Surg Hand Surg 1994; 28:95–105.

85. Cass DL, Bullard KM, Sylvester KG, Yang EY, Longaker MT, Adzick NS. Wound size and gestational age modulate scar formation in fetal wound repair. J Pediatr Surg 1997; 32:411.

13
Facts and Models of Induced Organ Regeneration: Skin and Peripheral Nerves

Ioannis V. Yannas

Massachusetts Institute of Technology, Cambridge, Massachusetts

I. INTRODUCTION

Although there is considerable evidence of spontaneous organ regeneration in fetal models, there is no evidence that the adult mammal can regenerate any of its organs spontaneously to any significant extent. There appear to be almost no exceptions. In spite of a widespread belief to the contrary, the liver does not regenerate spontaneously. An excised lobe does not regenerate by in situ restoration of the lost mass; instead, the entire organ undergoes compensatory hypertrophy, with a resulting restoration of organ function but not with restoration of the excised lobe (1,2). Even bone does not live up to its reputation for extensive spontaneous regeneration. Under controlled experimental conditions, a defect as small as 0.5 mm has healed by formation of lamellar bone; however, the new bone tissue that has formed has been deposited perpendicularly to the long axis of the bone and has originated from marrow and periosteal cells (gap healing) (3). Larger bone defects are known to heal by formation of nonmineralized connective tissue (soft callus); this tissue later becomes mineralized, forming hard callus (union) (4,5). In contrast, epithelial and endothelial cell layers, which have been removed from the surfaces of various organs, with care taken not to injure underlying mesenchymal tissues, are restored spontaneously.

There is an increasing number of reports with documentation that organ regeneration in the adult mammal can be induced by use of appropriate agents. In a volume devoted to the topic of scarless healing, the significance of these reports lies in the stark contrast between wound healing that leads to repair with scar formation, and healing that leads to regeneration without scar.

In this chapter, the facts of induced organ regeneration are presented first and are followed by hypotheses that outline the pathways through which an injured organ can be induced to restore its physiological structure and function. The emphasis is on induced regeneration of skin and peripheral nerves, the two organs about which the evidence has been by far the most extensively recorded.

II. FACTUAL BASIS OF INDUCED ORGAN REGENERATION IN THE ADULT MAMMAL

One of the stark realities faced by health workers in burn units or in the plastic surgery units of hospitals is that the adult mammalian dermis does not regenerate spontaneously (1,6–15). Studies initiated in the early 1970s have eventually shown, however, that a porous graft copolymer of type I collagen and chondroitin 6-sulfate (collagen–GAG copolymer) induces regeneration of the dermis in large areas of full-thickness skin loss in the guinea pig (16–20) and in the porcine model (21,22). This finding has been extended to humans (23–26). Induced regeneration of the dermis was demonstrated on the basis of conventional histological and ultrastructural studies (19,20,27,28), the use of small-angle laser light scattering studies from histological tissue (29), as well as on the basis of functional studies (19). The new integument was structurally and functionally competent but was totally lacking in hair follicles and other skin appendages (19,20).

Early studies with this analog of the extracellular matrix (ECM analog) emphasized keratinocyte seeding of the highly porous analog prior to grafting in order to achieve simultaneous regeneration of an epidermis as well as a dermis. It has since been recognized that, although seeding of the ECM analog with a minimal density of autologous, uncultured keratinocytes speeds up epidermal regeneration, cell seeding is not required for regeneration of the dermis (21,22). The combined evidence has served to identify a cell-free macromolecular network with highly specific structure, the dermis regeneration template (DRT), which has unprecedented morphogenetic activity (20).

Only one of several collagen–GAG matrices studied as described above was capable of preventing scar tissue formation and promoting dermal regeneration. The active ECM analog was characterized by a collagen/GAG ratio of 98/2 w/w, average pore diameter between 20 and 120 μm, and sufficiently high cross-link density to resist degradation by collagenases over about 10 days following grafting (average molecular weight between cross-links in the template, 12 kDa). Several other very closely related ECM analogs showed either significantly reduced activity or no activity at all (20). The ECM analogs that showed high activity in promoting dermal regeneration also delayed significantly the onset of wound contraction (20). The available evidence compels the conclusion that the activity of this insoluble network inside the wound bed depends critically on maintenance of a highly specific three-dimensional structure over a period of time between about 5 and 15 days. The active network has been referred to as skin or dermis regeneration template. The observed activity of DRT, consisting of drastic modification of the outcome of the skin wound healing process, has not been duplicated by application on the wound bed of solutions of one or more growth factors or by application of suspensions of keratinocytes or fibroblasts.

A different ECM analog, also possessing a highly specific network structure, has induced regeneration of a partially functional sciatic nerve across a transected gap of 15 mm in the rat sciatic nerve (30–32). In this animal model, the nerve stumps at either side of the gap are inserted in a silicone tube or, more recently, in a collagen tube (tubulation) (33); in the absence of a tube, regeneration is decidedly absent and neuroma formation is invariably reported. The silicone tube does not support regeneration as well as the collagen tube, and is therefore useful as a negative tubulation control (33).

It is well known that spontaneous regeneration through the unfilled silicone tube occurs reproducibly at a gap length of 5 mm, whereas regeneration across a 15-mm gap is not observed (30,34–36). The ECM analog that has been shown to possess the greatest activity so far, inducing regeneration across a 15-mm gap that was bridged by a tube that contained the ECM analog, is referred to as nerve regeneration template (NRT). It has an average pore diameter of 5 μm, an average molecular weight between cross-links of 30 to 40 kDa, a preferred orientation of pore channel axes in the direction of the nerve axis, and a 98/2 w/w ratio of type I collagen to GAG (31,32). The significant differences between the macromolecular network structure and pore structure of DRT and NRT are presented in Table 1.

Table 1 Structural Properties of Two Regeneration Templates

Structural characteristic of ECM analog	Dermis regeneration template	Nerve regeneration template
Collagen/GAG, w/w	98/2	98/2
Degradation half-life in vivo (wk)	1.5	6–8
Average pore diameter (μm)	20–120	5
Pore channel orientation	Random	Axial

A third ECM analog has been reported capable of inducing regeneration of the canine meniscus following 80% transection (37–39). The ECM analog used in these studies has been stated by the investigators (37,38) to be similar to one described earlier (18). However, its detailed structure was not reported.

In summary, evidence is accumulating that, under appropriate conditions, the adult mammal can be induced to regenerate, at least partially, certain organs, namely skin, peripheral nerves, and the knee meniscus, that are not regenerated spontaneously. However, many basic unanswered questions remain. Most pressing are questions on the detailed cell-biological mechanism by which active ECM analogs modify so spectacularly one or more of the processes of spontaneous wound healing.

III. CERTAIN CRITICAL EXPERIMENTAL PARAMETERS IN THE IDENTIFICATION OF A REGENERATION TEMPLATE

A. Anatomically Well-Defined Experimental Volume (40,41)

The study of organ synthesis in vivo is potentially beset by lack of reproducibility in conditions from one wound to another in the same animal or from a wound in one animal to that in another. The problem of wound-to-wound variability was dramatically minimized, even eliminated for many practical purposes, in the early experiments of Billingham and Medawar (6,7), who pioneered the concept of the anatomically constant wound. In their rodent models, skin was routinely excised down to the panniculus carnosus, a layer of muscle that lies under the dermis. Such a wound, including the exudate that flows into it, consists of a planar tissue substrate that is nearly identical over the plane.

The precise choice of dimensions of an anatomically constant wound varies with the goal of the investigator. In experiments in which the synthesis of peripheral nerve in rats has been studied, an anatomically constant wound has consisted of a gap, between 5 and 15 mm long, along the axis of the nerve fiber. This experimental configuration has been established following the ground-breaking studies of Lundborg et al. (34,42–47). The experimental ECM analog, in the form of a highly porous, rodlike matrix, has been placed inside a tube and the entire device has been grafted as a bridge for the experimental gap. The nerve stumps are placed inside the tube and are in full contact with the ECM analog (30–33).

Isolation of the experimental volume can be effected by bounding it with anatomically distinct tissues that belong to a neighboring organ, by an implanted device, or by the atmosphere. Examples are a gap in articular cartilage that is bounded by the bony end plate on one side and by synovial fluid on the other as a clinical model of a joint that has been compromised by osteoarthritis; a full-thickness skin lesion, bounded by muscle on the proximal side and by the atmosphere on the distal side, representing the massively burned patient; a gap in a peripheral nerve that is bounded tangentially by a silicone tube (tubulation) as a model of extensive trauma that typically leads to paralysis; a tubulated gap in Achilles tendon. Boundaries that are anatomically distinct from the organ under study provide a morphological and functional basis for separation of the synthetic events occurring inside the experimental volume from any acute or chronic events that may occur outside it.

An approach to the problem of isolating the experimental volume from the residual organ was approached in a study of skin regeneration induced by DRT by using the template in the form of an "island" graft. The island was located in the center of the full-thickness wound, sufficiently distant from the edges of the wound to eliminate the possibility of cell migration from tissues at the wound edges to the graft in the center of the wound (48). Island grafts were introduced by early investigators of skin wound healing (6,7).

B. Quantitative Analysis of Tissue Products (Scar and Neuroma)

Since the experimental volume is typically continuous with the residual organ, the question arises regarding the possibility of distinguishing newly synthesized tissue from mature tissue. A solution to this problem can, in principle, be based on the use of morphological techniques of sufficiently high resolution to distinguish between new and mature tissues of the same organ. The resolution requirements are obviously maximized, and the desired distinction becomes correspondingly more difficult, when the regenerate is mature and when it closely replicates physiological tissues adjacent to it. For example, although conventional histological methods have been used to distinguish dermis from scar, there is an acute need for new methodology that can be used to identify states that are intermediate between the extremes of physiological skin and scar. Without the benefit of new quantitative assays, it will not be possible to plan an experimental series that can lead the investigator efficiently away from scar and in the direction of the physiological organ. Precisely because tissues are normally such complicated states of matter, a very wide range of analytical principles can, in principle, be used to advantage as a basis for an assay.

A biochemical principle and a physical principle are among the several that can be used to distinguish quantitatively between dermis and scar. A potential biochemical method is based on the observation that the proteoglycan content in scar differs from that in the dermis, amounting, in essence, to a 16% higher content of dermatan sulfate and a 35% lower content of hyaluronic acid in scar (49,50). Making use of conventional histological sections, the physical method has been based on the realization that laser light scattering, previously employed in polymer physics to study macromolecular orientation, can be used to provide a quantitative measure of the degree of orientation of collagen fibers in scar relative to that in dermis (29).

Neuroma is formed when a peripheral nerve has been transected and no tubulation has been provided to ensheathe the resulting gap. Although the proximal and distal stumps heal in significantly different ways, both become capped with a tissue mass that comprises primarily connective tissue, blood vessels, Schwann cells, and several tangled axons, mostly unmyelinated and ending blindly (51–55). Electrophysiological study has established that the fine fibers are electrically excitable; however, the conduction velocity is very low, approximately 10% of normal (56). In principle, herefore, a quantitative analytical protocol for neuroma could be based either on a morphometric assay or on an electrophysiological study.

C. Template Identification

In the experimental model discussed here, the long-term experimental goal briefly consists in identifying a highly specific ECM analog that, when brought in contact with the exudate inside the experimental volume, blocks synthesis of scar and induces instead synthesis of a volume of physiological organ approximately equal to the experimental volume.

IV. MODELS OF THE MECHANISM OF REGENERATION (57)

A. Overview of Models That Constitute the Process of Regeneration

The evidence for regeneration described above requires the regeneration template to interact with components of the exudate (cells and cytokines) inside the experimental volume in such a way as to modify drastically the kinetics and mechanism of the spontaneous healing process that normally converts exudate to scar tissue. The processes by which such modification takes place are described below as a sequence of model steps that constitute a hypothetical mechanism for the observed regeneration. Each of these models is supported by one or more sets of data that are briefly mentioned. In summary, the desired mechanism requires the template surface to be adequately close and accessible to cells migrating from the exudate; migrating cells that have approached close enough require the template surface to be populated with the appropriate type and density of binding sites for certain cells and cytokines; such interaction must be allowed to proceed over the necessary time period; and finally, when the interaction has successfully modified the kinetics and mechanism of wound healing away from repair, it is required that the template remove itself even as new tissue is being synthesized adjacent to the surface of the template.

B. Proximity of Cells and Cytokines to Template Surface

Following implantation of the porous template into the wound bed, there is need for transfer of cells and cytokines present in the exudate to the surface of the template. The exudate is pulled inside the capillaries (pore channels) of the template by surface tension, as described by:

$$P = 2\gamma/r \tag{1}$$

where r is the radius of the pore channel in a template undergoing wetting by exudate with an air–liquid surface tension of γ in dynes/cm. According to Eq. (1), the suction pressure P increases, and wetting is promoted, as the pore radius decreases. For example, water with an air–liquid surface tension of $\gamma = 72$ dyn/cm is pulled inside a pore radius of 100 μm with a suction pressure of almost one-hundredth of one atmosphere; the pressure increases almost to one full atmosphere when the pore radius decreases to 1 μm. Following flow of exudate inside the pore channels of a template with average pore diameter of 100 μm, cells and cytokines are within a distance of less than 50 μm from the template surface, a distance that can be covered within no more than a few minutes by these components of the exudate.

C. Critical Cell Path Length, Maximum Dimension of Template

Cells from the solid-like tissue surrounding the experimental volume into the template require adequate nutrition during the entire time of residence in it. The complexity of nutritional requirements of the cell is simplified by defining a critical nutrient that is required for normal cell function; such a nutrient is assumed to be metabolized by the cell at a rate R mole/cm^3/sec. The nutrient is pictured being transported from the solid-like tissue, where the concentration of nutrient is assumed to be a constant C_0 due to the presence of vascular supply, over a distance L through the exudate until it reaches the cell. In the early days following implantation of the template there is as yet no angiogenesis and the nutrient is, therefore, transported exclusively by diffusion which is characterized by a diffusivity D cm^2/sec. Dimensional analysis readily yields the cell lifeline number:

$$S = RL^2/DC_0 \tag{2}$$

which can be used to compare the relative magnitude of the rate of nutrient consumption by the cell nutrient (numerator) and the rate of supply of nutrient to the cell by diffusion (denominator). If the rate of consumption of the critical nutrient exceeds greatly the rate of supply, $S \gg 1$; the cell must soon die. At steady state, the rate of consumption of nutrient by the cell just equals the rate of transport by diffusion over the distance L. Under conditions of steady state $S = O(1)$; at that point, the value of L becomes the critical cell path length, L_c the longest distance away from the wound bed boundary along which the cell can migrate without requiring nutrient in excess of that supplied by diffusion. Alternatively, L_c is defined as the distance of migration beyond which cells require the presence of a vascular supply. For many cell nutrients of low molecular weight, L_c is of order 100 μm. Use of S provides, therefore, an estimate of the maximum template dimension that can support cells (58).

D. Upper and Lower Bounds of Template Pore Diameter

Having successfully migrated onto the template surface, a host cell is visualized interacting with binding sites on the surface. The surface density of binding sites can be expressed as Φ_b, equal by definition to the number of sites N_b per unit surface of template. Another way of expressing Φ_b (more usefully expressed in terms of quantities measurable by optical microscopy) is in terms of the volume density of binding sites ρ_b (number of sites per unit volume porous template) and the specific surface of the template expressed in units of mm^2/cm^3:

$$\Phi_b = N_b/A = \rho_b/\sigma \tag{3a}$$

Assuming that each cell is bound to (an a priori unknown number of) χ binding sites, there will be N_b/χ bound cells per unit surface; the volume density of cells will be $\rho_c = \rho_b/\chi$ and the surface density σ of cells will be:

$$\Phi_c = \Phi_b/\chi = N_b/\chi A = \rho_b/\chi\sigma = \rho_c/\sigma \tag{3b}$$

Observations of myofibroblast density inside templates with pore diameters of about 10 μm have yielded typical values of the volume density, ρ_c, approximately 10^7 myofibroblasts per cm^3 porous template. For a template of average pore diameter 10 μm, the specific surface σ is calculated to be approximately $8 \times 10^4 \, mm^2/cm^3$ template; therefore, 1 cm^3 porous template is characterized by a cell surface density of $\Phi_c = \rho_c/\sigma = 10^7/8 \times 10^4 = 125$ cells/mm^2. For a template of identical composition but average pore diameter as large as 300 μm, Φ_c is the same as above; however, the specific surface is calculated to be only about $3 \times 10^3 \, mm^2/cm^3$ template. In this case, the volume density of cells is, accordingly, only $\rho_c = \Phi_c \cdot \sigma = 125 \times 3 \times 10^3 = 3.75 \times 10^5$ per cm^3 porous template. We conclude that the template that has the smaller average pore diameter (10 μm) accommodates a volume density of myofibroblasts that is about 27 times higher than with the template that has the larger pore diameter (300 μm). These considerations suggest a maximum pore diameter requirement for the template, simply to ensure a specific surface that is large enough to bind an appropriately large number of cells.

Additional reflection makes it obvious that cells originating in the wound bed cannot migrate inside the template and eventually reach binding sites on its surface unless the template has an average pore diameter large enough to allow this. There is, therefore, a requirement for a minimum pore diameter for the template, about equal to the characteristic diameter of the cells (approximately 5 μm). Thus, the pore diameter of the regeneration template is limited both by an upper bound and a lower bound. This conclusion is in agreement with the experimental evidence that shows that ECM analogs, identical in chemical composition but differing only in average pore diameter, show maximum activity (inhibition of onset of wound contraction, consistent with regeneration rather than scar formation) when the average pore diameter lies between 20 and 120 μm (20). Further evidence has shown that, when other structural parameters of the template remain constant, loss of the 20- to 120-μm porous structure of the template by simple evaporation at room temperature (a process that yields an ECM analog with average pore diameter of less than 1 μm) leads to synthesis of a scar capsule at the surface of the grafted analog, evidence of a barrier to cell migration inside an implant (58,59).

E. Template Residence Time

A template must be in place long enough to induce the appropriate synthetic processes to take place, but it must disappear in timely fashion so as not to interfere with these same processes that it induces. The time period necessary to induce synthesis will be taken to be of the same order as that required to complete the wound healing process at that anatomical site. In general, the rate of wound healing is quite different in tissues such as, for example, the dermis and the sciatic nerve. Since the template is an insoluble (and, therefore, nondiffusible) three-dimensional network, it follows that cells that are bound on it become immobilized and their migration is, accordingly, arrested. Not only cells are prevented from migration to locations that are appropriate for synthesis of a new organ but, in addition, the laying down of newly synthesized ECM by the cells in the space of the wound bed is probably blocked physically by the presence of the template. These considerations suggest strongly that the persisting insolubility of the template will increasingly interfere with the synthesis of the new organ at that site. The template is, accordingly, required to become diffusible (by degradation to small molecular fragments) and thereby remove itself from the wound bed in order not to interfere with cellular processes that lead to the emerging organ.

The simplest model that can accommodate these two requirements is one that requires synchronization of the two processes: organ synthesis and template degradation (58,59). This model leads directly to the hypothesis of *isomorphous tissue replacement*:

$$t_d/t_s = O(1) \tag{4}$$

In Eq. (4), t_d denotes a characteristic time constant for degradation of the template at the tissue site where a new organ is synthesized with a time constant of t_s. The degradation rate can be estimated by histological observation of the decrease in mass of template fragments at various times (21,27,60). A closer estimate of t_d has been obtained by measuring the kinetics of disintegration of the macromolecular network using rubber elasticity theory (16). An alternate procedure consists of monitoring the kinetics of mass disappearance of a radioactively labeled template. A rough estimate of t_s can be obtained by observing t_h, the timescale of synthesis of new tissue during healing (in the absence of a template) at the anatomical site (59). Using the latter approach, it has been estimated that t_s for the regenerating dermis is approximately 3 weeks (59) and approximately 6 weeks for the regenerating peripheral nerve (31). These estimates allow adjustment of t_d for the template, by adjustment of the cross-link density and GAG content, to levels that are approximately equal to the value of t_s, as the latter is dictated by the nature of the anatomical site.

The isomorphous tissue replacement hypothesis has received some experimental support from observations that when the ratio in Eq. (4) was adjusted to values much smaller than 1 (by implanting a rapidly degrading ECM analog, for which $t_d \ll t_s$), the wound healing process resulted in contraction and synthesis of scar, as would have been the case if the template was missing. It was also observed that when the ratio in Eq. (4) was much larger than 1 (by implanting an ECM analog that degraded very slowly, so that $t_d \ll t_s$), the ECM analog was surrounded by a capsule of scar tissue (58,59). Even though this limited evidence cannot be used to test the hypothesis of Eq. (4) conclusively, it is, at the least, compatible with a template half-life that has both lower and upper bounds. Direct experimental support for this conclusion is afforded by experimental evidence based on studies of inhibition of wound contraction by several ECM analogs with defined structure. These studies have shown that, of several ECM analogs studied, the dermal regeneration template was the analog that degraded at a rate corresponding to a half-life of about 1.5 to 2 weeks; ECM analogs that degraded at much slower or much faster rates were not active (20).

The simplest template structure that can participate in this disappearing act with minimum harm to the host is one in which the template undergoes degradation by enzymes of the wound bed to nontoxic low-molecular-weight fragments that diffuse rapidly away from the site of organ synthesis (58,59).

F. Chemical Composition of Template

Interactions that are developmentally significant are known to involve cells, growth factors, and ECM components. The last include the collagens, elastin, several proteoglycans, as well as cell adhesion molecules, such as fibronectin and laminin. Studies of organ development have established beyond doubt that specific ECM components are required during the process (61,62). Since development and induced regeneration have a common end point, we will assume that the required cell–matrix binding events in each case are similar; if so, the identity of matrix components in each case must also be similar. This presumptive similarity between developmental and regenerative mechanisms has been previously referred to briefly in terms of the hypothetical rule: regeneration recapitulates ontogeny (19); however, we emphasize the lack of detailed evidence for such an identity. In the dermis, as well as in the connective tissue of peripheral nerves, type I collagen is present in greatest abundance, whereas the most prominent glycosaminoglycans in the dermis are dermatan sulfate and chondroitin 6-sulfate; in peripheral nerves, type I collagen and sulfated proteoglycans have also been prominently observed (63).

Although quite richly endowed with undifferentiated cells and growth factors, the early exudate of a spontaneously healing skin wound or a peripheral nerve wound is free of ECM components and is, therefore, lacking in components that are known to be required for development. As pointed out above, this lack of ECM components is hypothetically associated with the absence of synthetic processes that lead to a physiological organ.

These hypothetical considerations are consistent with the choice of type I collagen and at least one of the proteoglycans or glycosaminoglycans as basic structural components of regeneration templates. Although several efforts have been made to replace the use of ECM analogs in templates with synthetic polymers, there is, at this time, no firm evidence that synthetic polymers can induce regeneration of the dermis or of a peripheral nerve in lesions in which the physiological structures are not regenerated spontaneously.

There is considerable experimental evidence linking the biological activity of the dermal regeneration template to the detailed features of its network structure features (see Table 1). Two ECM analogs, one of which was prepared with a GAG while the other was prepared with the corresponding proteoglycan, showed the same activity in an in vivo assay (inhibition of onset of wound contraction) that appears to predict dermal regeneration (64). This result suggested that the dermal regeneration template can be constructed using a GAG, rather than the corresponding proteoglycan, without loss of activity. The necessity for a covalently cross-linked network of collagen and the sulfated GAG derived from the observation that these two macromolecules form an ionic complex spontaneously at acidic pH; however, the complex is dissociated at neutral pH, i.e., under conditions that prevail following implantation (65). To preserve the chemical composition of the ECM analog in vivo over the period suggested by the residence time considerations discussed above, it was therefore necessary to introduce a certain density of covalent bonds between collagen chains and GAG molecules, i.e., to form a collagen–GAG graft copolymer (65). There is evidence that an increase in the fraction of GAG in the copolymer increases the resistance of the macromolecular network to degradation by mammalian collagenases (16). Such resistance also increases with the density of collagen–collagen cross-links and collagen–GAG cross-links (59,66).

A review of the effect of each of these structural features of the dermal regeneration template on its activity, especially in the inhibition of the onset of wound contraction, can be made based on the published evidence (20,64). Such a review suggests that the chemical composition of the macromolecular network and the detailed pore structure of the DRT contribute about equally to its activity. A similar study of the relation between structure and activity for the nerve regeneration template has not been made.

In spite of progress in understanding the biological significance of many of the structural features of DRT, there is still some uncertainty regarding the detailed molecular and cell biological mechanisms by which DRT or NRT induces regeneration, even partial, of the respective organs.

A modified version of the material in this chapter has appeared recently (57).

ACKNOWLEDGMENT

The author acknowledges support by National Institutes of Health Grant 61977, National Science Foundation Grant 61549, and Veterans' Administration Grant 60185.

REFERENCES

1. Goss RJ. Regeneration versus repair. In: Cohen IK, Diegelmann RF, Lindblad WJ, eds. Wound Healing. Philadelphia: Saunders, 1992:20–29.
2. Michalopoulos GK, DeFrances M. Liver regeneration. Science 1997; 276:60–66.
3. Shapiro F. Cortical bone repair. J Bone Joint Surg 1988; 70-A:1067–1081.
4. Ham AW. Histology. Philadelphia: Lippincott, 1965.
5. Hay ED. Regeneration. New York: Holt, Rinehart & Winston, 1966.
6. Billingham RE, Medawar PB. The technique of free skin grafting in mammals, J Exp Biol 1951; 28:385–402.
7. Billingham RE, Medawar PB. Contracture and intussusceptive growth in the healing of extensive wounds in mammalian skin. J Anat 1955; 89:114–123.
8. Ross R, Benditt EP. Wound healing and collagen formation. I. Sequential changes in components of guinea pig skin wounds observed in the electron microscope. J Biophys Biochem Cytol 1961; 11:677–700.
9. Ross R, Odland G. Human wound repair. II. Inflammatory cells, epithelial-mesenchymal interrelations, and fibrogenesis. J Cell Biol 1968; 39:152–168.
10. Dunphy JE, Van Winkle W. Repair and regeneration: The Scientific Basis for Surgical Practice. New York: McGraw-Hill, 1968.

11. Peacock EE Jr. Control of wound healing and scar formation in surgical patients. Arch Surg 1981; 116:1325–1329.

12. Peacock EE Jr. Wound healing and wound care. In: Schwartz SI, Shires GT, Spencer FC, Storer EH, eds. Principles of Surgery. 4th ed. New York: McGraw-Hill, 1984.

13. Peacock EE Jr, Van Winkle W Jr. Wound Repair. 2nd ed. Philadelphia: Saunders, 1976.

14. Madden JW. Wound healing: biologic and clinical features. In: Sabison D, ed. Textbook of Surgery. 10th ed. Philadelphia: Saunders, 1972.

15. Boykin JV, Molnar JA. Burn scar and skin equivalents. In: Cohen IK, Diegelmann RF, Lindblad WJ, eds. Wound Healing. Philadelphia: Saunders, 1992.

16. Yannas IV, Burke JF, Huang C, Gordon PL. Suppression of in vivo degradability and of immunogenicity by reaction with glycoaminoglycans. Polymer Rep Am Chem Soc 1975; 16:209–214.

17. Yannas IV, Burke JF, Warpehoski M, Stasikelis P, Skrabut EM, Orgill D., Giard DJ. Prompt, long-term functional replacement of skin. Trans Am Soc Artif Intern Organs 1981; 27:19–22.

18. Yannas IV, Burke JF, Orgill DP, Skrabut EM. Wound tissue can utilize a polymeric template to synthesize a functional extension of skin. Science 1982; 215:174–176.

19. Yannas IV, Orgill DP, Skrabut EM, Burke JF. Skin regeneration with a bioreplaceable polymeric template. In: C. G. Gebelein, ed. Polymeric Materials and Artificial Organs. American Chemical Society Symposium Series, No. 256, 1984:191–197.

20. Yannas IV, Lee E, Orgill DP, Skrabut EM, Murphy GF. Synthesis and characterization of a model extracellular matrix that induces partial regeneration of adult mammalian skin. Proc Natl Acad Sci USA 1989; 86:933–937.

21. Orgill DP, Butler CE, Regan JF. Behavior of collagen-GAG matrices as dermal replacement in rodent and porcine models. Wounds 1996; 8:151–157.

22. Butler CE, Orgill DP, Yannas IV, Compton CC. Effect of keratinocyte seeding of collagen-glycosaminoglycan membranes on the regeneration of skin in a porcine model. Plast Reconstr Surg 1998; 101:1572–1579.

23. Burke JF, Yannas IV, Quimby WC, Jr., Bondoc CC, Jung WK. Successful use of a physiologically acceptable artificial skin in the treatment of extensive burn injury, Ann Surg 1981; 194:413–428.

24. Heimbach D, Luterman A, Burke J, Cram A, Herndon D, Hunt J, Jordan M, McManus W, Solem L, Warden G, Zawacki B. Artificial dermis for major burns, Ann Surg 1988; 208:313–320.

25. Jaksic T, Burke JF. The use of "artificial skin" for burns. Annu Rev Med 1987; 38:107–117.

26. Tompkins RG, Hilton JF, Burke JF, Scoenfeld DA, Hegarty MT, Bondoc CC, Quinby WC, Jr, Behringer GE, Ackroyd FW. Increased survival after massive thermal injuries in adults: preliminary report using artificial skin. Child Care Med 1989; 17:734–740.

27. Murphy GF, Orgill DP, Yannas IV. Partial dermal regeneration is induced by biodegradable collagen-glycosaminoglycan grafts. Lab Invest 1990; 62:305–313.

28. Stern R, McPherson M, Longaker MT. Histologic study of artificial skin used in the treatment of full-thickness thermal injury. J Burn Care Rehabil 1990; 11:7–13.

29. Ferdman AG, Yannas IV. Scattering of light from histologic sections: a new method for the analysis of connective tissue. J Invest Dermatol 1993; 100:710–716.

30. Yannas IV, Orgill DP, Silver J, Norregaard TV, Zervas NT, Schoene WC. Regeneration of sciatic nerve across 15-mm gap by use of a polymeric template. In: Gebelein CG, ed. Advances in Biomedical Polymers. New York: Plenum, 1987:1–9.

31. Chang AS, Yannas IV, Perutz S, Loree H, Sethi RR, Krarup C, Norregaard TV, Zervas NT, Silver J. Electrophysiological study of recovery of peripheral nerves regenerated by a collagen-glycosaminoglycan copolymer matrix. In: Gebelein CG, ed. Progress in Biomedical Polymers. New York: Plenum, 1990:107–120.

32. Chang AS, Yannas IV. Peripheral nerve regeneration. In: Smith B, Adelman G, eds. Neuroscience Year (Supplement 2 to the Encyclopedia of Neuroscience). Boston: Birkhauser, 1992:125–126.

33. Chamberlain LJ, Yannas IV, Hsu HP, Spector M. Histological response to a fully degradable collagen device implanted in a gap in the rat sciatic nerve. Tissue Eng 1997; 3:353–362.

34. Lundborg G, Fahlin LB, Danielsen N, Gelberman RH, Longo FM, Powell HC, Varon S. Nerve regeneration in silicone model chambers: influence of gap length and of distal stump components. Exp Neurol 1982; 76:361–375.

35. Madison RD, Da Silva CF, Dikkes P. Entubulation repair with protein additives increases the maximum nerve gap distance successfully bridged with tubular prostheses. Brain Res 1988; 447:325–334.

36. Williams LR, Danielsen N, Muller H, Varon S. Exogenous matrix precursors promote functional nerve regeneration across a 15-mm gap within a silicone chamber in the rat. J Comp Neurol 1987; 264:284–290.

37. Stone KR, Rodkey WG, Webber RJ, McKineey L, Steadman JR. Collagen-based prostheses for meniscal regeneration. Clin Orthop 1990; 252:129–135.

38. Stone KR, Webber RJ, Rodkey WG, Steadman JR. Prosthetic meniscal replacement: In vitro studies of meniscal regeneration using copolymeric collagen prostheses. Arthroscopy 1989:5:152.

39. Stone KR, Steadman R, Rodkey WG, Li ST. Regeneration of meniscal cartilage with use of a collagen scaffold. J Bone Joint Surg 1997; 79-A:1770–1777.

40. Yannas IV. Regeneration templates. In: Bronzino JD, ed. The Biomedical Engineering Handbook. Boca Raton: CRC, 1995:1619–1635.

41. Yannas IV. In vivo synthesis of tissues and organs. In: Lanza RP, Langer RS, Chick WL. eds. Textbook of Tissue Engineering. New York: Landes/Academic Press, 1996.

42. Lundborg G, Dahlin LB, Danielsen N, Johannesson A, Hansson HA, Longo F, Varon S. Nerve regeneration across an extended gap: a neuronobiological view of nerve repair and the possible involvement of neuronotrophic factors. J Hand Surg 1982; 7:580–587.

43. Lundborg GR, Gelberman H, Longo FM, Powell HC, Varon S. In vivo regeneration of cut nerves encased in silicone tubes: growth across a six-millimeter gap. J Neuropathol Exp Neurol 1982; 41:412–422.

44. Williams LR, Longo FM, Powell HC, Lundborg G, Varon S. Spatial-temporal progress of peripheral nerve regeneration within a silicone chamber: parameters for a bioassay, J Comp Neurol 1983; 218:460–470.

45. Williams LR, Powell HC, Lundborg G, Varon S. Competence of nerve tissue as distal insert promoting nerve regeneration in a silicone chamber. Brain Res 1984; 293:201–211.

46. Williams LR, Varon S. Modification of fibrin matrix formation in situ enhances nerve regeneration in silicone chambers. J Comp Neurol 1985; 231:209–220.

47. Lundborg G. Nerve regeneration and repair: A review. Acta Orthop Scand 1987; 58:145–169.

48. Orgill DP, Yannas IV. Design of an artificial skin. IV. Use of island graft to isolate organ regeneration from scar synthesis and other processes leading to skin wound closure. J Biomed Mater Res 1997; 36:531–535.

49. Garg HG, Burd DAR, Swann DA. Small dermatan sulfate proteoglycans in human epidermis and dermis. Biomed Res 1989; 10:197–207.

50. Garg HG, Lippay EW, Burd DAR. Purification and characterization of iduronic acid-rich and glucuronic acid-rich proteoglycans implicated in human post-burn keloid scar. Carbohydr Res 1990; 207:295–305.

51. Cajal RY. Degeneration and regeneration of the nervous system. London: Oxford University Press, 1928; also, New York: Hafner press, 1981.

52. Weiss P. The technology of nerve regeneration: A review. Sutureless tubulation and related methods of nerve repair. J Neurosurg 1944; 1:400–450.

53. Young JZ. Growth and differentiation of nerve fibers. Symp Soc Exp Biol Growth 1948; 2:57–74.

54. Jenq CB, Coggeshall RE. Long-term patterns of axon regeneration in the sciatic nerve and its tributaries. Brain Res 1985; 345:34–44.

55. Chamberlain LJ, Yannas IV, Hsu HP, Strichartz G, Spector M. Collagen–GAG substrate enhances the quality of nerve regeneration through collagen tubes up to level of autograft. Exp Neurol 1998; 154:315–329.

56. Wall PD, Gutnick M. Ongoing activity in peripheral nerves: the physiology and pharmacology of impulses originating from a neuroma. Exp Neurol 1974; 43:580–593.

57. Yannas IV. Models of organ regeneration processes induced by templates. Ann NY Acad Sci 1997; 831:280–293.

58. Yannas IV, Burke JF. Design of an artificial skin. I. Basic design principles. J Biomed Mater Res 1980; 14:65–81.

59. Yannas IV. Use of artificial skin in wound management. In: Dineen P, ed. The Surgical Wound. Philadelphia: Lea & Febiger, 1981:171–190.

60. Yannas IV, Burke JF, Huang C, Gordon PL. Correlation of in vivo collagen degradation rate with in vitro measurements. J Biomed Mater Res 1975; 9:623–628.

61. Hay ED. Cell Biology of Extracellular Matrix. New York: Plenum, 1981.

62. Loomis WF. Developmental Biology. New York: Macmillan, 1986.

63. Rutka JT, Apodaca G, Stern R, Rosenblum M. The extracellular matrix of the central and peripheral nervous systems: structure and function, J Neurosurg 1988; 69:155–170.

64. Shafritz TA, Rosenberg LC, Yannas IV. Specific effects of glycosaminoglycans in an analog of extracellular matrix that delays wound contraction and induces regeneration. Wound Repair Regen 1994; 2:270–276.

65. Yannas IV, Burke JF, Gordon PL, Huang C, Rubenstein RH. Design of an artificial skin. Part II. Control of chemical composition. J Biomed Mat Res 1980; 14:107–131.

66. Yannas IV. Regeneration of skin and nerves by use of collagen templates. In: Nimni M, ed. Collagen: Biotechnology. Vol. III. Boca Raton: CRC, 1988:87–115.

14
Clinical Use of Skin Substitutes

Dennis P. Orgill, Christine Park, and Robert Demling
*Harvard Medical School, and Burn Center, Brigham and Women's
Hospital, Boston, Massachusetts*

I. STRUCTURE AND FUNCTION OF NORMAL SKIN

A. Functions

Skin is the largest organ in the body. The bilayer organ is composed of an outer thin epidermis attached to a thicker dermis at the dermal–epidermal junction. The average thickness of the bilayer is 1 to 2 mm. This bilayer, especially the dermal component, is considerably thinner in infants and the elderly, being under-developed in infants and atrophic in the elderly.

Skin serves a variety of vital functions (Fig. 1). As a barrier, it protects the organism from the external environment, including trauma, desiccation, and invasion by foreign organisms. It is strong yet supple and elastic, and responds to environmental stress by mechanisms of hypertrophy, callusing, or tanning. It provides *protection* against harmful environmental insults (e.g. temperature, chemicals, bacteria, mechanical trauma). Its *thermoregulatory* function combats excess heat loss and also eliminates excess heat gain. The skin contributes to maintenance of *fluid balance* by evaporative loss of fluids as well as a limited capacity to absorb. Furthermore, its *immunological* functions include immune surveillance by specialized cells residing in the skin, and the antibacterial nature of the keratin layer. It serves as a *neurosensory interface* via peripheral sensory nerve endings for pain, temperature, and touch. Its appearance is important for *social interactions* and identification.

B. Epidermis

Current knowledge of the structure and function of skin enables investigators to apply polymer chemistry, cell culture, and gene transfer techniques as prototypes

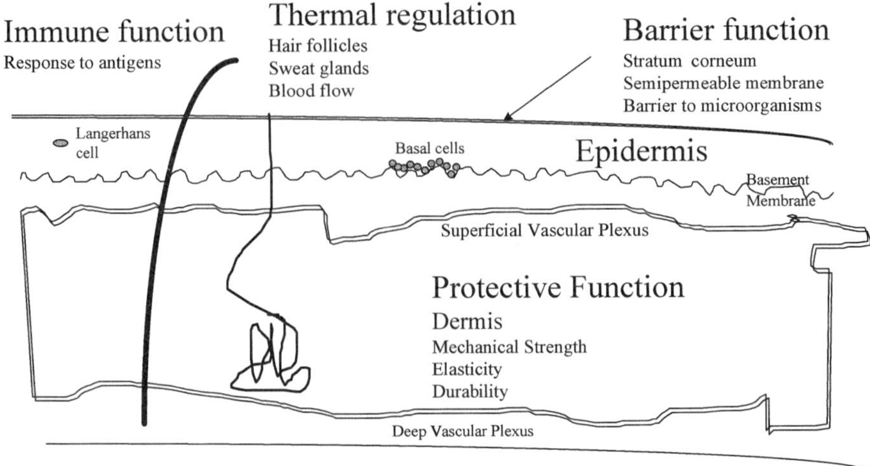

Figure 1   Basic structure and function of skin.

for tissue-engineered skin substitutes. Skin can be modeled as a bilaminate membrane with the outer layer referred to as the epidermis and the underlying layer referred to as the dermis. The avascular epidermis, a stratified squamous epithelium, is embryonically derived from the ectoderm. The epithelium has five morphologically distinct layers: the *stratum basale, stratum spinosum, stratum granulosum, stratum lucidum*, and the *stratum corneum*. Keratinocytes proliferate at the stratum basale and migrate upward as they terminally differentiate into anuclear, keratin-filled cells that form the semipermeable outermost layer, the stratum corneum. The epidermis is continually shed and replaced by new cells.

The basement membrane, or dermal–epidermal junction, separates the epithelium from the underlying dermis. This dermal–epidermal junction is an undulating surface with deep papillary projections called rete ridges, which contribute to the maintenance of dermal–epidermal integrity against shear forces. A number of proteins and substances synthesized by both dermis and epidermis are unique to the basement membrane, such as laminin and collagen type IV.

Other cell types contained in the epidermis are melanocytes and Langerhans cells. Melanocytes produce the pigment melanin that protects the skin from radiation from ultraviolet light. There can be a wide difference in pigmentation expressed in melanocytes, resulting in different degrees of pigmentation throughout the body. The Langerhans cell is a dendritic cell derived from the mesoderm that serves a role in the immunological function of the skin. It is rich in the proteins laminin and collagen VII. Adnexal organs, including hair follicles, sebaceous glands, and sweat glands, are epidermal derivatives that invaginate into the dermis. As such, they are avascular and have a basement membrane contiguous with normal skin. They are lined with keratinocytes that divide, mature, and undergo programmed cell death much as keratinocytes do on the skin's surface. Regeneration depends on [1] chemical stimuli mostly from dermal elements, particularly fibronectin and growth factors, and [2] contact orientation, again from the dermal surface.

The thickness and types of keratin expressed in the epithelium account for much of the texture of the skin and are dependent on the anatomical location and demands. For example, the palms and soles of the feet have a thick glabrous skin as contrasted with a thinner stratum corneum on the trunk. Areas subject to repeated pressures or minor trauma respond by localized hypertrophy of the horny layers of the skin, or callus.

C. Dermis

1. Structure

The dermis endows skin with resilience and substantial mechanical strength. It is a very dynamic, thick layer of connective tissue also in constant turnover, comprising a connective tissue of fibroblasts, extracellular matrix proteins, and ground substance, principally collagen and glycosaminoglycans, interlaced with elastin, a protein that contributes to the significant elastic recoil of the skin. The dermis is richly vascularized by a superficial and deep plexus of vessels. The superficial plexus provides blood supply in the vicinity of the basement membrane, from which the epidermis derives nourishment via diffusion. The degree of vascular supply to the skin varies throughout the body and is notably higher in the head and neck area than in the trunk. This, in addition to the effects of melanin, accounts for some of the difference in coloration throughout the body.

The superficial layer of dermis, or papillary dermis, forms an interdigitating, tight junction with the rete ridges of the epidermis. Disruption of the contiguity between the epidermis and dermis at this level results in serous fluid accumulation or blistering, which further separates the epidermis from the dermis. Lack of the normal undulating dermal–epidermal topography is a cause for the increased blistering and breakdown seen after some methods of skin replacement.

The extracellular matrix of the papillary dermis is composed largely of fine collagen and elastin fibers, with a preponderance of collagen type III. The reticular dermis underlies the papillary dermis, and is composed of a network of larger-diameter collagen and elastin fibers, with a preponderance of collagen type I. The skin appendages are formed by elements of both the epidermis and the dermis. Apocrine and eccrine sweat glands, hair follicles, and peripheral nerve endings are all found in the dermis. The rich nerve supply to the skin lies principally within the superficial dermis.

The typical morphology of the collagen fibers in the skin is crimped and oriented in multiple directions when the skin is at its resting length. A small force in any direction will result in a large displacement of skin until the fibers have straightened. At that point, skin becomes much stiffer, requiring a much higher force to effect a similar displacement. By contrast, in scar tissue, collagen fibers are closely packed and oriented not randomly but rather parallel to each other with a reduced amount of elastin (1). What makes scar tissue feel hard and stiff is this markedly reduced extensibility and elastic recoil.

2. Dermal Cells and Functions

a. Fibroblasts. The fibroblast, the primary dermal cell type, derives from the mesenchyme and produces key structural extracellular matrix proteins, collagen and elastin, as well as matrix proteins, such as fibronectin and tenascin. Fibronectin is a key fibroblast-derived signal protein for the orchestration of wound healing. In addition, these cells produce the adhesion proteins necessary for the attachment of epidermal cells to the basement membrane and for epidermal cell migration and replication. After injury, fibroblasts migrate into the wound and proliferate in order to produce increased quantities of these dermal proteins and matrix as well as cytokines and other growth stimulants.

The ground substance, also synthesized by fibroblasts, is made up of complex polysaccharide-proteins known as glycosaminoglycans and proteoglycans. The matrix provides a semifluid which allows for cell and connective tissue orientation as well as nutrient diffusion to the cells and a scaffolding for cell migration.

b. Endothelial Cells. These cells make up the lining of the microvessels and macrovessels, including the new capillaries produced after injury. Like fibroblasts, endothelial cells are mesenchymally derived and are attracted into a wound by local signals.

c. Macrophages. These cells, again of mesenchymal origin, are normally present in tissue but increase in number after injury, attracted by chemotactic factors released with the activation of inflammation. The long-lived cells themselves release chemical messages, growth factors, and stimulants that orchestrate healing.

d. Platelets. These factor-rich particles release a host of growth factors and adherence proteins during the initial postburn period.

e. Neutrophils. These short-lived cells are the first cells that migrate to the wound surface. Their role is to control bacteria or other toxic elements from surface penetration. Their release of proteases and oxidants kill bacteria, but also can result in injury of normal cells and tissue. The surface exudate is rich in dead and dying neutrophils with toxic protease activity, and excessive inflammation, as occurs with necrotic surface tissue and ongoing neutrophil sequestration, will impede healing.

3. Dermal Matrix Components and Functions

a. Collagen. This protein is the major building block of connective tissue, accounting for 30% of total body protein. The fibers are secreted in immature form by the fibroblast and are oriented by matrix signals and through proteoglycan contact. Collagen type I is the most abundant collagen in normal skin. Besides dermal structure, this collagen provides a contact orientation for dividing and migrating epithelial cells. Collagen type III is a less pliable collagen found more commonly in scar (2).

b. Fibronectin. This adhesion protein is a large glycoprotein found in all tissue and plasma. It is a major adherence protein for migrating epithelial cells via collagen type I, and cross-linking to fibrin and collagen causes adherence of

Table 1 Dermal Molecules and Growth Factors Involved in Wound Healing

Molecule	Source	Action
Basic fibroblast growth factor	Keratinocyte, fibroblast	Stimulates epidermal cell growth
Epiodermal growth factor	Salivary gland	Stimulates epidermal cell proliferation
Keratinocyte growth factor	Hypothalamus	Stimulates epidermal cell growth
Interleukin-1	Macrophage, epidermal 1 cm/cell	Stimulates epidermal growth and motility
Platelet-derived growth factor	Platelets, endothelium	Stimulates epidermal hyperplasia in combination with EGF
Transforming growth factor-β	Fibroblasts, platelets	All forms inhibit epidermal cell proliferation but stimulate motility
Collagen type I	Fibroblast	Supports epidermal cell attachment and spreading
Collagen type IV	Fibroblast, epidermal cell	Supports epidermal cell attachment and spreading
Collagen type V	Epidermal cell	Basement membrane zone
Fibronectin	Fibroblast, macrophage, serum	Supports epidermal cell adhesion and spreading
Laminin	Epidermal cell	Epidermal cell adherence
Vitronectin	Serum	Promotes cell adhesion and spreading

tissues to each other (3). A critical protein in wound healing, it is a chemoattractant, and it provides contact orientation for all cells in the healing process. When applied topically, it has been shown to increase the healing rate of chronic wounds (4).

c.   Ground Substance.   A large number of proteoglycans and glycosaminoglycans comprise the ground substance, which is the foundation for the deposition of dermal cells, collagen, and other proteins. In addition, it provides the scaffold for the epidermal basement membrane. The ground substance deactivates toxic proteases released by neutrophils, possesses adherence properties via cell–matrix interactions, and serves as a conduit to bring critical matrix proteins and growth factors into contact with each other (5).

d.   Growth Factors.   It is well recognized that the healing process is mediated by a group of macrophage-produced, and, to a lesser degree, epithelial cell–produced, polypeptides, whose interaction with a cell surface receptor leads to intracellular changes leading to cell proliferation, morphological changes, and synthesis of proteins (6) (Table 1). Growth factors can themselves possess chemoattractive ability. Once released, growth factors can be rapidly deactivated by wound proteases (e.g., those released by neutrophils). The burn wound is activated to contain excess protease likely to facilitate breakdown of surface dead tissue. This protease-rich environment can lead to delayed wound healing due to overinactivation of growth factors (7).

II. DEVELOPMENT OF SKIN SUBSTITUTES

A. Biology of Burns

Much of the impetus for the development of skin substitutes has stemmed from the loss of large areas of skin in burn victims. Burns can be classified by the depth of skin damaged. The skin's response to wounding is complex. It begins with the inflammatory phase, with initiation of the coagulation cascade at the time of wounding to achieve hemostasis, followed by an influx of inflammatory mediators and cells. In the cellular proliferation phase, fibroblasts and keratinocytes proliferate and migrate into the wound, ultimately restoring the integrity of the skin via processes of angiogenesis, wound contraction, and peripheral epithelialization. The final phase is one of connective tissue formation and scarring, which peaks at 4 weeks but can persist for months to years. During this phase, collagen, proteoglycans, and chondroitin sulfates are laid down and remodeled as the scar matures.

First-degree burns involve just the epidermis and are most frequently seen as a result of ultraviolet light exposure (sunburn). Although quite painful, these usually heal with good function and little to no functional sequelae. Second-degree burns involve the entire epidermis and a portion of the dermis. Because the basement membrane is disrupted in these burns, fluid enters the potential space between the epidermis and dermis, and blistering commonly occurs. Many of the nerve endings are damaged, but not necrosed, making these burns exquisitely painful. In superficial second-degree burns, keratinocytes that line the adnexal organs proliferate to quickly regenerate an overlying epidermis. By contrast, in deep second-degree burns, this process can take over 3 weeks to occur.

Third-degree, or full-thickness, burns result in death of the entire dermis and epidermis. Because the adnexal organs are destroyed, there is no possibility of epidermal regeneration from the wound. The dermis, having been permanently obliterated, is replaced by granulation tissue, which is fundamentally an inflammatory reaction. In small wounds left untreated, the wounds heal from the edges by processes of wound contraction, peripheral epithelialization, and scarring. In the case of large full-thickness burns, however, many centers have found that early surgical excision of severely burned tissue reduces recovery time and sepsis resulting from bacterial proliferation under the eschar. Because skin grafts are often in scant supply, the ensuing problem of immediate physiological and functional wound coverage has been a continuing dilemma, as with any condition leading to extensive skin loss.

B. Current Treatment for Large Burns

Excision and grafting with split-thickness skin grafts are now the standard of care in treating large, deep, second- and third-degree burns in most burn centers in the United States. A split-thickness skin graft is commonly taken with a machine that allows a thin layer of skin 0.04 to 0.20 inch to be taken from an uninjured area of the body. These grafts harvest the epidermis and a variable amount of dermis. The donor sites heal by epithelialization of the dermis analogous to the healing of a second-degree burn. To increase the area covered, the skin can be "meshed" to expand the donor skin. Although this reduces the donor site area, an often strong and unsightly meshed pattern persists on the recipient wound because scar tissue forms where meshed skin is absent. Furthermore, many patients are displeased with scars produced at the donor sites. For some wounds, autologous split-thickness skin grafting is sufficient, but it is often not feasible because of the limited availability of donor sites.

When adequate amounts of autograft skin are not available, temporary coverage may be achieved with cadaveric allograft, xenograft, or synthetic epidermal substitute, such as Biobrane™ (8,9). While this solves the problem of immediate wound closure following early excision, which is essential to the survival of extensive burns, permanent coverage must be eventually sought. In addition, the tissue formed beneath the epithelium following meshed split-thickness skin grafts onto full-thickness wounds is not dermis, but scar. Serious morbidity can follow, with severe functional limitations due to hypertrophic scarring, contractures, and the need for multiple reconstructive procedures.

As a result of these clinical problems, a number of strategies have been designed by investigators to improve reconstitution of skin in the severely burned patient. As we have gained experience treating burns, many of the techniques currently available have been applied to other areas of medicine in which skin loss has been a problem, including reconstructive surgery, ulcers, and genetic disorders of the skin.

C. Design Criteria of Tissue-Engineered Skin Substitutes

The evolution of biological dressings began with the recognition that burn wounds require a barrier protection to prevent infection and desiccation and to maximize healing. Such treatments included the application of various oils and salves as well as biological coverage using materials such as amniotic membrane and xenograft skin. In the United States, guinea pig, chicken, rabbit (10), porcine (11), and canine (12) skin were proposed as suitable xenograft transplant tissue. However, xenografts cannot become vascularized and incorporated by the host, so that they ultimately are sloughed.

Observations of the healing properties of epidermal replacements on partial-thickness wounds versus full-thickness wounds led to the bilayer concept of wound coverage, which recognizes that both dermal and epidermal components are necessary for a successful biological dressing and skin replacement (13). Because dermis cannot spontaneously regenerate in adult mammals, full-thickness wounds heal via ingrowth of granulation tissue, which epithelializes and scarifies. Kangesu et al. (14) confirmed the importance of both dermal and epidermal elements in closure of skin defects. Dermal elements are critical to optimize survival of keratinocytes. Keratinocytes themselves appear to play a pivotal role in inducing angiogenesis, vascular organization, and reinnervation of dermis (15,16).

Functional wound coverage should ideally provide a normalized equilibrium of heat exchange, fluid and electrolyte loss and absorption, restoration of barrier protection, and appropriate cues for the facilitation of healing (17) and restoration of normal tissue architecture (18). It should be bacteriostatic, noninflammatory, and nontoxic, with low antigenicity. Furthermore, an ideal skin substitute should be engineered with adequate drapability to maintain adherence to body contours. Long-term characteristics of a skin replacement should additionally include restoration of normal tissue architecture, an avoidance of scar contracture, restoration of mechanical strength and elasticity with function appropriate to anatomical site, and cosmetic acceptability.

Ideally, in replacing skin with tissue-engineered substitutes, we desire a perfect replication of normal skin. Based on the many functions of skin, the variation from person to person, and the variation depending on anatomical site, this is a very difficult problem. Various skin substitutes have been proposed to address skin replacement in the context of burn wounds. Treatments have focused on replacement of skin, as well as other organs, via autograft, allograft, xenograft, artificial implant, tissue synthesized in vitro, and, most recently, by the use of biomaterials engineering to facilitate in vivo regeneration (19).

Engineering design teaches one to prioritize the design criteria and predict the constraints on the design to arrive at a range of solutions to a particular problem. Tissue engineering, which has developed over the last 50 years, is an interdisciplinary approach that combines the principles of the biological sciences with engineering to develop biological constructs. As outlined by Langer and Vacanti (20), three general strategies exist for the creation of new tissues: [1] isolated cells or cell substitutes, [2] tissue-inducing substances, and [3] cells placed on or within matrices.

To fulfill all of the ideal design criteria (Table 2) would be very difficult at this time, given the state of our technology. However, there are currently a number of tissue-engineered skin substitutes available to clinicians that allow some of these design criteria to be met.

D. Market Demands of Tissue-Engineered Skin Replacements

There have been many prototypes for tissue engineered skin replacement (TESR) produced in the laboratory over the last 20 years. Only a few of these prototypes are available for clinical use today. The transfer of technology from the laboratory to the clinical arena can be an arduous process with a variety of pitfalls along the way. The difficulty and length of this process can frequently be underestimated even by experienced investigators.

A successful TESR must better solve a specific clinical problem. Because there are many different causes and clinical types of skin loss, it is unlikely that

Table 2   Design Criteria for Tissue-Engineered Bilayer Skin Substitute

Mechanical Properties	Biological Properties
Drapability	Control of fluid loss
Shear and tear strength	Nontoxic and noninflammatory
Modulus of elasticity	Antimicrobial
Handling and suturing ability	Nonimmunogenic
Control of degradation rate	Promotes angiogenesis and synthesis of
Adherent	neodermis
Structure compatible for ingrowth of cells	Scarless healing

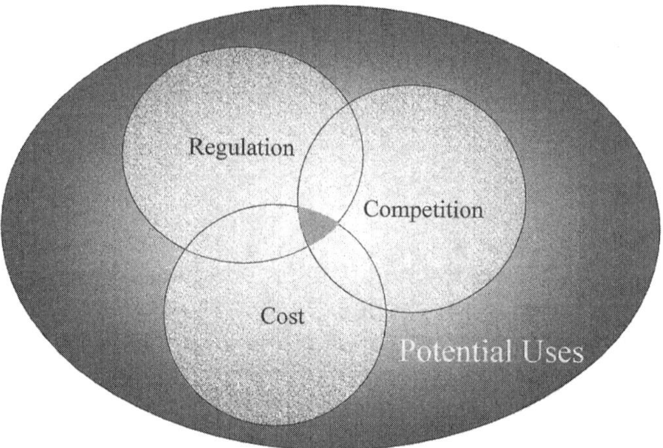

Figure 2 The actual usage of a product can be limited by regulation, competition, or cost considerations.

a single type of solution will be useful in all cases. For clinicians to adopt a new product, it must first be approved by the appropriate governmental regulatory body in the country in which it is sold. Additionally, in an era of cost containment, the product should solve the problem in a cost effective manner (Fig. 2).

In the United States, the Food and Drug Administration (FDA) approves tissue-engineered devices. It examines criteria related to safety and efficacy of the product to protect the public from faulty devices. Until recently, there was little regulation required for products produced primarily from patients own tissues. To be successful in today's marketplace, a TESR must solve a clinical problem, be approved by a governmental regulatory agency, and be financially viable for patients, clinicians, and the manufacturer.

III. TEMPORARY EPIDERMAL REPLACEMENTS

A. Temporary Skin Substitutes for Partial-Thickness Burns

The objective of this approach is to actively alter the quality and rate of healing of a partial-thickness burn. The approach is quite different from the standard treatment, in which the rate of healing usually seen with the degree of partial-thickness burn being treated is accepted as the norm. The bioengineering approach focuses on the two key controlling elements for tissue regeneration.

The first element is controlling the wound healing environment, mainly protecting the wound from external insults. A form of material-based skin cover is utilized for this purpose, which protects, but does not actively interact with, the wound repair.

The second element is the biological manipulation of the healing process. Key biological signals and cues, required for both rate and orchestration of healing, are ideally incorporated into a temporary skin substitute that directly interacts with a viable burn wound surface.

The behavior of the healing tissue can theoretically be improved as opposed to simply being protected from the environment, as seen with purely synthetic substitutes. This biological manipulation can lead to a more accurate duplication of lost epidermis and dermis. There are well-recognized growth factors and other proteins that activate cell proliferation, migration, and tissue organization. Keratinocytes exposed to a fibronectin matrix elect both a more active migration behavior and increased replication. In addition, matrix proteins, especially fibronectin and collagen type I, are known to act as cell guidance structures along which epithelial cells migrate and orient to regenerate a more normal epidermis.

Because the bioengineered skin membrane is also subject to environmental insults, an outer layer of nylon or other synthetic material can protect the bioactive properties of the inner contact membrane, resulting in the ideal synthetic skin substitute for the partial-thickness burn.

B. Biobrane™ (Bertek Pharmaceuticals, Sugarland, Texas)

This bilaminar skin substitute is mainly a material-based skin cover with excellent protection properties when used on a clean superficial dermal burn (21). The product consists of an outer impermeable thin silicone membrane that has minute pores incorporated to provide for drainage of fluid or exudate. The inner layer is an irregular nylon fabric mechanically bonded to the silicone. Collagen type IV from porcine skin is present in the nylon mesh to potentially bind to the wound surface. However, surface binding appears to be primarily through physical contact of the irregular nylon surface to a wet wound, producing hydrophobic bonding as well as fibrin entrapment from the wound in the nylon weave. There is no evidence for any direct biological activity. After several days, fibronectin, produced by wound fibroblasts, enhances the adherence by binding to the entrapped fibrin in the nylon mesh (22).

Adherence is excellent when used on a superficial burn, providing a protective barrier to surface desiccation, bacterial contamination, and water loss from the wound surface. The nylon-with-silicone material also provides flexibility. Prevention of a surface exudate decreases protease activity, thereby optimizing reepithelialization along the thin water layer on the surface. Histological studies have demonstrated that epithelium migrates along the nylon strands. Several studies have demonstrated increased reepithelialization compared with a standard gauze coverage or topical antibiotics. The product is drapable, permitting coverage on curved surfaces and appears not to produce any immune response. A long shelf-life (2 years) lends it an added advantage.

Contraindications to its use include a deeper dermal burn in which adherence is poor since the wound surface is dryer, not permitting adequate binding to the nylon inner layer. Significant bacterial contamination is another contraindication due to the lack of any direct antibacterial properties of the product.

Dressings manufactured from polyurethane films, such as Opsite™ and Tegaderm™ have similar properties, but appear to adhere less firmly and are less flexible.

C. Dermagraft-TC™ (Advanced Tissue Sciences, Inc., La Jolla, California)

This temporary skin substitute is a bilayer product that combines the material-based outer cover with a bioactive inner layer. The product is produced by placing human fibroblasts extracted from neonatal foreskins onto the inner layer of Biobrane in a culture medium. The fibroblasts proliferate and secrete the natural components of normal dermis on the inner layer. Large quantities of natural fibronectin, human collagen type I, glycosaminoglycans, and other matrix products are produced, as well as smaller amounts of growth factors (23).

The product is cryopreserved at the end of the 17-day growth cycle. This time period has been selected as peak fibroblast product content is present at this time. Cryopreservation destroys the fibroblasts but preserves the bioactivity of the fibroblast-derived products (24).

With the knowledge that cadaver-allografted wound beds demonstrate excellent take of subsequent skin grafts, as discussed above, this synthetic construct was designed to use tissue engineering principles and cell culture technology to produce a more readily available and superior means of temporary wound coverage in the deep second-degree burn. In clinical trials, the product was compared with cryopreserved cadaver allograft for the temporary coverage of excised burn wounds (24,25). Treatment with this product was at least equivalent to allograft in the context of the character of the wound bed and subsequent autograft "take." It was easier to remove the temporary coverage from the wound bed with less bleeding, and whereas cadaver allograft exhibited some evidence of immune rejection (i.e., epidermal sloughing), Dermagraft-TC–prepared wounds did not.

Dermagraft-TC (Temporary Cover) is marketed for use on mid-dermal to deep partial-thickness burns. These wounds are at a high risk for conversion to a deeper injury from surface inflammation or environmental insults.

The potential advantages of this product over synthetic skin substitutes is the presence of wound healing stimulants on the membrane itself. Fibronectin is a known healing stimulant. In addition, the dermal elements on the membrane can produce a biochemical bonding to surface fibrin and collagen, leading to more rapid and stronger adherence. Since a wet surface is not required for adherence, a deeper burn can thereby be protected. Dermagraft-TC has the same properties of Biobrane with the exception of the pores. Furthermore, there is a bioactive property present on its inner surface that is lacking in Biobrane. This bioactive quality can lead to more rapid reepithelialization, owing especially to the immediate availability of fibronectin, which otherwise requires several days for production by the wound itself.

Current studies have demonstrated minimal antigenicity of the product and a more rapid healing compared with topical antibiotics after transplantation to allogenic hosts (26). Comparison with pure synthetics like Biobrane have not yet been published. In general, however, Biobrane is not used on mid-dermal burns due to decreased adherence.

Since surface adherence is necessary for efficacy, Dermagraft-TC should not be placed over surface eschar as present on a nondebrided mid-dermal or on any deep-dermal burn. At present, this product is unique in that it is the only temporary skin substitute containing active human fibroblast products known to augment and orchestrate wound reepithelialization. Current studies also indicate less scar formation with the use of this product compared with topical antibiotics, reflecting a more organized tissue repair process.

Although the American Association of Tissue Banks has published standards for tissue banking and the Food and Drug Administration has specified quality control guidelines, adherence to these standards is not currently mandated. Therefore, it has been stated that the use of this tissue-engineered construct may depend on a cost–benefit analysis balancing the consequence of stiffening regulations for the already limited supply of cadaver allograft versus the costs of buying a biosynthetic product (27).

IV. PERMANENT EPIDERMAL REPLACEMENTS: CULTURED EPITHELIAL AUTOGRAFTS

In 1953, Billingham and Reynolds (28) performed the first transplants of trypsinized epidermal sheets and epidermal cell suspensions in rabbits. Although a confluent epithelium was produced, the grafts were fragile and underwent significant wound contraction. With the establishment of the standard for cell culturing (29) and the development of cultured human keratinocytes grafts (30) came a clinically applicable technique to address permanent epithelial regeneration. Using this technique, a small donor site can be expanded up to 10,000-fold and, over the course of several weeks, a multilayered, confluent epithelial sheet can be formed. These cultured epithelial autografts (CEAs) were applied directly onto excised full-thickness wounds of major burn victims (31). The resulting epidermis was noted to be fragile and prone to blistering and ulceration with minimal trauma. Compton et al. (32) performed a 5-year followup comparing CEA applied directly to wounds versus meshed split-thickness skin grafts. Cultured epithelial autograft did provide useful wound coverage with formation of a scar bed with some neodermal function and reduced scarring, but the histological data suggested compromised function for at least 1 to 2 years after wounding. The epidermal–wound junction following grafting of CEA is noted to exhibit incomplete basement membrane structures, abnormal anchoring fibrils, and rete ridge formation. Thus, the epidermis is weakened compared with normal skin with lower resistance to shear forces and increased susceptibility to breakdown.

The "take" rate of CEA has been related to the nature of the wound bed. Cultured epithelial autografts grafted onto chronic granulating wounds have a 15% take (33), freshly excised or early granulating wounds result in a 28 to 47% take (40), and wounds dressed with cadaveric allografts have a 45 to 75% take (32,34). Wound beds that have been prepared with allograft are highly vascular with connective tissue components, which has been postulated to contribute to superior take of CEA on wound beds previously covered with allograft. This led to the demonstration of the importance of epithelial–mesenchymal interactions in the fate of epithelial grafts. Cultured epithelial autograft combined with dermal autograft had a 10-fold higher take than CEA grafted onto granulation tissue in a study using a porcine model (14) and in clinical trials (35).

Clinically, the CEA take rate has been reported to be as low as 15% (36), to a more moderate range (37), to greater than 90% (38). Some workers cited increased infection rates (36), scar contracture (39), and a high failure rate compared with meshed split-thickness skin grafts (40,41). In contrast, others have been enthusiastic about its cosmetic and functional results (42,43), and a reduced incidence of hypertrophic scarring and keloid formation (44). In a prospective trial, the use of cultured epithelial autografts, grafted onto vascularized allodermis, partial-thickness wounds, or acellular cryopreserved dermis, was compared to standard burn wound care in a group of patients with greater than 50% body surface area burns. The investigator reported a reduced mortality with no significant difference between the two treatment methods with respect to other major complications or for readmissions due to breakdown of the graft (45). The final engraftment rates of the CEAs were not measured in this study. Some reports suggest, however, that the ultimate take rate of CEA may be 50% or less because of late graft loss. Mouse fibroblasts used to grow the CEA have been shown to persist and are capable of stimulating an immunological rejection, which could contribute to the continuing dilemma of late graft loss (46).

Because of the significant time delay required between harvesting of autologous keratinocytes until preparation of a CEA is complete, the use of "banked" cultured allogenic keratinocytes seemed to be a promising alternative and was proposed by Hefton et al. in 1983 (47). Despite initial positive reports (48), allogenic keratinocytes appeared to regain immunogenicity (49) and did not seem to persist after grafting (40).

Efforts to optimize in vitro methods of producing a cultured epithelial replacement are ongoing, and products such as Epicel-CEA™ (Genzyme Tissue Repair, Cambridge, Massachusetts) have made the production of cultured epithelial autografts commercially available. After creating a cell suspension from a skin biopsy, the suspension is plated, and colonies spread to form stratified confluent sheets of keratinocytes 2 to 8 cell layers thick. The grafts are prepared on company premises and delivered back to the hospital when ready. Technical improvements have reduced the time in culture from 3 to 4 weeks, the historical average, to an average of 16 days for sufficient amounts to cover 18% of the typical adult's body surface area. Twenty-one days are required to produce enough CEA to cover 45% body surface area.

Lifeskin™ (Culture Technology, Inc., Sherman Oaks, California) is another product that provides CEA. It differs from the standard CEA in that it is technically a composite graft. Separate in vitro cultures of autologous fibroblasts and keratinocytes are maintained after skin biopsy to produce confluent sheets of fibroblasts and keratinocytes that are then combined and cocultured for a period of another 6 days. The delivery time for this product, according to the company, is 17 to 21 days (50).

V. DERMAL REPLACEMENTS

A. Alloderm™ (LifeCell Corp., The Woodlands, Texas)

The first generation of allograft dermis used with epithelial replacements for permanent full-thickness wound coverage involved the initial application of full-thickness allograft using tissue-banked cadaver skin. This was followed by dermabrasion of the highly antigenic epidermal layer once the graft had become vascularized and attached to the wound bed. The remaining intact allodermis was then covered with an autologous skin graft.

Although fresh allograft skin, and, to a lesser degree, cryopreserved allograft skin, provides excellent adherence to the wound with rapid vascularization and control of bacterial growth, graft rejection and subsequent inflammation of the wound bed makes it vulnerable to infection. Due to widespread concerns for disease transmission (51) and the antigenicity of intact allogenic dermis, an acellular cryopreserved, lyophilized allodermis has subsequently been developed and is commercially available as Alloderm. Because the epidermal layer is destroyed, the product lacks the bilayer property of intact allogenic skin and functions strictly as a dermal transplant.

The preparation of the acellular cryopreserved allodermis from tissue-banked cadaver skin involves separation of the epidermis from the dermis, when applied topically, and sterilization of the dermis with detergents and freeze-drying. Staining for major histocompatibility complex (MHC) class I and II as markers for alloantigens after processing is negative. A characteristic feature of this permanent dermal replacement is that it retains the intrinsic ultrastructural features of dermis. The retention of these dermal components and their structure (i.e., papillary and reticular dermis) is therefore hypothesized to play an important role. Collagen and elastin bundle orientation particular to the papillary or reticular dermis are preserved, as well as basement membrane proteins, such as types IV and VII collagen and laminin, and are thought to facilitate attachment and re-formation of the dermal–epidermal junction (52).

Currently, the product is clinically used together with ultrathin (0.003 to 0.006 inch) meshed split-thickness autografts. Several clinical studies have been performed, reporting an equivalent 14-day take rate of this dermal matrix with traditional split-thickness autografting; followup to 6 months demonstrated equivalent clinical assessments for the Alloderm™-ultrathin autograft combination compared with traditional skin grafting (53,54). Lymphocyte proliferation assays did not demonstrate any evidence of immunological rejection, and the dermal matrix supported fibroblast ingrowth, angiogenesis, and keratinocyte migration from the overlying autograft (55).

In addition to the use of this product with ultra-thin split-thickness skin grafting, superior keratinocyte engraftment has been reported in an animal study employing the product in combination with cultured keratinocytes in a hydrophilic dressing (56). This finding is consistent with the finding of durable skin replacement in humans employing allogenic dermal replacement in combination with CEA (32,34). Such bilayer grafts demonstrate a significantly higher take rate than those achieved on granulation tissue alone, and histological evidence suggests that the epithelial components become well integrated with the allogenic dermis (57).

Langdon and Cuono (58) support the use of this combination, reporting textural and histological qualities similar to wound healing in normal skin. However, in this study, the basement membrane zones of the dermal–epidermal junction and microvasculature were not complete until 124 days. Munster (45) did utilize Alloderm with CEA in several patients in a prospective trial evaluating CEA, but no direct comparison of the product versus standard allografting in the context of CEA was performed. The Cuono group (59) has constructed a composite graft, consisting of acellular dermis, cultured human fibroblasts, and cultured human keratinocytes, and transplanted these composites onto athymic mice. Retention of ultrastructural features and rapid repopulation of the dermis with fibroblasts was reported.

B. Extracellular Matrix Analogs

1. Integra™ (Integra LifeSciences Corp., Plainsboro, New Jersey)

Other than the optimization of the technology of allografting, bioengineering research has also sought to create fully synthetic, biocompatible skin substitutes. Use of collagenous materials was first attempted as early as 1943 for wound dressings (60). Building on this precedent, Yannas and Burke (60–62) developed a skin substitute consisting of an acellular, biodegradable collagen–glycosaminoglycan (CG) copolymer matrix coated with a thin polysiloxane (silicone) elastomer. This extracellular matrix analog (ECMA) is commercially available as Integra. Type I collagen, the most abundant collagen in the dermis, and chondroitin 6-sulfate, one of the major glycosaminoglycans, are co-precipitated, freeze-dried, and cross-linked with a dehydrothermal process and with glutaraldehyde. The pore size has been precisely determined to maximize ingrowth of cells, and the degree of cross-linking as well as glycosaminoglycan composition has been defined to control the rate of matrix degradation. Recapitulating two of the most abundant substances found in the extracellular matrix, the product functions as a dermal analog and scaffold for the infiltration of fibroblasts and neovascularization. The silicone membrane, through which water flux is approximately that of epidermis (63), functions as a synthetic epidermis during the period of vascularization and neodermal formation.

This ECMA induced formation of a neodermis in clinical trials (64). In animal studies, when this matrix was seeded with autologous keratinocytes, collagen fiber orientation and elastin fiber structure resembled native dermis (65). Small-angle light scattering measurements quantitatively confirmed the presence of a low degree of collagen fiber orientation in normal dermis, and a high degree of orientation in scar; as could be predicted, dermis regenerated with the CG matrix contained a moderate degree of collagen finer orientation (66). The neodermis resulting from grafting of the CG matrix exhibited less myofibroblast differentiation than in ungrafted wounds (67), and wounds grafted with the CG matrix underwent significantly reduced contraction (68). A transient giant cell inflammatory reaction is observed, which ultimately results in the complete degradation of the matrix as the neodermis is formed.

The product is marketed in the United States for use in large full-thickness and deep second-degree burns and is currently clinically used with very thin split-thickness skin grafts, which are applied after a period of vascularization and tissue ingrowth to the CG matrix. It has received approval in Europe for use in reconstructive surgery. It is stored in 70% isopropyl alcohol or in freeze-dried form. The silicone layer acts as a temporary ''epidermis'' during the period before skin grafting, providing barrier protection and mechanical strength. The subsequent skin coverage, in a multicenter randomized trial, was equivalent in quality to conventional split-thickness skin grafting with the benefit of more rapid healing of the donor site (69). The CG copolymer has also been used for peripheral nerve regeneration, and its various applications have been recently reviewed (70). However, infection has been cited as one of the main limitations encountered with Integra (64), and research is ongoing to modify the product.

Further experimentation in animal models has demonstrated that the CG matrix provides a favorable substrate for CEA when CEA is applied 10 days after grafting of the CG matrix to full-thickness wounds (71). The matrix can also be seeded with cultured, isolated autologous cells and grafted in a one-step procedure resulting in a confluent epidermis in a porcine model within 19 days of grafting and a resulting skin with a normal maturation and differentiation sequence after 2 weeks (72). The epidermal component is thereby accomplished in vivo rather than in vitro. The seeding density used for the keratinocytes in this model is a critical variable, with 50,000 cells/cm^2 graft as the minimum dilution to achieve a consistent and rapidly confluent epidermis (73). Isolation of the seeded grafts from the surrounding normal epidermis by means of island grafting confirmed that the neoepidermis originates from the seeded keratinocytes and is adherent to the underlying vascularized neodermis (74).

2. Collagen Matrices

a. Collagen Split Graft. A number of variations on the CG matrix dermal analog exist that are collagen-only constructs without the glycosaminoglycan component. One such example is a collagen split graft, which is a cross-linked collagen matrix with separated top and bottom layers. Using a rat model, Dutch investigators noted that the bottom layer functioned as a matrix for the formation of a neodermis and inhibition of wound contraction, while the top layer facilitated proliferation and reepithelialization of full-thickness wounds (75).

b. Terudermis® (Terumo Co., Kanagawa, Japan). This product, which is marketed in Japan but not commercially available in the United States, is a collagen matrix dermal analog that is fabricated from dehydrothermally cross-linked bovine fibrillar collagen and denatured collagen gelatin (76). The product induces neodermal formation with persistence of the grafted collagen fibers for up to 20 weeks in a rat model (77). This product may be used for the treatment of full-thickness wounds together with split-thickness skin grafting.

c. Pelnac® (Neomatrix, Kowa, Japan). Another modification on the Burke and Yannas CG matrix includes this product, which employs porcine collagen for the matrix, and a silicone membrane (78,79). Investigators have devised a method by which to allow a sustained release of antibiotics just beneath the silicone sheet (80). Fibroblasts have also been experimentally placed in the pores of the uppermost layer of the collagen sponge, overlaid with keratinocytes, and subsequently cultured at the air–liquid interface to produce a composite graft.

VI. COMPOSITE GRAFTS

A. Dermagraft™ (Advanced Tissue Sciences, Inc., San Diego, California)

Another approach to the design of bilayer skin replacement incorporates cultured allogenic cells into synthetic materials to form bilayer, simultaneous epidermal and dermal replacements known as "composite grafts." Related to Dermagraft-TC, Dermagraft uses Vicryl (lactic acid–glycolic acid copolymer) mesh instead of nylon as the scaffold for the allogenic cultured fibroblasts, but is otherwise prepared in a similar fashion to the nylon mesh construct. Unlike its counterpart, however, the Vicryl-based construct is biodegradable over time and is not meant for temporary epithelial coverage. Rather, it is approved for a different indication—that of the treatment of full-thickness diabetic ulcers.

As opposed to the CG matrix, which is designed to degenerate by about 14 days and is associated with a giant-cell inflammatory response, degradation of the polyglycolic acid/polylactic acid (PGA/PLA) meshes is observed from day 15 onward, persists for up to 99 days, and is associated with only a minimal inflammatory response. The original investigators of this product, citing these factors as well as a concern for the susceptibility of collagen to enzymatic digestion and elevated levels of collagenase in a wound, replaced their initial use of a CG membrane with the PGA/PGL construct (81–83).

This dermal analog is also cryopreserved after preparation, yet the metabolic activity of the fibroblasts is preserved in order to provide a "living" graft that continues to secrete extracellular matrix and growth factors to the ulcer bed (84). The product was used with meshed split-thickness skin grafts in an athymic mouse model, which allowed cellular infiltration and vascularization of the grafts with complete incorporation into the wounds. The presence of viable fibroblasts is critical for the reepithelialization of the wound when utilizing split-thickness skin grafts (STSGs) with this product. Control grafts without fibroblasts resulted in poor take of the STSG and poor neodermal formation (85).

B. Apligraf™, Living Skin Equivalent (Organogenesis, Inc., Canton, Massachusetts)

While Dermagraft uses synthetic materials as the scaffolding for fibroblasts, Apligraf, formerly known as Graftskin, is a composite graft based on investigations pioneered by Bell et al. (86), who described a collagen matrix contracted by fibroblasts and overlaid with keratinocytes. The living skin equivalent (LSE) is a bilayered, viable skin replacement consisting of a collagenous dermal matrix populated with fibroblasts and a separate layer consisting of a stratified differentiated epidermis. Both fibroblasts and keratinocytes are derived from neonatal foreskins. The stratum corneum is induced by organotypic culture conditions (raising the construct to the air–liquid interface) after a period of time in standard culture (87).

In studies on athymic mice, the basement membrane is noted to be continuous by 15 days with a distinct lamina lucida and lamina densa, and a dense array of anchoring fibrils and hemidesmosomes are evident by 30 days. The epidermal cells synthesize basement membrane components and provide functional, biological barrier protection (88). In the dermis, thick, tightly packed bundles of collagen are observed by 30 days with extracelluar matrix proteins, such as collagen, glycosaminoglycans, decorin, and tenascin (89). Surprisingly, stains for human involucrin are positive even at 60 days, suggesting persistence of the human cells in the graft (90). In order to expand the product's availability and life span, the LSE has been cryopreserved using a method to preserve viability. Followup studies have demonstrated that the LSE maintains viability as measured by graft take and confirmed using anti–human involucrin staining (91).

In a clinical study, the LSE was tested on 15 patients that had acute surgical wounds as a result of skin cancer excisions, with 12 of 15 resulting in clinical takes (92). All patients tested negative for HLA antibodies against antigens expressed on the cells of the LSE. Failures were due to infection in one case, self-removal by the patient in one case, and was unexplained in the third case. Although the usefulness of the LSE in the context of burns and large wounds has been postulated, data from clinical trials are awaited. The use of this product for chronic venous ulcers has been clinically studied using a protocol that involves repeated applications of the LSE over time. Healing of the ulcers occurs by promotion of healing by secondary intention by creating a favorable wound environment as well as healing by frank graft take (93).

C. Composite Cultured Skin (Ortec International, New York, New York)

Composite cultured skin (CCS) is a composite skin substitute that was initially developed for application in patients with skin defects caused by epidermolysis bullosa. Its indications were [1] as a biological coverage for medium split-thickness donor sites and [2] as a graft to cover tissue-deficient sites on the palmar and digital surfaces after contracture release in these patients. The basic construct is that of keratinocytes and fibroblasts cocultured in cross-linked bovine collagen sponges. This sponge is coated on one surface with nonporous collagen. The fibroblasts are seeded on the porous aspect of the sponge, whereas the keratinocytes are sequentially seeded on the nonporous aspect, which functions as an engineered "basement membrane" for the developing composite graft, which requires a 10- to 14-day production time, after which the product is cryopreserved. Keratinocytes and fibroblasts are allogenic cells and are derived from neonatal foreskins that have undergone serological and microbiological testing according to FDA standards.

In an initial clinical trial of seven patients with deep dermal burns, a mature epidermis was observed histologically at 14 days with full adherence of dermis to epidermis and reestablishment of an intact basement membrane and rete ridge pattern. Examination of regeneration and organization of elastin fibers revealed no quantitative difference between CCS and autograft (94). A multiple-center clinical trial is underway to investigate the safety and efficacy of this product in comparison with split-thickness autograft in the treatment of deep partial-thickness as well as full-thickness burns.

D. Fibrin Glue

Fibrin glue has been proposed as a matrix in which to suspend autologous cultured, nonconfluent keratinocytes. Kaiser et al. (96,97) have employed the keratinocyte-culture-in-fibrin-matrix (KFGS) for deep partial thickness burns and in conjunction with allogenic, glycerine-preserved split-thickness cadaver skin (95) in several patients with full-thickness burn wounds. The investigators report satisfactory adherence of the KFGS to the wound bed, a confluent epithelial layer within 4 days, and histological evidence of a stratified neoepidermis. KFGS grafted in conjunction with the allogenic graft resulted in a superior, more stable skin than KFGS grafted alone. Although the clinical and histological evidence suggested partial incorporation of the dermal allograft into the new skin, the epidermis of the allogenic dermal grafts was noted for desquamation within several days. A larger series will be necessary to more fully evaluate the benefit of the KFGS for use in skin replacement.

E. Combined Collagen Sponge and Gel

Japanese investigators have devised a composite graft of autologous cultured fibroblasts and keratinocytes within a collagen matrix. The collagenous portion of the graft consists of a spongy sheet in a honeycomb structure that is then filled with collagen gel. This structure allows for diffusion of nutrients to the cultured keratinocytes on the surface of the matrix after grafting. A limited clinical trial demonstrated development of mature epidermis and dermis (98).

VII. SUMMARY

Skin is the first tissue-engineered organ. There have been several successful approaches to this difficult problem that have led to advances in tissue engineering in many other organs and tissues. Most tissue-engineered skin substitutes available today address issues of epidermal and dermal regeneration with a goal of providing safe and expedient wound coverage and durable, functional reconstruction of the integument. Nevertheless, even the best results obtained today do not compare to the outcome of a carefully applied full-thickness autograft. Clearly, this technology is in its infancy.

During the course of the next millennium, increasingly complex strategies will employ the continuing evolution of biotechnology to create new generations of products (Fig. 3). Growth factors can be seeded into skin replacements in order to further direct neovascularization, innervation, and the progression of healing. Antibiotics can be delivered via these products to reduce infection rates. Principles of genetic engineering and gene therapy can be used to modify either the cells that are added to the constructs or cells that are already present in the wound bed. Color match is very important to patients and work on melanocyte cultures and melanin expression will be necessary for an optimal cosmetic result. Skin texture is related to keratin expression and is site-specific within the body. Regeneration of site-specific skin would permit improvements in appearance and function. The ability to accommodate adnexal structures within skin substitutes will be extremely beneficial, particularly in areas such as the scalp. Finally, the development of donor-independent keratinocytes would be a major step toward perfecting a tissue-engineered skin replacement.

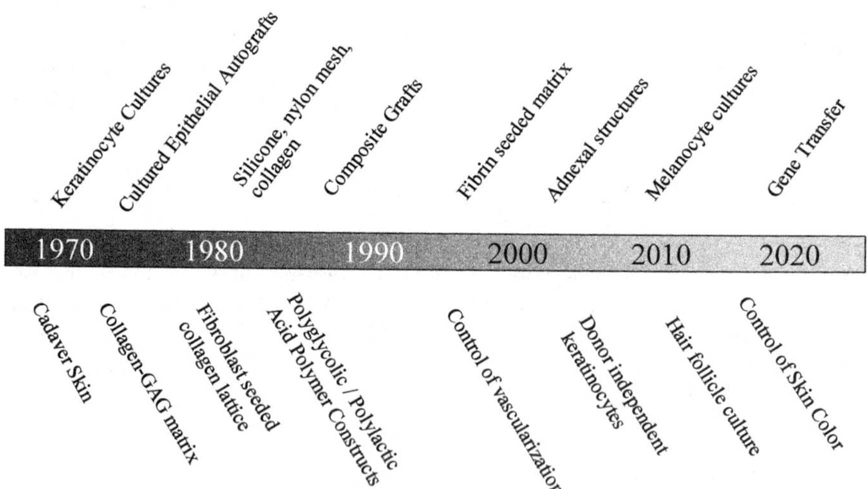

Figure 3 Possible timeline for advances in clinical skin substitutes. Times are not exact, but show many of the contributions to this field.

Patients and physicians alike desire a skin replacement that mimics normal skin; thus, efforts will continue toward the achievement of that goal.

REFERENCES

1. Doillon C, Dunn M, Bender E, Silver FH. Collagen fiber formation in repair tissue: development of strength and toughness. Coll Relat Res 1985; 5:481–492.
2. Clore J, Cohen I, Diegelmann R. Quantitation of collagen types I and III during wound healing. Proc Soc Exp Biol Med 1979; 161:337–341.
3. Git M, Toda K, Grinnell F. Activation of human keratinocyte migration on type I collagen and fibronectin. J Cell Sci 1990; 96:197–205.
4. Litvinov R, Izmailov SG, Zinkevich OD, Kocher OS, Ermolin GA. Effect of exogenes fibronectin on the healing of skin wounds. Bull Exp Biol Med 1987; 12:727–730.
5. Ragshow R. The role of extracellular matrix in post inflammatory wound healing and fibrosis. FASEB J 1994; 8:823–850.
6. Falanger V. Growth factors and wound healing. J Dermatol 1993; 19:711–718.
7. Neely A, Brown R, Chendening C. Proteolytic activity in human burn wounds. Wound Repair Regen 1997; 5:302–309.
8. Purdue GF, Hunt JL, Gillespie RW, Hansbrough JF, Dominic WJ, Robson MC, Smith DJ, Macmillan BG, Waymac JP, Herndon DN. Biosynthetic skin substitute versus frozen human cadaver allograft for temporary coverage of excised burn wounds. J Trauma 1987; 27:155–157.
9. Zawacki BE. Temporary wound closure after burn excision. J Burn Care Rehabil 1986; 7:138–143.
10. Sneve H. The treatment of burns and skin grafting. JAMA 1905; 45:1–8.
11. Bromberg BE, Song JC, Mohn MP. The use of pig skin as a temporary biologic dressing. Plast Reconstr Surg 1965; 36:80–90.
12. Switzer WE, Moncrief JA, Mills W Jr, Order SE, Lindberg RB. The use of canine heterografts in the therapy of thermal injury. J Trauma 1966; 6:391–395.
13. Pruitt BA Jr, Levine NS. Characteristics and uses of biologic dressings and skin substitutes. Arch Surg 1984; 119:312–322.
14. Kangesu T, Navasaria HA, Manek S, Fryer PR, Leigh IM, Green CJ. Keratodermal grafts: the importance of dermis for the in vivo growth of cultured keratinocytes. Br J Plast Surg 1993; 46:401–409.
15. Kangesu T, Manek S, Terenghi G, Gu XH, Navasaria HA, Polak JM, Green CJ, Leigh IM. Nerve and blood vessel growth in response to grafted dermis and cultured keratinocytes. Plast Reconstr Surg 1998; 101:1029–1038.
16. Gu XH, Terenghi G, Kangesu T, Navasaria HA, Springall DR, Leigh IM, Green CJ, Polak JM. Regeneration pattern of blood vessels and nerves in cultured keratinocyte grafts assessed by confocal laser scanning microscopy. Br J Dermatol 1995; 132:376–383.
17. Brown RA, Smith KD, McGrouther A. Strategies for cell engineering in tissue repair. Wound Repair Regen 1997; 5:212–221.

18. Gumbiner B. Cell adhesion: the molecular basis of tissue architecture and morphogenesis. Cell 1996; 84:345–357.

19. Putnam AJ, Mooney DJ. Tissue engineering useing synthetic extracellular matrices. Nature Med 1996; 2:824–826.

20. Langer R, Vacanti JP. Tissue Engineering. Science 1993; 260:920–926.

21. Frank D, Wachtel T, Frank N. Comparison of Biobrane, procine and human allograft as biologic dressings for burn wounds. Surg Forum 1980; 31:552–558.

22. Tavis M, Thornton J, Bartlett R, Woodroof E. A new composite skin substitute prosthesis. Burns 1980; 7:123–128.

23. Hansbrough JF, Morgan J, Greenleaf G, Underwood J. Development of a temporary living skin replacement composed of human fibroblasts cultured in Biobrane, a synthetic dressing material. Surgery 1994; 115:633–644.

24. Hansbrough JF, Mozingo DW, Kealey GP, Davis M, Gidner A, Gentzkow GD. Clinical trials of a biosynthetic temporary skin replacement, Dermagraft-Transitional Covering, compared with cryopreserved human cadaver skin for temporary coverage of excised burn wounds. J Burn Care Rehabil 1997; 18:43–51.

25. Purdue GF, Hunt JL, Still JM Jr, Law EJ, Hernson DN, Goldfarb IW, Schiller WR, Hansbrough JF, Hickerson WK, Himel HN, Kealey GP, Twomey J, Missavage AE, Solem LD, Davis M, Totoritis M, Gentzkow GD. A multicenter clinical trial of a biosynthetic skin replacement, Dermagraft-TC, compared with cryopreserved human cadaver skin for temporary coverage of excised burn wounds. J Burn Care Rehabil 1997; 18:52–57.

26. Sher SE, Hull BE, Rosen S, Church D, Friedman L, Bell E. Acceptance of allogenic fibroblasts in skin equivalent transplants. Transplantation 1983; 36:552–557.

27. Herndon DN. Perspectives in the use of allograft. J Burn Care Rehabil 1997; 18: S6.

28. Billingham RE, Reynolds J. Transplantation studies on sheets of pure epidermal epithelium and on epidermal cell suspensions. Br J Plast Surg 1953; 5:25.

29. Rheinwald JG, Green H. Serial cultivation of strains of human epidermal keratinocytes: the formation of keratinizing colonies from single cells. Cell 1975; 6:331–343.

30. Banks-Schlegel S, Green H. Formation of epidermis by serially cultivated human epidermal cells transplanted as epithelium to athymic mice. Transplantation 1980; 29:308–313.

31. Gallico G III, O'Connor NE, Compton CC, Kehinde O, Green H. Permanent coverage of large burn wounds with autologous cultured human epithelium. N Engl J Med 1984; 311(7):448–451.

32. Compton CC, Gill JM, Bradford DA, Regauer S, Gallico G, O'Connor NE. Skin regenerated from cultured epithelial autografts on full-thickness burn wounds from 6 days to 5 years after grafting. Lab Invest 1989; 60(5):600–612.

33. Teepe RGC, Kreis RW, Koebrugge EJ, Kempenaar JA, Vloemans AF, Hermans RP, Boxma H, Dokter J, Hermans J, Ponce M, et al. The use of cultured autologous epidermis in the treatment of extensive burn wounds. J Trauma 1990; 30:269–275.

34. Cuono CB, Langdon R, Birchall N, Barttelbort S, McGuire J. Composite autologous-allogenic skin replacement: development and clinical application. Plast Reconstr Surg 1987; 80:626–637.

35. Compton CC, Hickerson W, Nadire K, Press W. Acceleration of skin regeneration from cultured epithelial autografts by transplantation to homograft dermis. J Burn Care Rehabil 1993; 14:653–662.

36. Blight A, Mountford EM, Cheshire IM, Clancy JM, Levick PL. Treatment of full skin thickness burn injury using cultured epithelial grafts. Burns 1991; 17:495–498.

37. Still JM Jr, Orlet HK, Law EJ. Use of cultured epidermal autografts in the treatment of large burns. Burns 1994; 20:539–541.

38. Hickerson WL, Compton C, Fletchall S, Smith LR. Cultured epidermal autografts and allodermis combination for permanent burn wound coverage. Burns 1994; 20 1:S52–S55.

39. Warden G. The fifth quinquennium: 1989–1993. J Burn Care Rehabil 1993; 14:247–251.

40. DeLuca M, Albanese E, Bondanza S, Meana M, Ugozzoli L, Molina E, Cancedda R, Santi PL, Bormioli M, Stella M, et al. Multicentre experience in the treatment of burns with autologous and allogeneic cultured epithelium, fresh or preserved in a frozen state. Burns 1989; 15:303–309.

41. Clugston PA, Snelling CF, MacDonald IB, Maledy HL, Boyle JC, Germann E, Courtemanche A, Wirtz P, Fitzpatrick DJ, Kester DA, et al. Cultured epithelial autografts: three years of clinical experience with eighteen patients. J Burn Care Rehabil 1991; 12:533–539.

42. Sheridan RL, Tompkins RG. Cultured autologous epithelium in patients with burns of ninety percent or more of the body surface. J Trauma 1995; 38:48–50.

43. Haith LR Jr, Patton ML, Goldman WT. Cultured epidermal autograft and the treatment of the massive burn injury. J Burn Care Rehabil 1992; 13:142–146.

44. McAree KG, Klein RL, Boeckman CR. The use of cultured epithelial autografts in the wound care of severely burned patients. J Ped Surg 1993; 28:166–168.

45. Munster AM. Cultured skin for massive burns: A propective, randomized trial. Ann Surg 1996; 224(3):372–375.

46. Cairns BA, deSerres S, Brady LA. Xenogeneic mouse fibroblasts persist in human cultured epidermal grafts: a possible mechanism of graft loss. J Trauma 1995; 39(1):75–79.

47. Hefton JM, Madden MR, Finkelstein JL, Shires GT. Grafting of burn patients with allografts of cultured epidermal cells. Lancet 1983; 2:428–430.

48. Thivolet J, Faure M, Demidem A, Maduit G. Long-term survival and immunological tolerance of human epidermal allografts produced in culture. Transplantation 1986; 42:274–280.

49. Wikner NE, Huff CJ, Norris DA, Boyce ST, Cary M, Kissinger M, Weston WL. Studies of HLA-DR synthesis in cultured human keratinocytes. J Invest Dermatol 1986; 87:559–564.

50. Morgan JR, Yarmush ML. Bioengineered skin substitutes. Science and Med 1997; 4:6–15.

51. Kealey GP, Aguiar J, Lewis RW II, Rosenquist MD, Strauss RG, Bale JF Jr. Cadaver skin allografts and trannsmission of human cytomegalovirus to burn patients. J Am Coll Surg 1996; 182:201–205.

52. Wainwright D, Nag A, Call T, Griffey S, Atkinson Y, Livesey S. Normal histological

features persist in an acellular dermal transplant grafted in full-thickness burns. FASEB Summer Research Conference, 1994.

53. Wainwright D, Madden M, Luterman A, Hunt J, Monato W, Heimbach D, Kagan R, Sitting K, Dimick A, Herndon D. Clinical evaluation of an acellular allograft dermal matrix in full-thickness burns. J Burn Care Rehabil 1996; 17:124–136.

54. Lattari V, Jones LM, Varcelotti JR, Latenser BA, Sherman HF, Barrette RR. The use of a permanent dermal allograft in full-thickness burns of the hand and foot: a report of three cases. J Burn Care Rehabil 1997; 18:147–155.

55. Livesey SA, Herndon DA, Hollyoak MA, Atkinson YH, Nag A. Transplanted acellular allograft dermal matrix. Transplantation 1995; 60:1–9.

56. Rennekampff HO, Kiessig V, Griffey S, Greenleaf G, Hansbrough JF. Acellular human dermis promotes cultured keratinocytes engraftment. J Burn Care Rehabil 1997; 18:535–544.

57. Oddesey R. Addendum: Multicenter experiences with cultured epidermal autograft for treatment of burns. J Burn Care Rehabil 1992; 13:174–180.

58. Langdon RC, Cuono CB, Birchall N, Madri JA, Kuklinska E, McGuire J, Moellmann GE. Reconstitution of structure and cell function in human skin grafts derived from cryopreserved allogeneic dermis and autologous cultured keratinocytes. J Invest Dermatol 1988; 91:478–485.

59. Krejci NC, Cuono CB, Langdon RC, McGuire J. In vitro reconstitution of skin: fibroblasts facilitate keratinocyte growth and differentiation on acellular reticular dermis. J Invest Dermatol 1991; 97(5):843–848.

60. Yannas IV, Burke JF. Deisgn of an artificial skin. I. Design principles. J Biomed Mater Res 1980; 14:65–81.

61. Yannas IV, Burke JF, Gordon PL, Huang C, Rubinstein RH. Design of an artificial skin. II. Control of chemical composition. J Biomed Mater Res 1980; 14:107–132.

62. Dagalakis N, Flink J, Stasikelis P, Burke JF, Yannas IV. Design of an artificial skin. III. Control of pore structure. J Biomed Mater Res 1980; 14:511–528.

63. Yannas IV, Burke JF, Orgill DP, Skrabut EM. Wound tissue can utilize a polymeric template to synthesize a functional extension of skin. Science 1982; 215:174–176.

64. Burke JF, Yannas IV, Quinby WC Jr, Bondoc CC, Jung WK. Successful use of a physiologically acceptable artificial skin in the treatment of extensive skin injury. Ann Surg 1981; 194:413–428.

65. Yannas IV, Lee E, Orgill DP, Skrabut EM, Murphy GF. Synthesis and characterization of a model extracellular matrix that induces partial regeneration of adult mammalian skin. Proc Natl Acad Sci USA 1989; 86:933–937.

66. Ferdman AG, Yannas IV. Scattering of light from histologic sections: a new method for the analysis of connective tissue. J Invest Dermatol 1993; 100(5):710–716.

67. Murphy GF, Orgill DP, Yannas IV. Partial dermal regeneration is induced by biodegradable collagen-glycosaminoglycan grafts. Lab Invest 1990; 63(3):305–313.

68. Orgill DP, Butler CE, Regan JF, Barlow MS, Yannas IV. Behavior of collagen-GAG matrices as dermal replacement in rodent and porcine models. Wounds 1996; 8(5):151–157.

69. Heimbach D, Luterman A, Burke J, Cram A, Herndon D, Hurt J, Jordan M, McManus W, Solem L, Warden G, et al. Artificial dermis for major burns: a multicenter randomized trial. Ann Surg 1988; 208:313–320.

70. Ellis DL, Yannas IV. Recent advances in tissue synthesis in vivo by use of collagen-glycosaminoglycan copolymers. Biomaterials 1996; 17:291–299.
71. Orgill DP, Butler CE, Regan JF, Barlow MS, Yannas IV, Compton CC. A vascularized collagen-GAG matrix provides a dermal substrate and improves take of cultured epithelial autografts. J Plast Reconstr Surg. Accepted.
72. Compton CC, Butler CE, Yannas IV, Warland G, Orgill DP. Organized skin structure is regenerated in vivo from collagen-GAG matrices seeded with autologous keratinocytes. J Invest Dermatol 1998; 110:908–916.
73. Butler CE, Orgill DP, Yannas IV, Compton CC. The effect of keratinocyte seeding of collagen-glycoaminoglycan membranes on the regeneration of skin in a porcine model. Plast Reconstr Surg 1998; 6:1572–1579.
74. Orgill DP, Yannas IV. Design of an artificial skin. IV. Use of island graft to isolate organ regeneration from scar synthesis and other processes leading to skin wound closure. J Biomed Mater Res 1998; 39:531–535.
75. VanLuyn MJ, Verheul J, VanWachem PB. Regeneration of full-thickness wounds using collagen split grafts. J Biomed Mater Res 1995; 29:1425–1436.
76. Koide M, Osaki K, Konishi J, Oyamada K, Katakura T, Takahashi A, Yoshizato K. A new type of biomaterial for artificial skin: dehydrothermally cross-linked composites of fibrillar and denatured collagens. J Biomed Mater Res 1993; 27:79–87.
77. Matsui R, Okura N, Osaki K, Konishi J, Ikegami K, Koide M. Histological evaluation of skin reconstruction using artificial dermis. Biomaterials 1996; 17:995–1000.
78. Matsuda K, Suzuki S, Isshiki N, Yoshioka K, Okada T, Ikada Y. Influence of glycosaminoglycans on the collagen sponge component of a bilayer artificial skin. Biomaterials 1990; 11:351–355.
79. Suzuki S, Matsuda K, Maruguchi T, Nishimura Y, Ikada Y. Further applications of ''bilayer artificial skin.'' Br J Plast Surg 1995; 48:222–229.
80. Matsuda K, Suzuki S, Isshiki N, Yoshioka K, Hyon SH, Ikada Y. A bilayer ''artificial skin'' capable of sustained release of an antibiotic. Br J Plast Surg 1991; 44:142–146.
81. Cooper ML, Andree L, Hansbrough JF, Zapata-Sirvent RL, Spielvogel RL. Direct comparison of a cultured composite skin substitute containing human keratinocytes and fibroblasts to an epidermal sheet graft containing human keratinocytes on athymic mice. J Invest Dermatol 1993; 101:811–819.
82. Hansbrough JF, Boyce ST, Cooper ML, Foreman TJ. Burn wound closure with cultured autologous keratinocytes and fibroblasts attached to a collagen glycosaminoglycan substrate. JAMA 1989; 262:2125–2130.
83. Boyce ST, Foreman TJ, English KB, Stayner N, Cooper ML, Sakabu S, Hansbrough JF. Skin wound closure in athymic mice with cultured human cells, biopolymers, and growth factors. Surgery 1991; 110:866–876.
84. Naughton G, Mansbridge J, Gentzkow G. A metabolically active human dermal replacement for the treatment of diabetic foot ulcers. Artif Organs 1997; 21(11):1203–1210.
85. Hansbrough JF, Cooper ML, Cohen R, Spielvogel R, Greenleaf G, Bartel RL, Naughton G. Evaluation of a biodegradable matrix containing cultured human fibroblasts as a dermal replacement beneath meshed skin grafts on athymic mice. Surgery 1992; 111:438–446.

86. Bell E, Ehrlich P, Buttle DJ, Nakatsuji T. Living tissue formed in vitro and accepted as skin-equivalent of full thickness. Science 1981; 221:1052–1054.

87. Nolte CJM, Oleson MA, Bilbo PR, Parenteau NL. Development of a stratum corneum and barrier function in an organotypic skin culture. Arch Dermatol Res 1993; 285:466–474.

88. Parenteau NL, Bilbo P, Nolte CJ, Mason VS, Rosenberg M. The organotypic culture of human skin keratinocytes and fibroblasts to achieve form and function. Cytotechnology 1992; 9:163–171.

89. Nolte CJM, Oleson MA, Hansbrough JF, Morgan J, Greenleaf F, Wilkins L. Ultrastructural features of composite skin cultures grafted onto athymic mice. J Anat 1994; 185:325–333.

90. Hansbrough JF, Morgan J, Greenleaf G, Parikh M, Nolte C, Wilkins L. Evaluation of Graftskin composite grafts on full-thickness wounds on athymic mice. J Burn Care Rehab 1994; 15:346–353.

91. Wilkins LM, Watson SR, Prosky SJ, Meunier SF, Parenteau NL. Development of a bilayered living skin construct for clinical applications. Biotechnol Bioeng 1994; 43:747–756.

92. Eaglstein WH, Iriondo M, Laszlo K. A composite skin substitute (Graftskin) for surgical wounds: a clinical experience. Dermatol Surg 1995; 21:839–843.

93. Sabolinski ML, Alvarez O, Auletta M, Mulder G, Parenteau NL. Cultured skin as a 'smart material' for healing wounds: experience in venous ulcers. Biomat 1996; 17(3):311–320.

94. Salzberg CA, Norris J, Carr J. Use of a biological dressing for the early treatment of deep partial thickness burns. American Burn Association Meeting, New York, NY: March, 1997.

95. Mackie DP. The Euro Skin Bank: Development and application of glycerol-preserved allografts. J Burn Care Rehabil 1997; 18 Suppl 1:7–9.

96. Kaiser HW, Stark GB, Kopp J, Balcerkiewicz A, Spilker G, Kreysel HW. Cultured autologous keratinocytes in fibrin glue suspension, exclusively and combined with STS-allograft (preliminary clinical and histological report of a new technique). Burns 1994; 20(1):23–29.

97. Stark GB, Kaiser HW. Cologne Burn Centre experience with glycerol-preserved allogeneic skin. Part II. Combination with autologous cultured keratinocytes. Burns 1994; 20 Suppl 1:S34–S38.

98. Kuroyanagi Y, Kenmochi M, Ishihara S, Takeda A, Shiraishi A, Ootake N, Uchinuma E, Torikai K, Shioya N. A cultured skin substitute composed of fibroblasts and keratinocytes with a collagen matrix: preliminary results of clinical trials. Ann Plast Surg 1993; 31:340–349.

15

Hyaluronan-Based Membrane for the Prevention of Postsurgical Adhesions

James W. Burns and Kevin J. Barry
Genzyme Corporation, Cambridge, Massachusetts

I. INTRODUCTION

Postsurgical adhesions are abnormal unions of normally separated internal tissue and organ surfaces. Adhesions are reported to develop in 55 to 97% of surgical procedures in the abdominal and pelvic cavities (1,2). Although they do not always result in clinical problems requiring reoperation, adhesions are responsible for approximately 74% of small-bowel obstructions (3), and are a primary factor in postsurgical infertility in women (4,5). An estimated 5% of all abdominal surgical procedures will require reoperation due to complications caused by adhesion (6). The cost of treating adhesions surgically is extraordinary. In 1994, there were 303,836 surgical procedures in the United States for lysis of adhesions at a total hospitalization and surgical cost of $1.3 billion (7). Successfully limiting postsurgical adhesion development could significantly improve patient morbidity and, in the long term, lower health care costs.

II. PERITONEAL REPAIR AND ADHESION FORMATION

The general events in peritoneal wound healing injury that lead to adhesion development are shown in Figure 1. The peritoneum is a serous membrane that lines the wall of the abdomen and is reflected over the viscera (8–11). It consists of mesothelial cells in a continuous layer that rests upon loose mesenchymal tissue,

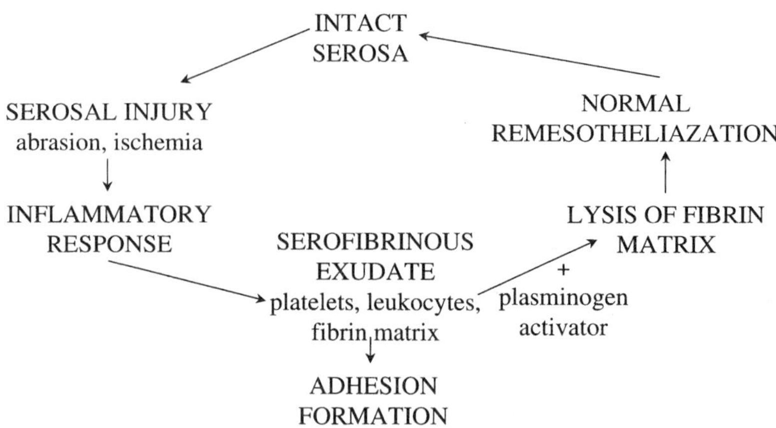

Figure 1 Schematic of peritoneal repair process following surgical injury.

basal lamina, and basement membrane. The loose mesenchymal tissue contains blood vessels, collagen and elastin fibers, fibroblasts, macrophages, lymphocytes, plasma cells, mast cells, adipocytes, and blood vessels. Peritoneal healing occurs differently from that of skin. As early as 1919, Hertzler (12) noticed that peritoneal defects heal uniformly throughout the defect and not just from the borders. Tissue injury, the initial step in adhesion formation, results in release of chemical mediators that affect vasopermeability and chemotaxis of tissue repair cells. These mediators include activating factors, such as prostaglandins, lymphokines, and lysozymes; chemotactic agents, which induce collagen formation and activate macrophages that attract leukocytes and lymphocytes to the injured area; permeability factors, such as bradykinin, serotonin, and histamine, which increase the passage of fibrinous exudate onto the damaged tissue surface; and tissue thromboplastin, which initiates the clotting cascade. These substances cause an increase in capillary permeability that leads to the formation of a serosanguineous exudate, which in turn results in fibrin deposition. Fibrinolysis is vital to remove the fibrin matrix and to allow normal remesothelialization to occur. In the absence of normal mesothelial cells or under ischemic conditions, the tissue's inherent fibrinolytic capacity is significantly diminished. As a result, the fibrin structure persists and becomes infiltrated with fibroblasts, which synthesize collagen to form permanent adhesions.

The various therapeutic approaches aimed at preventing postsurgical adhesion formation have focused on the different stages of adhesion development, outlined in Figure 1, and have included the use of pharmacological agents, such as antihistamines, heparin, corticosteroids, tissue plasminogen activator, nonsteroidal antiinflammatories, and barriers, such as polymer solutions and bioresorbable membranes.

Barriers present distinct advantages over pharmacological agents when used for adhesion prevention. Pharmacological agents are typically applied in solution to the general surgical field at the end of the procedure. When used in this manner, the agent affects wound healing in a non–site-specific manner. While pharmacological agents may mitigate adhesion formation at severely injured sites, they may adversely affect normal wound healing in less traumatized areas. In addition, the systemic activity of a pharmacological agent is difficult to control. It can also be difficult to maintain a concentration of a pharmacological agent sufficient to prevent adhesion formation, which may account for the ambiguous results often seen with their use in animal studies.

III. BARRIER METHODS FOR ADHESION PREVENTION

Barrier methods for preventing surgical adhesions are intended to separate damaged tissue surfaces during the critical early days of tissue repair when adhesions form. In animal models of peritoneal repair, reperitonealization appears to be substantially complete by 8 days after injury (10,11). It appears that adhesions permanently develop by 3 days following injury. Thus, the likelihood of forming permanent interconnecting fibrous bands between tissue surfaces is significantly reduced after approximately 3 days. For barriers to adhesion formation to be effective, they should not resorb substantially prior to 3 days after placement.

Natural and synthetic materials have been developed to mechanically separate visceral and parietal peritoneum during reperitonealization, such as oxidized regenerated cellulose (ORC), and GORE-TEX® (polytetrafluoroethylene [PTFE]). Early in the development of barriers, allograft amniotic membranes and free grafts of omentum were investigated for decreasing intraabdominal adhesion formation (13,14). These barriers were ineffective, and in some cases increased adhesion formation.

GORE-TEX Surgical Membrane (W.L. Gore, Flagstaff, Arizona), specifically designed to discourage cellular penetration and tissue attachment, has been used as a pericardial membrane substitute in cardiovascular surgery (15,16). At reoperation, the Surgical Membrane limited the adhesion formation to the epicardial–pericardial surfaces and induced no foreign body response. In a multicenter clinical study treating moderate to severe pelvic adhesions in women, adhesions were lysed and the GORE-TEX Surgical Membrane was implanted over the peritoneal defect. At a second-look laparoscopy, adhesion formation at the healed defect was reduced (17).

Interceed® (TC7) barrier (Ethicon, Rariton, New Jersey), is formulated from oxidized regenerated cellulose and is indicated as an adjuvant in gynecological surgery for reducing the incidence of adhesion formation. In a prospective, randomized, well-controlled, multicenter clinical trial, Interceed (TC7) was shown to be effective in reducing the incidence, extent, and severity of adhesions in 134 women with bilateral pelvic sidewall adhesions undergoing reproductive pelvic surgery (18).

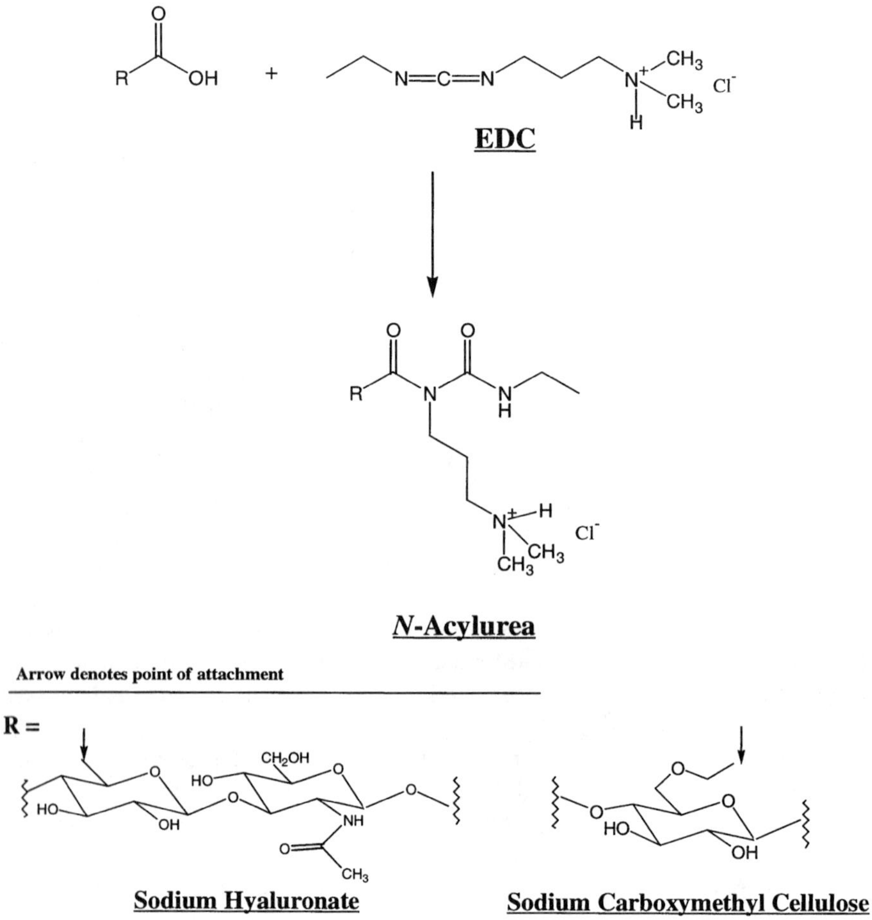

Figure 2 Chemical modification of sodium hyaluronate and CMC. The reaction with 1-(3-dimethylaminopropyl)-3-ethylcarbodiimide and subsequent rearrangement to *N*-acylurea renders a proportion of the carboxylate groups cationic. An ionic association between the negatively charged carboxylate groups and the positively charged *N*-acylurea groups slows down gel resorption from the peritoneum.

Seprafilm® Bioresorbable Membrane (Genzyme Surgical Products, Cambridge, MA) is composed of a matrix of sodium hyaluronate (HA) and carboxymethylcellulose (CMC) that has been chemically modified with 1-(3-dimethyl-aminopropyl)-3-ethyl-carbodiimide (EDC) (Fig. 2). Hyaluronate is a naturally occurring anionic polysaccharide consisting of repeat units of 1,3-linked *N*-acetyl-D-glucosamine and 1,4-linked D-glucuronic acid. Hyaluronate is found throughout mammalian extracellular matrix and has a number of biological functions involved in cell migration, angiogenesis, and wound repair (19–21). Carboxymethylcellulose, also an anionic polysaccharide, is a derivatized form of cellulose in which the glucosidic hydroxyl groups have been carboxymethylated, rendering the polymer water-soluble. Hyaluronate and CMC, when chemically modified by reaction with EDC, associate in such a way as to form a water-insoluble complex (22). The insoluble HA/CMC complex can be formed into a membrane suitable for placement on injured tissue surfaces. Although Seprafilm has reduced water solubility compared with native hyaluronic acid and carboxymethylcellulose, it bioresorbs in vivo within 28 days after implantation (23).

IV. PRECLINICAL STUDIES OF SEPRAFILM

A. Preclinical Efficacy

Preclinical studies have shown that Seprafilm significantly reduces the incidence and severity of postsurgical adhesions following a variety of surgical trauma. The ability of Seprafilm to reduce adhesion development was evaluated in a number of different in vivo efficacy studies that present a range of peritoneal injuries that could occur during abdominopelvic surgery.

The first study employed a rat cecal abrasion model (23). In this model, the cecum of each rat was abraded with surgical gauze in a standardized fashion to induce mesothelial damage and petechial bleeding. This model consistently causes significant adhesions in control animals. Seprafilm was applied to the ceca of treatment animals, while control animals received no treatment. The results of this study showed that the use of Seprafilm resulted in fewer significant adhesions and fewer adhesions of all grades, as well as a greater number of animals with no adhesions (Table 1).

A second study addressed a potential clinical situation by evaluating the effects of residual irrigation solutions on the adhesion reduction efficacy of Seprafilm. Although it is not recommended to leave irrigation fluid in the abdominal cavity when using Seprafilm, we wished to determine whether excess fluid might increase the resorption rate of Seprafilm and decrease its effectiveness. Four milliliters of saline or lactated Ringer's solution were instilled into the abdominal cavity following a standardized cecal abrasion procedure. In the appropriate treatment groups, Seprafilm was applied to the ceca. The results of this study showed

Table 1 Efficacy of Seprafilm Bioresorbable Membrane in a Rat Cecal Abrasion Model

	Control group (n = 39)[a,b]	Seprafilm group (n = 40)[a,b]
Mean (SEM) incidence of adhesions	1.9 (0.2)	0.2 (0.1)
No adhesions	3 (8)	32 (80)
Adhesions grades 2–4	36 (92)	3 (8)

[a] Figures are number (%) of animals with adhesions unless otherwise stated.
[b] All comparisons are significant ($P < 0.0001$).

that the presence of two common surgical irrigants following surgery did not adversely affect the efficacy of the Seprafilm adhesion barrier in a cecal abrasion model (Table 2).

Adhesion re-formation following adhesiolysis may be more difficult to prevent due to a more aggressive inflammatory response than occurs following de novo peritoneal injury. We therefore have examined the effect of Seprafilm on adhesion re-formation employing the rat cecal abrasion model. This study involved a modified cecal abrasion procedure in a three-stage experiment, which allowed for 1) the formation of adhesions as a result of cecal abrasion, followed by 2) lysis and placement of Seprafilm, and finally 3) evaluation of adhesion re-formation. The results of this study indicated that, following adhesiolysis, Seprafilm effectively reduced the mean incidence of adhesions of all types as well as the percentage of animals with significant adhesions compared with the non-

Table 2 Efficacy of the Seprafilm Bioresorbable Membrane in the Presence of 0.9% Saline Solution

	No treatment[a,b]	Seprafilm alone[a,b]	Seprafilm + saline[a,b]	Saline alone[a,b]
Mean (SEM) incidence of adhesions	1.9 (0.3)	0.3 (0.2)[c]	0.3 (0.2)[c]	1.9 (0.3)
No adhesions	0	7[d]	7[d]	2
Adhesions grades 2–4	10	2[e]	1[f]	8

[a] Figures are number of animals with adhesions unless otherwise stated.
[b] n = 10.
[c] $P < 0.001$ v. control or saline alone (Tukey-Kramer test).
[d] $P = 0.003$ v. no treatment and 0.07 v. saline alone.
[e] $P = 0.0007$ v. no treatment and 0.02 v. saline alone.
[f] $P = 0.001$ v. no treatment and 0.0055 v. saline alone (Fisher's exact test).

Table 3 Effect of Seprafilm Bioresorbable Membrane on Adhesion Re-Formation in the Rat Cecal Abrasion Model

Treatment group	Mean incidence ± SEM (n = 18)	% Animals with no adhesions (n = 18)
Group assignment following scoring seven days after cecal abrasion		
Control	1.6 ± 0.2[a]	0 (0/18)
Seprafilm	1.7 ± 0.2[a]	0 (0/18)
Adhesions scored following adhesiolysis and Seprafilm placement		
Control	1.3 ± 0.2[b]	28 (5/18)[c]
Seprafilm	0.3 ± 0.1[b]	72 (13/18)[c]

[a] $P > 0.05$ Mann Whitney rank sum analysis and chi square analysis.
[b] $P < 0.003$ Mann Whitney rank sum analysis.
[c] $P = 0.007$ chi square analysis.

treated control (Table 3). Seprafilm also significantly increased the percentage of treated animals with no adhesions.

In addition to adhesiolysis, another potent stimulus to adhesion development is tissue ischemia. We therefore developed a peritoneal wall defect model, which included placing nonabsorbable sutures around the 1- × 1-cm raw deperitonealized surface of the lateral abdominal wall of rats. Following tissue injury, animals randomly received either Seprafilm over the defect or nothing. Adhesions were scored based on extent, type, and tenacity 1 week following the procedure. The results of this study showed that the use of Seprafilm adhesion barrier significantly reduced the composite adhesion score of extent, type, and severity, and significantly increased the percentage of animals with no adhesions in the treated group relative to the nontreated controls (Table 4).

Other investigators have evaluated Seprafilm membrane in more aggressive models involving hernia repair. The presence of a persistent foreign body, such as a polypropylene mesh, is a potent stimulator to inflammation and adhesion

Table 4 Effect of Seprafilm Bioabsorable Membrane on Adhesion Reduction in the Rat Sidewall Injury Model

Group	Mean composite score ± SEM (n = 15)	% Animals with no adhesions (n = 15)
Control	6.3 ± 1.0	20.0 (3/15)
Seprafilm	1.8 ± 0.8[a]	73.3[b] (11/15)

[a] $P < 0.01$ chi square analysis.
[b] $P < 0.005$ Wilcoxon's rank sum analysis.

formation. In studies by Alponat et al. (24) and Hooker et al. (25), Seprafilm was placed between a polypropylene mesh used to repair abdominal wall defects and the underlying viscera. In the Hooker study, animals were reoperated and adhesions to the mesh scored at 4 to 8 weeks after surgery. Seprafilm significantly reduced adhesion development to the mesh (Fig. 3); additionally, Hooker et al. showed that Seprafilm had no adverse effect on tissue incorporation into the mesh. Interestingly, this effect persisted well after the Seprafilm was gone, indicating that the hernia repair mesh does not continue to stimulate adhesion development beyond the initial period of inflammation.

B. Preclinical Safety

Seprafilm has been evaluated in a standard battery of device safety studies, which have demonstrated that Seprafilm membrane is nontoxic, nonimmunogenic, and biocompatible (Table 5). Because HA is ubiquitous throughout the extracellular matrix and is involved in the normal wound repair process, we have examined the potential effect that Seprafilm might have on peritoneal repair.

Employing the rat cecal abrasion model, we studied histologically the effect of Seprafilm on injured peritoneum over 28 days. Seprafilm was placed on the abraded cecum, and the cecum was returned to the abdominal cavity. Ceca were harvested from 2 to 28 days after abrasion, fixed in formalin, and stained with hematoxylin and eosin. At 2 days, large numbers of inflammatory cells were apparent in animals treated with Seprafilm as well as the abraded control animals, although there may have been more macrophages present in the Seprafilm group

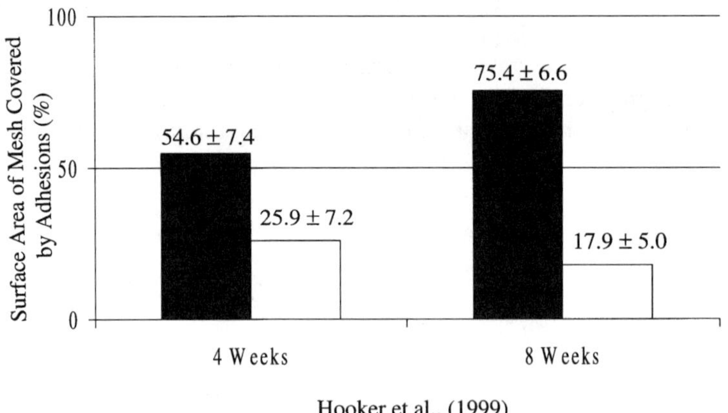

Figure 3 Effect of Seprafilm on adhesion formation to Marlex mesh in rat hernia models. (From Ref. 25.)

Table 5 Seprafilm Bioresorbable Membrane, Nonclinical Safety Studies

Study	Results
Ames mutagenicity	Not mutagenic
USP pyrogen	Not mutagenic
Intracutaneous toxicity	Nonirritant/not toxic
Acute toxicity—Intraperitoneal	Not toxic
Systemic toxicity	Not toxic
Maximization/dermal sensitization	Not a sensitizer
Systemic antigenicity	Non antigenic
Muscle implantation (7-day and 30-day)	Slight irritant
Hemolysis	Non hemolytic
Complement activation	Unreactive
Cytotoxic response in agar overlay and muscle implant studies	Not toxic unreactive
Cytotoxicity of Seprafilm	Not toxic
Disposition and excretion of radioactivity after peritoneal injection	> 90% of Seprafilm cleared in 28 days following IP implantation
Chromosomal aberration	No effect
Sister chromatid exchange	No effect
Effect on healing of bowel anastomosis	No effect

due to phagocytosis of the HA/CMC (Fig. 4). At day 7, granulation tissue began to develop in both treated and untreated tissues with no foreign body giant cells observed (Fig. 5). However, granulation in the untreated tissue group tended to be more organized. By 28 days, abraded ceca were healed in both untreated and Seprafilm-treated tissues (Fig. 6). Again, the granulation tissue of the untreated animals appeared denser than that of the Seprafilm-treated animals.

One of the most significant concerns for abdominal surgeons in using an adhesion prevention product that might affect wound healing is the integrity of intestinal anastomoses. The safety of Seprafilm was therefore evaluated in a rabbit large-bowel anastomosis model employing a complete (100%) anastomosis with minimal contamination, and a partial (90%) anastomosis with resulting leak in bacterial contamination (26). Sixty-four New Zealand white rabbits were randomly divided into two equal groups. Each of these groups was further subdivided into a treated group that had Seprafilm membrane wrapped around the anastomosis prior to closure and an untreated control group. Animals were sacrificed and assessed at either 7 or 14 days following surgery. The potential effect of Seprafilm was determined by measuring the hydrostatic bursting pressures of the anastomotic repairs. The results of the study showed that Seprafilm had no significant effect on bowel bursting pressure among the membrane-treated anasto-

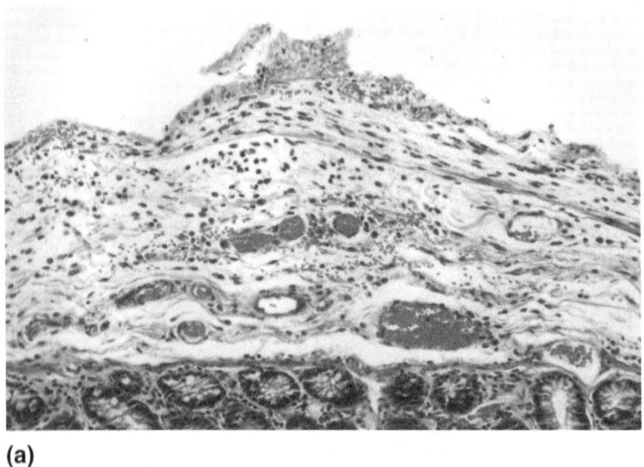

(a)

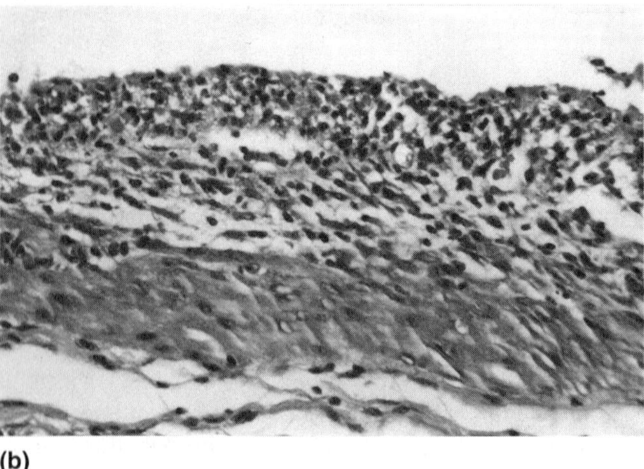

(b)

Figure 4   (a) Micrograph of peritoneum from untreated sidewall two days after injury.
(b) Micrograph of peritoneum from the HA/CMC bioresorbable membrane-treated sidewall two days after injury. (Magnification $\times$ 100.)

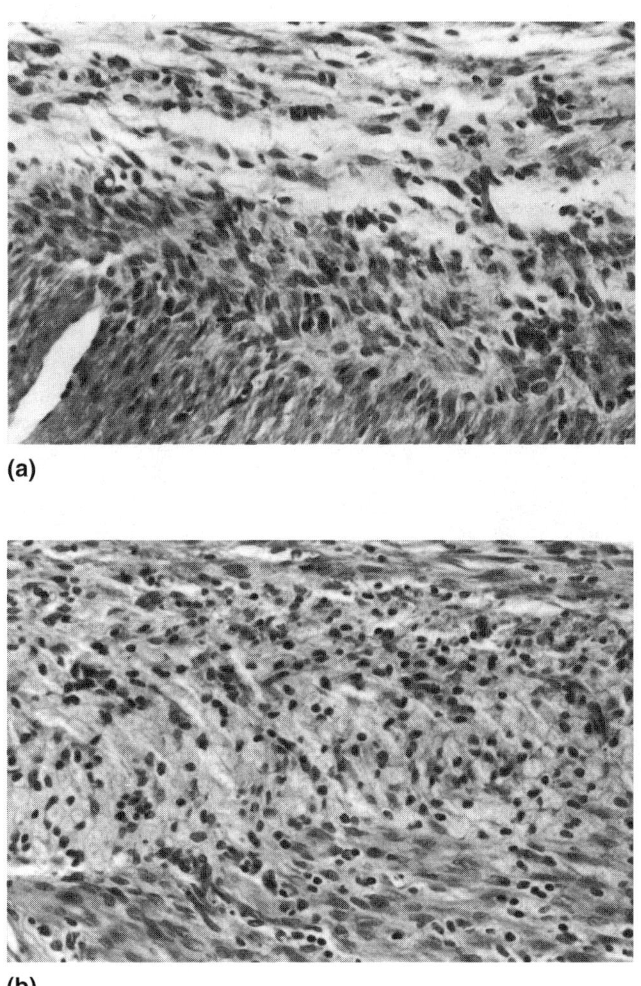

(a)

(b)

Figure 5 (a) Micrograph of peritoneum from untreated sidewall seven days after injury. (Bottom) Micrograph of peritoneum from HA/CMC bioresorbable membrane-treated sidewall seven days after injury. (Magnification $\times$ 100.)

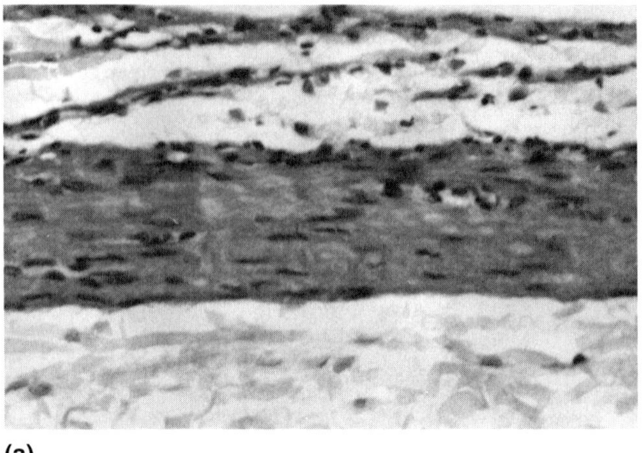

(a)

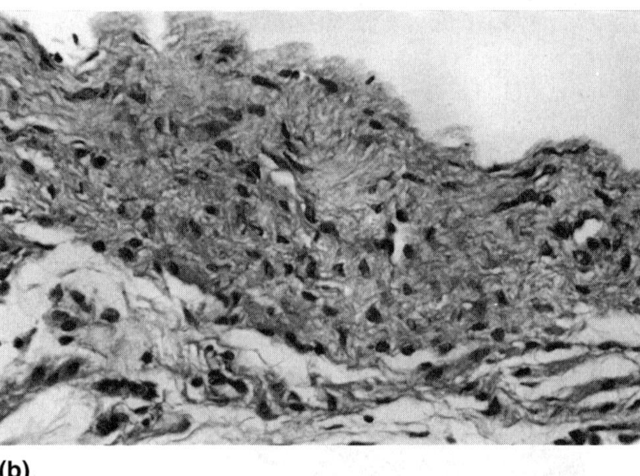

(b)

Figure 6   (a) Micrograph of peritoneum from untreated sidewall 28 days after injury. (b) Micrograph of peritoneum from HA/CMC bioresorbable membrane-treated sidewall 28 days after injury. (Magnification × 100.)

moses in either the complete or partial anastomoses groups at 7 and 14 days. Additionally, in the complete anastomoses group, Seprafilm reduced the incidence of anastomotic adhesions, however, it had no effect on adhesion reduction at the anastomoses that had been closed only 90%. Thus, in the situation in which the bowel does leak, inducing a highly inflammatory response, Seprafilm does not prevent the "good" adhesions that might contain the bacterial contamination locally.

IV. CLINICAL EVALUATIONS OF SEPRAFILM

To date, Seprafilm has been evaluated in two prospective randomized, masked, multicenter clinical studies involving patients undergoing either a total colectomy for Crohn's disease or familial polyposis (abdominal surgery model) or myomectomy (pelvic surgery model).

A. Abdominal Study

A total of 183 patients, 91 Seprafilm and 92 nontreatment patients, with either ulcerative colitis or familial polyposis, were enrolled in this study (27). Overall, the demographic characteristics of both Seprafilm and nontreatment groups were comparable. In the Seprafilm group, the membrane was applied on the omentum and viscera directly under the abdominal midline incision just before abdominal cavity closure. The mean total quantity of Seprafilm membrane applied in the treatment patients was 406.9 cm^2. One or more adverse events were reported by 82 of 91 patients (90%).

The most commonly reported adverse events in both groups were nausea, abdominal pain, and fever (Table 6). No adverse events were judged as directly related to Seprafilm. Sixty serious adverse events were reported and were judged as not related to the use of Seprafilm. Comparison of the incidence of specific adverse events between the treatment groups did not identify a significant difference ($P > 0.05$ Fisher's exact test). Changes in postoperative vital signs and laboratory values were reported in both the Seprafilm treatment and nontreatment groups. Most abnormal values were consistent with the effects of surgery or the patient's medical condition.

The number of patients who had adhesions at the site of membrane use was reduced by 45% in those treated with Seprafilm. No adhesions were observed in 51% of patients treated with Seprafilm, while only 6% of nontreated patients had no adhesions to the midline incision (Table 7). The incidence of patients with one or more adhesions to the midline incision was significantly reduced from 94% in the nontreatment patients, to 49% in the Seprafilm group ($P < 0.0001$, Fisher's exact test). The overall mean extent of adhesion (percentage of the incision length involved) among Seprafilm patients was 23%, significantly less than in the nontreatment group, 63% ($P < 0.0001$, Student's t-test). In addition, the evaluation of severity of adhesions demonstrated that 90% of the nontreatment patients, as compared with only 35% of the Seprafilm patients, had one or more adhesions that was assessed as grade 2 or 3, on a standardized grading

Table 6 Incidence of Adverse Events

Adverse event	Control group (n = 92)		Seprafilm group (n = 91)	
	n	%	n	%
Overall	86	93.5	82	90.1
Nausea	41	44.6	31	34.1
Abdominal pain	23	25.0	26	28.6
Fever	22	23.9	22	24.2
Rash	16	17.4	17	18.7
Vomiting	12	13.0	14	15.4
Nausea and vomiting	17	18.5	13	14.3
Gastrointestinal distress	12	13.0	11	12.1
Dehydration	13	14.1	11	12.1
Pruritus	13	14.1	11	12.1
Infection	9	9.8	10	11.0
Pain	16	17.4	10	11.0
Small-bowel obstruction	11	12.0	9	9.9
Paresthesia	10	10.9	8	8.8
Abscess	2	2.2	7	7.7
Ileus	6	65	6	6.6
Deep vein thrombosis	2	2.2	3	3.3
Pulmonary embolis	0	0.0	4	4.3
Sepsis	1	1.1	1	1.1
Death	0	0.0	1	1.1

scale of 1 (filmy, avascular), 2 (moderate thickness, limited vascularity), or 3 (dense thickness, vascularized). Overall, if adhesions were present in the Seprafilm group at all, they were significantly less severe than in the nontreatment group ($P < 0.0001$, Wilcoxon rank sum). Not surprisingly, the omentum was the most frequent structure adhered to the midline incision. Of significant interest is that even with the presence of the omentum, 65% of control patients had small bowel adhered to the midline incision. Importantly, Seprafilm reduced small-bowel adhesion to the midline to only 26% (Table 8).

B. Pelvic Study

The second clinical study with Seprafilm was conducted in female infertility patients having a myomectomy by laparotomy (28). Following myomectomy, patients underwent second-look laparoscopy and were subsequently evaluated via video for postoperative adhesion formation by an evaluator without knowledge

Table 7 Incidence, Extent, and Severity of Postoperative Adhesion Formation to the Midline Incision

	Control group (n = 90)		Seprafilm group (n = 85)		
	n	%	n	%	P value
Incidence					
No adhesions	5	6	43	51	<0.0001[a]
Adhesions	85	94	42	49	
Extent[b]					
All patients	90	63 ± 34	85	28 ± 34	<0.0001[c]
Patients with adhesions	85	67 ± 31	42	48 ± 34	=0.0008[c]
Severity[d]					
No adhesions	5	6	43	51	<0.001[e]
Grade 1	4	4	12	14	
Grade 2	29	32	17	20	
Grade 3	52	58	13	15	

[a] Fisher's exact test.

[b] The proportion of the total length of the initial surgery midline incision associated with any adhesions, as determined by dividing the length associated with adhesions (cm) by the overall length of the initial midline incision (cm). Data are reported as mean ± SD.

[c] Student's t-test.

[d] Grade 1, filmy thickness, avascular; grade 2, moderate thickness, limited vascularity; grade 3, dense thickness, vascularized.

[e] Wilcoxon's rank sum test.

of treatment status. Efficacy was assessed by a masked expert independent observer using videotapes obtained by laparoscopy at second-look surgery.

The total patient population in this study was 127 patients, 59 Seprafilm and 68 nontreatment patients. All of the 127 patients enrolled in the study had a history of uterine fibroids. One or more adverse events were reported in 58 of the 59 (98.3%) Seprafilm patients and in 67 of the 68 (98.5%) nontreatment patients. Pain (unspecified), fever, abdominal pain, and nausea were the most frequently reported adverse events in both treatment groups. There were no statistically significant differences in the overall incidence of adverse events between the treatment groups when evaluated by specific term. All adverse events listed are recognized complications of the surgical procedure and/or existing comorbid disease. No adverse event was considered to be definitely related to the study device. Five patients, two (3.4%) Seprafilm patients (patients 0112 and 0603) and three (4.4%) nontreatment patients (patients 0703, 0705, and 1102) had a total of six serious adverse events.

There were no significant differences between the patients treated with

Table 8 Distribution of Midline Adhesions to Intraabdominal Sites

	Control group (n = 90)		Seprafilm group (n = 85)		
	n	%	n	%	P value[a]
Omentum	71	79	33	39	0.00000005
Small bowel	57	63	21	25	0.0000002
Abdominal sidewall, left	19	21	2	2	0.00008
Bladder	11	12	3	4	0.031
Ileostomy	15	17	6	7	0.041
Stomach	12	13	4	5	0.041
Ileal pouch	5	6	1	1	0.119
Abdominal sidewall, right	12	13	8	9	0.283
Fallopian tube, right	4	4	2	2	0.368
Fallopian tube, left	4	4	2	2	0.368
Ovary, left	4	4	2	2	0.368
Ovary, right	3	3	2	2	0.527
Liver	7	8	6	7	0.543
Other	1	1	5	6	0.988

[a] Fisher's exact test.

Seprafilm and those in the untreated group at baseline in either demographic or intraoperative factors. The mean time to evaluation at second-look surgery was identical in both groups (23 postoperative days). Studies have suggested that no change in adhesion incidence, extent, or severity occurs after 7 postoperative days (29). In this clinical study, no difference in adhesion incidence or severity was witnessed between days 7 and 70. Adhesion extent on the posterior uterine surface was found to be affected but the treatment effect of Seprafilm was unchanged.

Of 119 women who completed the trial and were eligible for analysis, Seprafilm patients (n = 54) had an overall significant reduction in uterine adhesion versus nontreatment patients (n = 65) as determined by incidence, extent, severity, and area (Fig. 7). The mean number of sites adherent to the uterine surface in the Seprafilm group was 4.98 compared with 7.88 in the nontreatment group ($P < 0.0001$). The mean severity score was reduced to 1.9 in Seprafilm patients versus 2.43 in the nontreatment group ($P = 0.0022$). The mean extent score was 1.23 among the Seprafilm patients and 1.68 in nontreatment patients ($P = 0.0025$). The mean area involved with adhesions at second look was more than a third greater in nontreatment patients (18.7 cm^2) than in Seprafilm patients (13.2 cm^2, $P = 0.0113$). Importantly, significant reductions in adhesions for each of

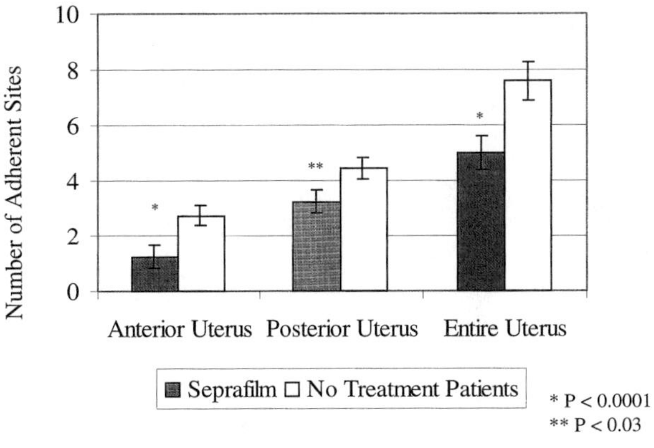

(a)

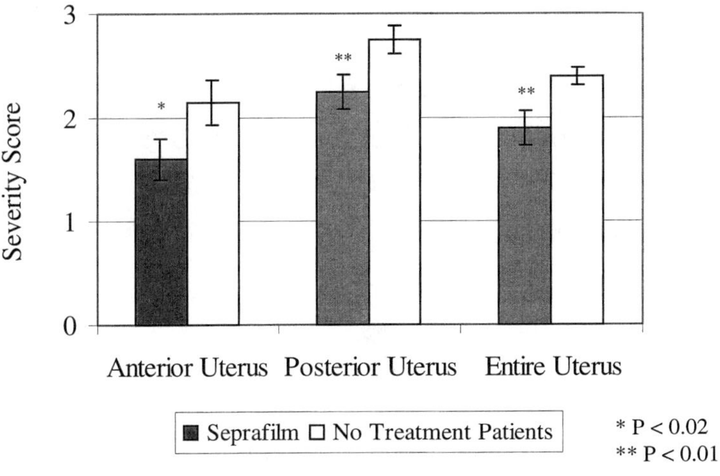

(b)

Figure 7 Adhesions at second-look laparoscopy. (a) Number of adherent sites, mean ± SEM. (b) Severity of adhesion formation, mean ± SEM. (c) Extent of adhesion formation, mean ± SEM. (d) Area of uterine surface involved with adhesions, mean ± SEM.

these determinations were present on both the anterior and posterior aspects of the uterus.

The dramatic reduction of incisional adhesions to the anterior uterus as confirmed by the reviewer and the principal investigators more accurately demonstrates the efficacy of Seprafilm in preventing adhesion formation. As determined

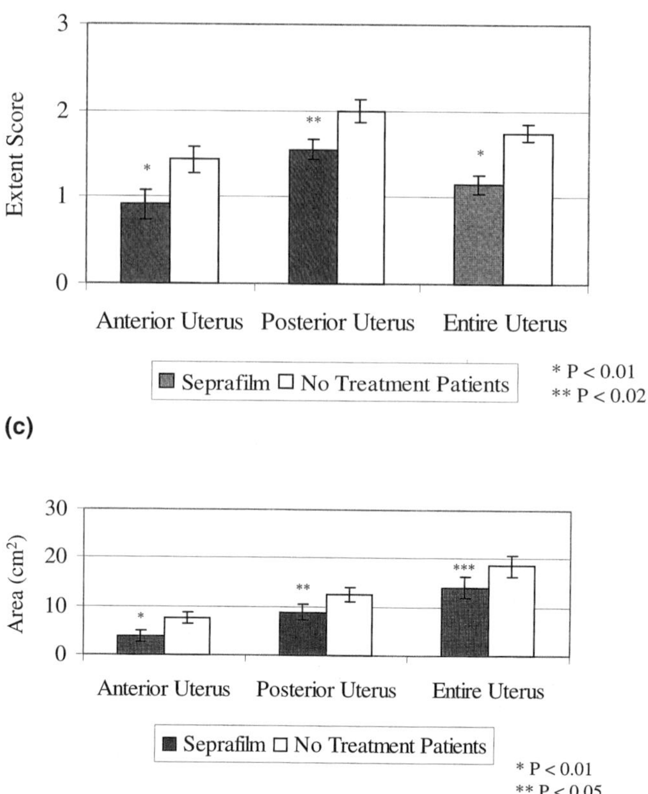

(c)

(d)

Figure 7 Continued

by the reviewer, only 6 of 51 (11.8%) nontreatment patients had no adhesions to anterior uterine incisions compared with 26 of 49 (53.1%) patients who had received Seprafilm ($P < 0.0001$). This finding persisted when both incisional and nonincisional adhesions were analyzed together (6.5% vs. 38.8%, $P < 0.0001$). The significant reduction in adhesion formation on the anterior uterine surface potentially reduces risks associated with future surgeries and the likelihood of postoperative bowel obstruction. The difference in the number of patients without adhesions to posterior uterine incisions between the two groups was not significant when determined by the reviewer but was significant in favor of Seprafilm when assessed by the principal investigators (12.5% vs. 27.8%, $P = 0.0320$). These differences may likely be related to the difficulties inherent in videoscopic assessment of the posterior uterine incisions.

VI. SUMMARY

Seprafilm membrane has been shown in two randomized clinical trials to prevent adhesions at specific sites of surgical trauma. These studies, for the first time, established efficacy for an adhesion prevention product in a nongynecological clinical population, and one undergoing a major abdominal surgical procedure. Preclinical studies have provided further support of the product's effectiveness and safety for use in abdominal and pelvic surgical procedures.

Adhesion prevention was the primary clinical end point in these studies, but future studies should examine specific clinical benefit to patients, such as a reduction in small-bowel obstructions.

REFERENCES

1. Operative Laparoscopy Study Group. Postoperative adhesions development after operative laparoscopy: evaluation at early second look procedures. Fertil Steril 1991; 55:700–705.
2. Trimbos-Kemper TCM, Trimbos JB, van Hall EV. Adhesion formation after tubal surgery: results of the eighth-day laparoscopy in 188 patients. Fertil Steril 1985; 43: 395–400.
3. Bizer LS, Liebling RW, Delany HM, Gliedman ML. Small bowel obstruction. The role of non-operative treatment in simple intestinal obstruction and predictive criteria for strangulation obstruction. Surgery 1981; 89:407–413.
4. Monk BJ, Berman ML, Montz FJ. Adhesions after extensive gynecologic surgery: clinical significance, etiology, and prevention. Am J Obstet Gynecol 1994; 170: 1396–1403.
5. Holtz G, Kling OR. Effect of surgical technique on peritoneal adhesion reformation after lysis. Fertil Steril 1982; 37:494–496.
6. Menzies D. Peritoneal adhesions: incidence, cause and prevention. Surg Annu 1992; 1:27–45.
7. Ray NF, Denton WG, Thamer M, Henderson SC, Perry S. Abdominal adhesiolysis: inpatient care and expenditures in the United States in 1994. J Am Coll Surg 1998; 186:1–9.
8. diZerega GS and Rodgers KE. The Peritoneum. New York: Springer-Verlag, 1992.
9. Pfeiffer CJ, Pfeiffer DC, Misra HP. Enteric serosal surface in the piglet. A scanning and transmission electron microscopic study of the mesothelium. J Submicrosc Cytol 1987; 19:237–246.
10. Raftery AT. Regeneration of parietal and visceral peritoneum. Br J Surg 1973; 60: 293–299.
11. Raftery AT. Regeneration of parietal and visceral peritoneum: an electron microscopical study. J Anat 1973; 115:375–392.
12. Hertzler AE. The Peritoneum. St. Louis: Mosby, 1919.

13. Muralidharan S, Gu J, Laub GW, Cichon R, Daloisio C, McGrath LB. A new biological membrane for pericardial closure. J Biomed Mater Res 1991; 25:1201–1209.

14. Nussbaum CE, McDonald JV, Baggs RB. Use of Vicryl (polyglactin 910) mesh to limit epidural scar formation after laminectomy. Neurosurgery 1990; 26:649–654.

15. Revuelta J, Garcia-Rinaldi R, Val F, Crego R, Duran CM. Expanded polytetrafluoroethylene surgical membrane for pericardial closure. J Thorac Cardiovasc Surg 1985; 89:451–455.

16. Heydorn WH, Daniel JS, Wade CE. A new look at pericardial substitutes. J Thorac Cardiovasc Surg 1987; 94:291–296.

17. Surgical Membrane Group. Prophylaxis of pelvic sidewall adhesions with Gore-Tex surgical membrane: a multicenter clinical investigation. Fertil Steril 1992; 57:921–923.

18. Surgical Membrane Group. Prophylaxis of pelvic sidewall adhesions with Gore-Tex surgical membrane: a multicenter clinical investigation. Fertil Steril 1992; 57:921–923.

19. Toole BP. Hyaluronan in morphogenesis. J Intern Med 1997; 242:35–40.

20. West DC, Hampson IN, Arnold F, Kumar S Angiogenesis induced by degradation products of hyaluronic acid. Science 1985; 228:1324–1326.

21. Abatangelo G, Martelli M, Vecchia P. Healing of hyaluronic acid-enriched wounds: histological observations. J Surg Res 1983; 35:410–416.

22. Burns JW, Cox S, Walts AE. Water insoluble derivatives of hyaluronic acid. U.S. Patent Number 5,017,229, 1991.

23. Burns JW, Colt MJ, Burgess LS, Skinner KC. Preclinical evaluation of Seprafilm™ bioresorbable membrane. Eur J Surg Supp 1997; 577:40–48.

24. Alponat A, Lakshminarasappa SR, Teh M, Rajnakova A, Moochhala S, Goh PM, Chan ST. Effects of physical barriers in prevention of adhesions: an incisional hernia model in rats. J Surg Res 1997; 68:126–132.

25. Hooker GD, Taylor BM, Driman DK. Prevention of adhesion formation with use of sodium hyaluronate-based bioresorbable membrane in a rat model of ventral hernia repair with polypropylene mesh—a randomized, controlled study. Surgery 1999; 125:211–216.

26. Medina M, Paddock HN, Connolly RJ, Schwaitzberg SD. Novel antiadhesion barrier does not prevent anastomotic healing in a rabbit model. J Invest Surg 1995; 8:179–186.

27. Becker JM, Dayton MT, Fazio VW, Beck DE, Stryker SJ, Wexner SD, Wolff BG, Roberts PL, Smith LE, Sweeney SA, Moore M. Prevention of postoperative abdominal adhesions by a sodium hyaluronate-based bioresorbable membrane: a prospective, randomized, double-blind multicenter study. J Am Coll Surg 1996; 183:297–306.

28. Diamond MP and The Seprafilm Adhesion Study Group. Reduction of adhesions after uterine myomectomy by seprafilm membrane (HAL-F): a blinded, prospective, randomized, multicenter clinical study. Fertil Steril 1996; 66:904–910.

29. Diamond MP, Daniell JF, Feste J, Surrey MW, McLaughlin DS, Friedman S, Vaughn WK, Martin DC. Adhesion reformation and de novo adhesion formation after reproductive pelvic surgery. Fertil Steril 1987; 47:864–866.

Index

About the Editors

HARI G. GARG is Associate Biochemist at Massachusetts General Hospital and Principal Associate in the Department of Medicine at the Harvard Medical School, Boston, Massachusetts. He is the author or coauthor of over 200 articles, abstracts and book chapters, the holder of one U.S. patent, and member of the Society for Glycobiology, the American Chemical Society, the Indian Chemical Society, and the Royal Society of Chemistry. Dr. Garg received the B.Sc. (1950), M.Sc. (1952), Ph.D. (1960), and the D.Sc. (1969) degrees from Agra University, India.

MICHAEL T. LONGAKER is John Marquis Converse Professor of Plastic Surgery Research, and Director of Plastic Surgical Research, New York University School of Medicine, New York. Dr. Longaker is the recipient of the 1999 Academic Scholar Award from the American Association of Plastic Surgeons and the 1999 Dr. Bernd Spiessl Award from the American Society of Maxillofacial Surgeons, and is the author or coauthor of over 475 articles and book chapters. He received the B.S. degree (1980) from Michigan State University, East Lansing, and the M.D. degree (1984) from the Harvard Medical School, Boston, Massachusetts.